THE INTERNATIONAL PHARMACOPOEIA

THIRD EDITION

VOLUME 3

QUALITY SPECIFICATIONS

THE INTERNATIONAL PHARMACOPOEIA

THIRD EDITION

PHARMACOPOEA INTERNATIONALIS

EDITIO TERTIA

Volume 3

Quality Specifications

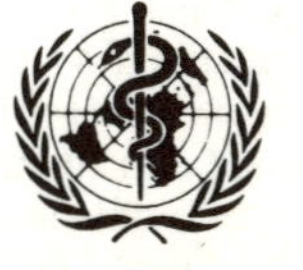

WORLD HEALTH ORGANIZATION

GENEVA

1988

ISBN 92 4 154215 2

PRINTED IN SWITZERLAND

85/6578 — Presses Centrales — 7000

CONTENTS

	Page
Preface	8
Acknowledgements	10
Monographs	13
List of reagents, test solutions, and volumetric solutions	337
Amendments and corrigenda to Vols. 1 and 2	371
Index	387

MONOGRAPHS
(Latin names)

Page

Aluminii hydroxidum	15	Chlorhexidini dihydro-chloridum	71
Amikacinum	17	Chlortetracyclini hydro-chloridum	73
Amikacini sulfas	18	Cimetidinum	76
Amiloridi hydrochloridum	21	Clofaziminum	78
Amodiaquinum	23	Clomifeni citras	80
Amphotericinum B	25	Colchicinum	82
Argenti nitras	28	Cyclophosphamidum	84
Azathioprinum	29	Cytarabinum	86
Bacitracinum	31	Deferoxamini mesilas	88
Bacitracinum zincum	33	Dehydroemetini dihydro-chloridum	90
Barii sulfas	35	Dexamethasoni natrii phosphas	91
Beclometasoni dipropionas	37	Dextromethorphani hydro-bromidum	94
Benzathini benzylpenicillinum	39	Dicloxacillinum natricum	96
Betamethasoni valeras	42	Diloxanidi furoas	99
Biperidenum	45	Dimercaprolum	100
Biperideni hydrochloridum	46	Diphenoxylati hydrochloridum	102
Bleomycini hydrochloridum	48	Dopamini hydrochloridum	103
Bleomycini sulfas	52	Doxorubicini hydrochloridum	105
Busulfanum	55	Doxycyclini hyclas	107
Calcii carbonas	57	Edrophonii chloridum	109
Calcii folinas	59	Emetini hydrochloridum	111
Carbamazepinum	61		
Carbidopum	63		
Chlorambucilum	65		
Chloramphenicoli palmitas	67		
Chlorhexidini diacetas	69		

Ephedrinum 113	Natrii nitroprussidum . . . 199
Ephedrini hydrochloridum . 115	Natrii stibogluconas 201
Ephedrini sulfas 117	Natrii sulfas 203
Ergocalciferolum 119	Natrii sulfas anhydricus . . 205
Erythromycinum 121	Natrii thiosulfas 207
Erythromycini ethylsuccinas . 123	Natrii valproas 209
Erythromycini stearas . . . 125	Neomycini sulfas 211
Ether anaesthesicus 128	Neostigmini metilsulfas . . 213
Ethionamidum 129	Nifurtimoxum 216
Ferrosi fumaras 131	Niridazolum 218
Flucytosinum 133	Nitrazepamum 220
Fludrocortisoni acetas . . . 135	Nitrofurantoinum 222
Fluoresceinum natricum . . 138	Noscapinum 224
Fluorouracilum 141	Noscapini hydrochloridum . 226
Gallamini triethiodidum . . 143	Nystatinum 228
Gentamicini sulfas 145	Oxamniquinum 229
Glibenclamidum 147	Oxytetracyclini dihydras . . 231
Homatropini hydrobromidum 149	Oxytetracyclini hydrochloridum 234
Hydralazini hydrochloridum . 150	Paracetamolum 237
Hydrocortisoni natrii succinas 152	Paromomycini sulfas . . . 239
Hydroxocobalaminum . . . 154	Penicillaminum 241
Hydroxocobalamini chloridum 158	Pentamidini isetionas . . . 243
Hydroxocobalamini sulfas . 158	Pentamidini mesilas 245
Ipecacuanhae radix 161	Pethidini hydrochloridum . . 247
Kalii citras 164	Phytomenadionum 249
Levonorgestrelum 166	Pix lithanthracis 251
Levothyroxinum natricum . 168	Praziquantelum 252
Loperamidi hydrochloridum . 170	Prednisoloni acetas 254
Magnesii hydroxidum . . . 172	Probenecidum 256
Magnesii oxidum 174	Procaini benzylpenicillinum . 258
Mebendazolum 176	Procarbazini hydrochloridum 260
Methotrexatum 178	Promethazini hydrochloridum 262
Methylthioninii chloridum . 180	Protionamidum 264
Metoclopramidi hydro-	Pyranteli embonas 265
chloridum 182	Pyrazinamidum 268
Metrifonatum 184	Pyrimethaminum 269
Miconazoli nitras 186	Quinidini sulfas 271
Naloxoni hydrochloridum . . 188	Quinini bisulfas 273
Natrii calcii edetas 190	Quinini dihydrochloridum . 276
Natrii citras 192	Rifampicinum 278
Natrii cromoglicas 194	Salbutamolum 280
Natrii fluoridum 196	Salbutamoli sulfas 282
Natrii nitris 197	Sennae folium 284

Sennae fructus 286	Tetracaini hydrochloridum . 314
Spectinomycini hydro-	Thiamini hydrobromidum . 316
chloridum 288	Thiamini hydrochloridum . 318
Spironolactonum 290	Thiamini mononitras . . . 319
Stibii natrii tartras . . . 293	Thioacetazonum 321
Sulfacetamidum 294	Tiabendazolum 323
Sulfacetamidum natricum . . 296	Trihexyphenidyli hydro-
Sulfadimidinum 298	chloridum 325
Sulfadimidinum natricum . . 300	Tubocurarini chloridum . . 326
Sulfadoxinum 302	Verapamili hydrochloridum . 328
Sulfasalazinum 305	Vincristini sulfas 330
Suraminum natricum . . . 307	Warfarinum natricum . . . 332
Suxamethonii chloridum . . 310	Zinci oxydum 335
Testosteroni enantas . . . 312	

PREFACE

The International Pharmacopoeia is published by the World Health Organization by virtue of resolution WHA3.10[1] of the Third World Health Assembly. Information on the publication of the first and second editions of *The International Pharmacopoeia* and on the preparatory work for the third edition will be found in the prefaces to volumes 1 and 2 of the third edition.[2]

Volume 1 of the third edition contains the description of general methods of analysis, and volume 2 gives quality specifications for 126 essential drug substances. Volume 3 is a continuation of volume 2 and contains quality specifications for the remaining 157 substances in the WHO Model List of Essential Drugs,[3] some of which have not previously been included in any national or international compendia.

Future volumes will contain quality standards for widely used finished dosage forms as well as for pharmaceutical aids and packaging materials employed in their manufacture and packing.

In accordance with the above-mentioned resolution, *The International Pharmacopoeia* constitutes a collection of recommended methods and specifications that are not intended to have a legal status as such in any country, unless expressly introduced for that purpose by appropriate legislation, but are offered to serve as reference so that national requirements can be established on a similar basis in any country. It should be noted that, in general, the quality of pharmaceutical products cannot be adequately established on the basis of specifications alone, and that they should invariably be produced in accordance with Good Manufacturing Practices.[4]

Many national or regional pharmacopoeias rely increasingly on complex techniques of analysis that, while time-saving, require expensive equipment and highly specialized personnel. These methods are therefore inapplicable in countries lacking such resources.

Since *The International Pharmacopoeia* aims primarily at accommodating the needs of developing countries, it offers instead sound, simplified, and classical chemical methods. Moreover, the selection of methods is correlated with the WHO recommendations concerning equipment for small and medium-sized drug quality control laboratories.[5]

---

[1] *WHO Handbook of Resolutions and Decisions,* vol. 1, 1973, p. 127.

[2] WORLD HEALTH ORGANIZATION. *The International Pharmacopoeia,* third edition, Geneva, vol. 1, 1979; vol. 2, 1981.

[3] WHO Technical Report Series, No. 722, 1985.

[4] WHO Official Records, No. 226, 1975, p. 35 and Annex 12, p. 88 (regularly revised and reissued as unpublished WHO document, PHARM/82.4).

[5] WHO Technical Report Series, No. 704, 1984.

The production of *The International Pharmacopoeia* helps *inter alia* to advance the setting of pharmacopoeial standards at national level in that it fosters a valuable exchange of experiences gained in a wide variety of countries.

The International Pharmacopoeia provides general methods of analysis that would be applicable not only to materials included in the pharmacopoeia, but also to new products submitted for registration.

The International Pharmacopoeia accommodates, where appropriate, a measure of flexibility into methods and requirements in order to facilitate its use on a global basis. Thus, in line with several national compendia, *The International Pharmacopoeia* allows compliance with its requirements to be determined by the use of alternative methods so as to make better use of the analytical equipment and expertise available. Alternative identification methods are included in several monographs, permitting the use of classical analytical methods in place of physicochemical tests calling for expensive apparatus. Alternative assay methods previously validated against a pharmacopoeial method may also be employed. However, in the event of a dispute, only the results obtained by the procedure given in *The International Pharmacopoeia* are conclusive.

General notices and methods of analysis included in previous volumes of this edition are also applicable to this volume.

As in volume 2, for substances used in more than one form (e.g., anhydrous and hydrated, or non-injectable and sterile) the requirements for the relevant forms have already been collected together in a single monograph, but separate tests have been provided, as required for each specific form.

In spite of the above-mentioned policy of relying on classical analytical methods, cases arise where certain complex materials (e.g., bleomycins) can be adequately controlled only by searching techniques, such as "high-pressure liquid chromatography". Accordingly, this method has been included in several of the monographs to be found in the present volume. In this connection, an expanded version of the description of the method given in volume 1 has been included in the Amendments to Volumes 1 and 2, pages 373-387. Following recent trends in analytical terminology, the title of this method has been changed to "High performance liquid chromatography".

The monograph on praziquantel is deemed to be in need of further revision, since the assay method employed, infrared quantitative spectrophotometry, is not considered to be a suitable method for the purpose of *The International Pharmacopoeia*. However, it has been decided to publish the monograph as it stands, taking into consideration the importance of praziquantel for the schistosomiasis control programmes in a number of countries and the fact that there is no official monograph so far for this substance in any other pharmacopoeia. Specialists in the field are specifically requested to take note of this monograph (which could be regarded as *provisional*) with a view to developing an alternative assay method.

Further work is needed to implement the recommendations contained in the twenty-ninth report of the WHO Expert Committee on Specifications for

Pharmaceutical Preparations[1] concerning the replacement of toxic reagents and solvents presently employed in several tests and assays, such as the use of mercuric acetate in some non-aqueous titrations of hydrochlorides. However, the opinion has been expressed during several informal consultations that when developing assay procedures for replacement priority should be accorded to precision and reliability of analytical methods.

No monographs on medicinal gases are provided in volumes 2 and 3 of *The International Pharmacopoeia,* though some such gases are included in the WHO Model List of Essential Drugs (oxygen, nitrogen oxide, etc.). The reason for this is that, unlike other drug substances (in powder or liquid form), gases cannot be offered for sale or distributed through the pharmaceutical supply system unless presented in special containers. In this they are closer to finished pharmaceutical forms and will be described among such in a future volume of *The International Pharmacopoeia.*

In accordance with general analytical practice, the symbol for specific extinction ($E_{1\,cm}^{1\,\%}$) in spectrophotometric measurements has been replaced by the symbol for absorbance ($A_{1\,cm}^{1\,\%}$).

ACKNOWLEDGEMENTS

The process of establishing and revising the quality specifications included in volume 3 of the third edition was carried out during the period 1980–85 with the help of members of the WHO Expert Advisory Panel on the International Pharmacopoeia and Pharmaceutical Preparations and other specialists.

The following specialists participated both in person and by correspondence in the preparation of volume 3: Dr H.Y. Aboul-Enein, Drug Development Laboratory, King Faisal Specialist Hospital and Research Centre, Riyadh, Saudi Arabia; Professor E.A. Babayan, Department of New Drug Evaluation, Ministry of Health, Moscow, USSR; Mr J.Y. Binka, Medicines Board, Medical and Health Department, Banjul, Gambia; Dr H.R. Bolliger, F. Hoffmann-La Roche & Co., Basle, Switzerland; Mr J.R. Buriánek, State Institute for the Control of Drugs, Prague, Czechoslovakia; Dr D. Cook, Drug Research Laboratories, Ottawa, Ontario, Canada; Professor Y.M. Dessouky, Cairo, Egypt; Dr L.F. Dodson, National Biological Standards Laboratory, Canberra, Australia; Dr I. Elverdam, Dumex, Copenhagen, Denmark; Dr K. Florey, The Squibb Institute for Medical Research, New Brunswick, NJ, USA; Dr S. Fusari, Warner-Lambert Research Institute, Morris Plains, NJ, USA; Dr L.T. Grady, The United States Pharmaco-

---

[1] WHO Technical Report Series, No. 704, 1984, p. 49.

peia, Rockville, MD, USA; Dr J. Gutzwiller, F. Hoffmann-La Roche & Co., Basle, Switzerland; Dr S. Haghighi, Food and Drug Control Laboratories, Teheran, Islamic Republic of Iran; Dr A. Häussler, Hoechst AG, Frankfurt, Federal Republic of Germany; Mr A. Holbrook, Imperial Chemical Industries PLC, Macclesfield, England; Miss S. Johansson, WHO Collaborating Centre for Chemical Reference Substances, Stockholm, Sweden; Dr C.A. Johnson, British Pharmacopoeia Commission, London, England; Mr O. Karlsson, Apothekernes Laboratorium, Oslo, Norway; Mrs P. Kashemsant, Department of Medical Sciences, Ministry of Public Health, Bangkok, Thailand; Mr R.H. King, The United States Pharmacopeia, Rockville, MD, USA; Professor Y.F. Krylov, State Research Institute for Standardization and Quality Control of Drugs, Ministry of Health, Moscow, USSR; Miss E. Lamsdon, UN Division of Narcotic Drugs, Vienna, Austria; Professor C.L. Lapière, Institute of Pharmacy, University of Liège, Liège, Belgium; Professor J. Laszlovszky, National Institute of Pharmacy, Budapest, Hungary; Dr J.W. Lightbown, National Institute for Biological Standards and Control, Potters Bar, England; Dr K.L. Loening, Chemical Abstracts Service, Columbus, OH, USA; Dr K. Lingner, Ciba-Geigy AG, Basle, Switzerland; Professor R. Moreau, René Descartes University, Paris, France; Dr Ng Tju Lik, Department of Scientific Services, Singapore; Professor E. Nieminen, National Control Laboratory for Medicines, Helsinki, Finland; Dr T. Nonnenmann, F. Hoffmann-La Roche & Co., Basle, Switzerland; Mr B. Öhrner, WHO Collaborating Centre for Chemical Reference Substances, Stockholm, Sweden; Professor A.A. Olaniyi, Faculty of Pharmacy, University of Ibadan, Ibadan, Nigeria; Dr V. Parrák, State Institute for the Control of Drugs, Bratislava, Czechoslovakia; Dr H. Partenheimer, Ciba-Geigy AG, Basle, Switzerland; Dr M. Pesez, Roussel Uclaf SA, Romainville, France; Professor S. Philianos, National Pharmacopoeia Commission, Athens, Greece; Professor J. Richter, Institute of Drugs of the German Democratic Republic, Berlin, German Democratic Republic; Dr N. Rofael, National Organization for Drug Control and Research, Cairo, Egypt; Dr S.K. Roy, Central Drugs Laboratory, Calcutta, India; Dr K. Satiadarma, Department of Pharmacy, Institute of Technology, Bandung, Indonesia; Dr P. Schorn, European Pharmacopoeia Commission, Strasbourg, France; Professor St. Škramovský, Czechoslovak Pharmacopoeia Commission, Prague, Czechoslovakia; Professor S.D. Sokolov, Department of New Drugs and Medical Equipment, Ministry of Health, Moscow, USSR; Dr I. Suzuki, National Institute of Hygienic Sciences, Tokyo, Japan; Professor Tu Guoshi, National Institute for the Control of Pharmaceutical and Biological Products, Ministry of Health, Beijing, China; Dr V. Usieli, Institute for the Standardization and Control of Pharmaceuticals, Ministry of Health, Jerusalem, Israel; Professor H. Vanderhaeghe, Rega Pharmaceutical Institute, Leuven, Belgium; Dr M.J. Vernengo, WHO/PAHO Drug Quality Project, Rio de Janeiro, Brazil; Dr E. Weisenberg, Institute for the Standardization and Control of Pharmaceuticals, Ministry of Health, Jerusalem, Israel; Mrs M. Westermark, WHO Collaborating Centre for Chemical Reference Substances, Stockholm, Sweden; Dr W. Wieniawski, Institute of Drug Research and

Control, Warsaw, Poland; Dr W.W. Wright, The United States Pharmacopeia, Rockville, MD, USA.

Furthermore, comments were obtained from several Pharmacopoeia Commissions, national institutes for the quality control of drugs and drug research laboratories. The World Health Organization takes this opportunity to express its gratitude to all those persons and institutions.

MONOGRAPHS

ALUMINII HYDROXIDUM

Aluminium hydroxide

Molecular formula. $Al(OH)_3$

Relative molecular mass.   78.00

Chemical name.   Aluminium hydroxide; CAS Reg. No. 21645-51-2.

Description.   A white, fine, amorphous powder; odourless.

Solubility.   Practically insoluble in water and ethanol ($\sim$750 g/l) TS; soluble in hydrochloric acid ($\sim$70 g/l) TS and sodium hydroxide ($\sim$80 g/l) TS.

Category.   Antacid.

Storage.   Aluminium hydroxide should be kept in a tightly closed container.

REQUIREMENTS

General requirement.   Aluminium hydroxide contains not less than 71.9% and not more than 94.9% of $Al(OH)_3$.

Identity test

Dissolve 0.10 g by heating in 5 ml of sodium hydroxide ($\sim$80 g/l) TS. To the clear solution add 0.5 g of ammonium chloride R; a white, gelatinous precipitate is produced.

Heavy metals.   For the preparation of the test solution dissolve 0.5 g, while heating, in 5 ml of acetic acid ($\sim$300 g/l) TS, dilute to 10 ml with water and filter. Adjust the pH of the filtrate to 3–4, dilute to 40 ml with water and mix. Determine the heavy metals content as described under "Limit test for heavy metals", according to Method A (vol. 1, p. 119); not more than 60 µg/g.

Arsenic.   Use a solution of 3.3 g in 20 ml of sulfuric acid ($\sim$100 g/l) TS and 35 ml of water and proceed as described under "Limit test for arsenic" (vol. 1, p. 122); the arsenic content is not more than 5 µg/g.

Ammonium salts.   Transfer 5.0 g to an ammonia distillation apparatus, add 25 ml of sodium hydroxide ($\sim$200 g/l) TS and 200 ml of water, distil about 100 ml, collecting the distillate in 25.0 ml of hydrochloric acid (0.1 mol/l) VS.

Titrate the excess acid with sodium hydroxide (0.1 mol/l) VS using methyl red/ethanol TS as indicator; not less than 22.5 ml of sodium hydroxide (0.1 mol/l) VS is required.

Chlorides.   Dissolve 0.10 g in 2 ml of nitric acid ($\sim$130 g/l) TS, boil, cool, dilute to 10 ml with water and filter. Proceed with 5 ml of the filtrate as described under "Limit test for chlorides" (vol. 1, p. 116); the chloride content is not more than 10 mg/g.

Sulfates.   Dissolve 0.10 g in 5 ml of hydrochloric acid ($\sim$70 g/l) TS, boil, cool, dilute to 10 ml with water and filter. Proceed with the filtrate as described under "Limit test for sulfates" (Vol. 1, p. 116); the sulfate content is not more than 5 mg/g.

Neutralizing capacity.   Pass a sufficient quantity of the test substance, triturated if necessary, through a sieve of nominal mesh aperture 150 μm, add 0.50 g to 200 ml of hydrochloric acid (0.05 mol/l) VS previously heated to 37 °C, and stir continuously, maintaining the temperature at 37 °C; the pH of the solution at 37 °C, after 10, 15, and 20 minutes, is not less than 1.8, 2.3, and 3.0, respectively, and at no time more than 4.0. Add 10 ml of hydrochloric acid (0.5 mol/l) VS previously heated to 37 °C, stir continuously for 1 hour, maintaining the temperature at 37 °C. Titrate the solution with sodium hydroxide (0.1 mol/l) VS to pH 3.5. The neutralizing capacity is not less than 83.3 % of the theoretical amount when calculated by the formula $(1000)(150\text{-}y)/A \times W \times 38.46$, in which y is the number of ml of sodium hydroxide (0.1 mol/l) VS required, A is the percent of $Al(OH)_3$ obtained in the assay, W is the quantity, in g, of test substance taken, and 38.46 is the theoretical value of each g of $Al(OH)_3$.

Alkaline impurities.   The pH of a 0.04 g/ml suspension in carbon-dioxide-free water R is not more than 10.0.

Assay.   Proceed with about 0.15 g, accurately weighed, as described under "Complexometric titrations" for aluminium (vol. 1, p. 128). Each ml of disodium edetate (0.05 mol/l) VS is equivalent to 3.900 mg of $Al(OH)_3$.

AMIKACINUM

Amikacin

Molecular formula. $C_{22}H_{43}N_5O_{13}$

Relative molecular mass. 585.6

Graphic formula.

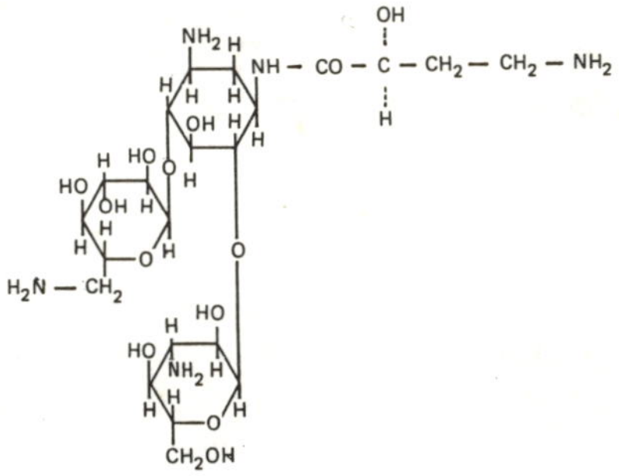

Chemical name. *O*-3-Amino-3-deoxy-*a*-D-glucopyranosyl-(1→4)-*O*-[6-amino-6-deoxy-*a*-D-glucopyranosyl-(1→6)]-*N*³-(4-amino-L-2-hydroxybutyryl)-2-deoxy-L-streptamine; (*S*)-*O*-3-amino-3-deoxy-*a*-D-glucopyranosyl-(1→6)-*O*-[6-amino-6-deoxy-*a*-D-glucopyranosyl-(1→4)]-*N*¹-(4-amino-2-hydroxyoxobutyl)-2-deoxy-D-streptamine; CAS Reg. No. 37517-28-5.

Description. A white, crystalline powder; almost odourless.

Solubility. Sparingly soluble in water.

Category. Antibacterial drug.

Storage. Amikacin should be kept in a tightly closed container.

REQUIREMENTS

General requirement. Amikacin contains not less than 900 µg of $C_{22}H_{43}N_5O_{13}$ per mg, with reference to the anhydrous substance.

Identity tests

A. Dissolve 10 mg in 1 ml of water, add 1 ml of sodium hydroxide (~80 g/l) TS and mix, then add 2 ml of cobalt(II) nitrate (10 g/l) TS; a violet colour is produced.

B. Dissolve 0.05 g in 3 ml of water and add 4 ml of anthrone TS; a bluish violet colour is produced.

Specific optical rotation. Use a 20 mg/ml solution and calculate with reference to the anhydrous substance: $[a]_D^{20\,°C} = +97$ to $+105°$.

Sulfated ash. After ignition moisten the residue with 2 ml of nitric acid (~1000 g/l) TS and about 0.2 ml of sulfuric acid (~1760 g/l) TS; not more than 10 mg/g.

Water. Determine as described under "Determination of water by the Karl Fischer method", Method A (vol. 1, p. 135), using about 0.2 g of the substance; the water content is not more than 85 mg/g.

pH value. pH of a 10 mg/ml solution in carbon-dioxide-free water R, 9.5–11.5.

Assay. Carry out the assay as described under "Microbiological assay of antibiotics" (vol. 1, p. 145), using either (*a*) *Bacillus subtilis* (ATCC 6633) as the test organism, culture medium Cm1 with a final pH of 6.5–6.7, sterile phosphate buffer pH 6.0 TS1, TS2 or TS3, an appropriate concentration of amikacin (usually 5–20 µg/ml), and an incubation temperature of 32–35 °C, or (*b*) *Staphylococcus aureus* (ATCC 29737) as the test organism, the same culture medium and phosphate buffer, an appropriate concentration of amikacin (usually 10 µg/ml), and the same incubation temperature. The precision of the assay is such that the fiducial limits of error of the estimated potency ($P = 0.95$) are not less than 95% and not more than 105% of the estimated potency. The upper fiducial limit of error of the estimated potency ($P = 0.95$) is not less than 900 µg per mg, calculated with reference to the anhydrous substance.

AMIKACINI SULFAS

Amikacin sulfate

Amikacin sulfate (non-injectable)
Amikacin sulfate, sterile

Molecular formula. $C_{22}H_{43}N_5O_{13},2H_2SO_4$

Relative molecular mass. 781.8

Graphic formula.

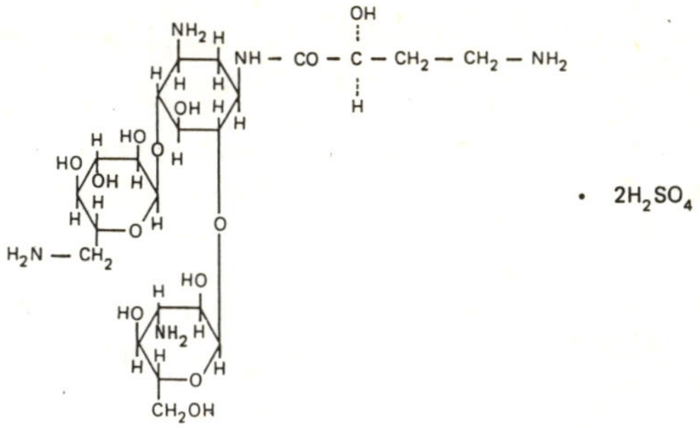

Chemical name. O-3-Amino-3-deoxy-α-D-glucopyranosyl-(1→4)-O-[6-amino-6-deoxy-α-D-glucopyranosyl-(1→6)]-N^3-(4-amino-L-2-hydroxybutyryl)-2-deoxy-L-streptamine sulfate (1:2) (salt); (S)-O-3-amino-3-deoxy-α-D-glucopyranosyl-(1→6)-O-[6-amino-6-deoxy-α-D-glucopyranosyl-(1→4)]-N^1-(4-amino-2-hydroxy-1-oxobutyl)-2-deoxy-D-streptamine sulfate (1:2) (salt); CAS Reg. No. 39831-55-5.

Description. A white to yellowish white, crystalline powder; almost odourless.

Solubility. Very soluble in water; practically insoluble in methanol R, acetone R, ether R, or chloroform R.

Category. Antibacterial drug.

Storage. Amikacin sulfate should be kept in a tightly closed container.

Labelling. The designation sterile Amikacin sulfate indicates that the substance complies with the additional requirements for sterile Amikacin sulfate and may be used for parenteral administration or for other sterile applications.

REQUIREMENTS

General requirement. Amikacin sulfate contains not less than 650 International Units per mg, with reference to the anhydrous substance.

Identity tests

A. Dissolve 10 mg in 1 ml of water, add 1 ml of sodium hydroxide (~80 g/l) TS and mix, then add 2 ml of cobalt(II) nitrate (10 g/l) TS; a violet colour is produced.

B. Dissolve 0.05 g in 3 ml of water and add 4 ml of anthrone TS; a bluish violet colour is produced.

C. A 20 mg/ml solution yields reaction A described under "General identification tests" as characteristic of sulfates (vol. 1, p. 115).

Specific optical rotation. Use a 10 mg/ml solution and calculate with reference to the anhydrous substance; $[a]_D^{20\,°C} = +69$ to $+79°$.

Sulfated ash. After ignition moisten the residue with 2 ml of nitric acid ($\sim$1000 g/l) TS and about 0.2 ml of sulfuric acid ($\sim$1760 g/l) TS; not more than 10 mg/g.

Water. Determine as described under "Determination of water by the Karl Fischer method", Method A (vol. 1, p. 135), using about 0.2 g of the substance; the water content is not more than 50 mg/g.

pH value. pH of a 10 mg/ml solution in carbon-dioxide-free water R, 6.0–7.5.

Assay. Carry out the assay as described under "Microbiological assay of antibiotics" (vol. 1, p. 145), using either (a) *Bacillus subtilis* (ATCC 6633) as the test organism, culture medium Cml with a final pH of 6.5–6.7, sterile phosphate buffer pH 6.0 TS1, TS2 or TS3, an appropriate concentration of amikacin (usually 5–20 IU per ml), and an incubation temperature of 32–35 °C, or (b) *Staphylococcus aureus* (ATCC 29737) as the test organism, the same culture medium and phosphate buffer, an appropriate concentration of amikacin (usually 10 IU per ml), and the same incubation temperature. The precision of the assay is such that the fiducial limits of error of the estimated potency ($P = 0.95$) are not less than 95% and not more than 105% of the estimated potency. The upper fiducial limit of error of the estimated potency ($P = 0.95$) is not less than 650 IU per mg, calculated with reference to the anhydrous substance.

Additional Requirements for Sterile Amikacin Sulfate

Storage. Sterile Amikacin sulfate should be kept in a hermetically closed container.

Undue toxicity. Carry out the test as described under "Test for undue toxicity" (vol. 1, p. 154), using 0.5 ml of a solution in sterile water R containing 1.6 mg of the substance being examined per ml.

Sterility. Complies with the "Sterility testing of antibiotics" (vol. 1, p. 152), applying the membrane filtration test procedure.

AMILORIDI HYDROCHLORIDUM

Amiloride hydrochloride

Amiloride hydrochloride, anhydrous
Amiloride hydrochloride dihydrate

Molecular formula. $C_6H_8ClN_7O,HCl$ (anhydrous); $C_6H_8ClN_7O,HCl,2H_2O$ (dihydrate).

Relative molecular mass. 266.1 (anhydrous); 302.1 (dihydrate).

Graphic formula.

NH
Cl
CO—NH—C—NH$_2$
N
. HCl . nH$_2$O
H$_2$N
N
NH$_2$
n = 0 (anhydrous)
n = 2 (dihydrate)

Chemical name. *N*-Amidino-3,5-diamino-6-chloropyrazinecarboxamide mono-hydrochloride; 3,5-diamino-*N*-(aminoiminomethyl)-6-chloropyrazinecarboxa-mide monohydrochloride; 3,5-diamino-6-chloro-*N*-(diaminomethylene)pyra-zinecarboxamide monohydrochloride; CAS Reg. No. 2016-88-8 (anhydrous).
N-Amidino-3,5-diamino-6-chloropyrazinecarboxamide monohydrochloride di-hydrate; 3,5-diamino-*N*-(aminoiminomethyl)-6-chloropyrazinecarboxamide monohydrochloride dihydrate; 3,5-diamino-6-chloro-*N*-(diaminomethylene)-pyrazinecarboxamide monohydrochloride dihydrate; CAS Reg. No. 17440-83-4 (dihydrate).

Description. A pale yellow to greenish yellow powder; odourless or almost odourless.

Solubility. Slightly soluble in water and ethanol ($\sim$750 g/l) TS; practically in-soluble in chloroform R and ether R.

Category. Diuretic.

Storage. Amiloride hydrochloride should be kept in a well-closed container, protected from light.

REQUIREMENTS

General requirement. Amiloride hydrochloride contains not less than 98.0 % and not more than 101.0 % of $C_6H_8ClN_7O,HCl$, calculated with reference to the dried substance.

Identity tests

● Either tests A and C or tests B and C may be applied.

A.   Carry out the examination as described under "Spectrophotometry in the infrared region" (vol. 1, p. 40). The infrared absorption spectrum is concordant with the spectrum obtained from amiloride hydrochloride RS or with the *reference spectrum* of amiloride hydrochloride.

B.   The absorption spectrum of a 5.0 µg/ml solution in hydrochloric acid (0.1 mol/l) VS, when observed between 230 nm and 380 nm, exhibits maxima at about 285 nm and 361 nm; the absorbances of a 1-cm layer at the maximum wavelength of 285 nm and 361 nm are about 0.28 and 0.31, respectively.

C.   A 5 mg/ml solution yields reaction A described under "General identification tests" as characteristic of chlorides (vol. 1, p. 112).

Sulfated ash.   Not more than 1.0 mg/g.

Water.   Determine as described under "Determination of water by the Karl Fischer method", Method A (vol. 1, p. 135), using about 0.2 g of the substance; for the dihydrate the water content is not less than 110 mg/g and not more than 130 mg/g.

Free acid.   Dissolve 1.0 g in a mixture of 50 ml of methanol R and 50 ml of water, and titrate with sodium hydroxide (0.1 mol/l) VS determining the endpoint potentiometrically; not more than 0.3 ml is required.

Related substances.   Carry out the test as described under "Thin-layer chromatography" (vol. 1, p. 83), using silica gel R1 as the coating substance and a mixture of 15 volumes of tetrahydrofuran R and 2 volumes of ammonia ($\sim$50 g/l) TS as the mobile phase. Apply separately to the plate 5 µl of each of 2 solutions in a mixture of 4 volumes of methanol R and 1 volume of chloroform R containing (A) 0.40 mg of the test substance per ml, (B) 4.0 µg of the test substance per ml. After removing the plate from the chromatographic chamber, allow it to dry in air and examine the chromatogram in ultraviolet light (365 nm). Any spot obtained with solution A, other than the principal spot, is not more intense than that obtained with solution B.

Assay.   Dissolve about 0.45 g, accurately weighed, in a mixture of 100 ml of glacial acetic acid R1, 15 ml of dioxan R, and 10 ml of mercuric acetate/acetic acid TS, and titrate with perchloric acid (0.1 mol/l) VS, determining the endpoint potentiometrically as described under "Non-aqueous titration", Method A (vol. 1, p. 131). Each ml of perchloric acid (0.1 mol/l) VS is equivalent to 26.61 mg of $C_6H_8ClN_7O,HCl$.

AMODIAQUINUM

Amodiaquine

Molecular formula. $C_{20}H_{22}ClN_3O$

Relative molecular mass.   355.9

Graphic formula.

CH$_2$N(C$_2$H$_5$)$_2$
N
NH
OH
Cl

Chemical name.   4-[(7-Chloro-4-quinolyl)amino]-*a*-(diethylamino)-*o*-cresol; 4-[(7-chloro-4-quinolinyl)amino]-2-[(diethylamino)methyl]phenol; CAS Reg. No. 86-42-0.

Description.   A yellow, crystalline powder; odourless.

Solubility.   Practically insoluble in water; soluble in chloroform R.

Category.   Antimalarial drug.

Storage.   Amodiaquine should be kept in a tightly closed container.

REQUIREMENTS

General requirement.   Amodiaquine contains not less than 97.0% and not more than 103.0% of $C_{20}H_{22}ClN_3O$, calculated with reference to the anhydrous substance.

Identity tests

● Either test A or tests B and C may be applied.

A.   Carry out the examination as described under "Spectrophotometry in the infrared region" (vol. 1, p. 40). The infrared absorption spectrum is concordant with the spectrum obtained from the free base of amodiaquine hydrochloride RS or with the *reference spectrum* of amodiaquine.

B.   Dissolve 20 mg in 1.0 ml of water and add 0.5 ml of ammonium thiocyanate/cobalt(II) nitrate TS; a green precipitate is produced.

C.   See the test described below under "Related substances". The principal spot obtained with solution A corresponds in position, appearance, and intensity with that obtained with solution B.

Sulfated ash.   Not more than 2.0 mg/g.

Water.   Determine as described under "Determination of water by the Karl Fischer method", Method A (vol. 1, p. 135), using about 0.8 g of the substance; the water content is not more than 5.0 mg/g.

Related substances.   Carry out the test as described under "Thin-layer chromatography" (vol. 1, p. 83). Prepare a solution of chloroform saturated with ammonia by shaking chloroform R with ammonia (~260 g/l) TS and separate the chloroform layer. Use silica gel R2 as the coating substance and a mixture of 9 volumes of chloroform, saturated with ammonia, and 1 volume of dehydrated ethanol R as the mobile phase. For the preparation of the test solution dissolve 0.15 g of the substance being examined in 10 ml of chloroform saturated with ammonia (solution A). For the preparation of the reference solutions transfer 40 mg of amodiaquine hydrochloride RS to a glass-stoppered test-tube, add 2.0 ml of chloroform saturated with ammonia, and shake vigorously for 2 minutes. Allow the solids to settle, and decant the solution to a second test-tube (solution B). Dilute 1.0 ml of solution B to 200 ml with chloroform saturated with ammonia (solution C). Apply separately to the plate 10 µl of each of solutions A, B and C. After removing the plate from the chromatographic chamber, allow it to dry in air and examine the chromatogram in ultraviolet light (254 nm). Any spot obtained with solution A, other than the principal spot, is not more intense than that obtained with solution C.

Assay.   Dissolve about 0.3 g, accurately weighed, in sufficient hydrochloric acid (0.1 mol/l) VS to produce 200 ml; dilute 10.0 ml of this solution to 1000 ml with the same medium. Separately prepare a reference solution containing 15 µg of amodiaquine hydrochloride RS per ml of hydrochloric acid (0.1 mol/l) VS. Measure the absorbance of a 1-cm layer of both solutions at the maximum at about 342 nm against a solvent cell containing hydrochloric acid (0.1 mol/l) VS. Calculate the quantity, in mg, of $C_{20}H_{22}ClN_3O$ in the substance being examined using the formula $(355.9/428.8)(20C)(A_u/A_s)$, in which 355.9 and 428.8 are the relative molecular masses of amodiaquine and anhydrous amodiaquine hydrochloride, respectively, C is the concentration, in µg per ml, calculated with reference to the anhydrous substance of amodiaquine hydrochloride RS in the reference solution, and A_u and A_s are the absorbances of the solution of the substance being examined and the reference solution, respectively.

AMPHOTERICINUM B

Amphotericin B

Amphotericin B for parenteral use

Molecular formula. $C_{47}H_{73}NO_{17}$

Relative molecular mass.   924.1

Graphic formula.

Chemical name. (1R,3S,5R,6R,9R,11R,15S,16R,17R,18S,19E,21E,23E,25E,
27E,29E,31E,33R,35S,36R,37S)-33-[(3-Amino-3,6-dideoxy-β-D-mannopyra-
nosyl)-oxy]-1,3,5,6,9,11,17,37-octahydroxy-15,16,18-trimethyl-13-oxo-14,39-
dioxa-bicyclo[33.3.1]nonatriaconta-19,21,23,25,27,29,31-heptaene-36-carboxy-
lic acid; [1R-(1R*,3S*,5R*,6R*,9R*,11R*,15S*,16R*,17R*,18S*,19E,21E,23E,
25E,27E,29E,31E,33R*,35S*,36R*,37S*)]-33-[(3-amino-3,6-dideoxy-β-D-man-
nopyranosyl)oxy]-1,3,5,6,9,11,17,37-octahydroxy-15,16,18-trimethyl-13-oxo-
14,39-dioxabicyclo[33.3.1]nonatriaconta-19,21,23,25,27,29,31-heptaene-36-
carboxylic acid; (3R,5R,8R,9R,11S,13R,15S,16R,17S,19R,34S,35R,36R,37S)-
19-(3-amino-3,6-dideoxy-β-D-mannopyranosyloxy)-16-carboxy-3,5,8,9,11,13,15,
35-octahydroxy-34,36-dimethyl-13,17-epoxyoctatriaconta-20,22,24,26,28,30,
32-heptaen-37-olide; CAS Reg. No. 1397-89-3.

Description.   A yellow to orange powder; odourless or almost odourless.

Solubility.   Practically insoluble in water, ethanol ($\sim$750 g/l) TS, toluene R and
ether R; soluble in 200 parts of dimethylformamide R and in 20 parts of dimethyl
sulfoxide R, slightly soluble in methanol R.

Category.   Antifungal drug.

Storage.   Amphotericin B should be kept in a tightly closed container, protected
from light, and stored at a temperature between 2 and 8 °C.

Labelling.   The designation Amphotericin B for parenteral use indicates that the substance complies with the altered and additional requirements for Amphotericin B and may be used for parenteral administration.

Additional information.   Even in the absence of light, Amphotericin B is gradually degraded on exposure to a humid atmosphere, the decomposition being faster at higher temperatures. In diluted solutions it is sensitive to light and is inactivated at low pH values.

REQUIREMENTS

General requirement.   Amphotericin B contains not less than 750 µg per mg, calculated with reference to the dried substance.

Identity tests

A.   Dissolve 25 mg in 5 ml of dimethyl sulfoxide R, add sufficient methanol R to produce 50 ml, and dilute 2.0 ml to 200 ml with methanol R.   The absorption spectrum of the resulting solution, when observed between 300 nm and 450 nm, exhibits 3 maxima at about 362 nm, 381 nm, and 405 nm.   The ratio of the absorbance of a 1-cm layer at 362 nm to that at 381 nm is about 0.6; the ratio of the absorbance at 381 nm to that at 405 nm is about 0.9.

B.   Dissolve about 1 mg in 2.0 ml of dimethyl sulfoxide R and introduce 5 ml of phosphoric acid (~1440 g/l) TS to form a lower layer; a blue ring is immediately formed at the interface of the two liquids. Mix the two liquids; a strong blue colour is produced. Add 15 ml of water and mix; the colour of the solution changes to pale yellow.

Sulfated ash.   Not more than 30 mg/g.

Loss on drying.   Dry to constant weight at 60 °C under reduced pressure (not exceeding 0.6 kPa or about 5 mm of mercury); it loses not more than 50 mg/g.

Content of tetraenes.   Dissolve 0.05 g, accurately weighed, in 5 ml of dimethyl sulfoxide R, and add sufficient methanol R to produce 50 ml; dilute 4 ml to 50 ml with methanol R (solution A).   For the reference solutions dissolve similarly 0.05 g, accurately weighed, of amphotericin B RS instead of the substance being examined (solution B).   Further prepare a solution of 25 mg of nystatin RS, accurately weighed, in 25 ml of dimethyl sulfoxide R, and add sufficient methanol R to produce 250 ml; dilute 4 ml to 50 ml with methanol R (solution C). Measure the absorbances of a 1-cm layer of solutions A, B, and C at the maxima at about 282 nm and 304 nm, using as a blank a solution of 5 ml of dimethyl sulfoxide R diluted to 50 ml with methanol R, 4 ml of which are diluted once again to 50 ml with methanol R.

Calculate the $A_{1\ cm}^{1\ \%}$ of solutions A, B, and C at both wavelengths and then apply the following formula: $F+1000(B_1A_2-B_2A_1)/(C_2B_1-C_1B_2)$, where A_1 and A_2 are the $A_{1\ cm}^{1\ \%}$ of the substance being examined at 282 nm and 304 nm, respectively, B_1 and B_2 are the $A_{1\ cm}^{1\ \%}$ of amphotericin B RS at 282 nm and 304 nm, respectively, C_1 and C_2 are the $A_{1\ cm}^{1\ \%}$ of nystatin RS at 282 nm and 304 nm, respectively, and F is the declared content of tetraenes in amphotericin B RS; the content of tetraenes in the substance examined is not more than 150 mg/g.

Assay. Triturate 0.060 g with dimethylformamide R and add, with shaking, sufficient dimethylformamide R to produce 100 ml. Dilute 10 ml to 100 ml with dimethylformamide R and carry out the assay as described under "Microbiological assay of antibiotics" (vol. 1, p. 145), using *Saccharomyces cerevisiae* (NCTC 10716, or ATCC 9763) as the test organism, culture medium Cm3 with a final pH of 6.1, sterile phosphate buffer pH 10.5, TS1, an appropriate concentration of amphotericin B (usually between 0.5 and 10.0 µg/ml), and an incubation temperature of 29–33 °C. The precision of the assay is such that the fiducial limits of error of the estimated potency ($P = 0.95$) are not less than 95 % and not more than 105 % of the estimated potency. The upper fiducial limit of error of the estimated potency ($P = 0.95$) is not less than 750 µg per mg, calculated with reference to the dried substance.

Altered and additional requirements for Amphotericin B for parenteral use

Sulfated ash. Not more than 5.0 mg/g.

Content of tetraenes. Not more than 100 mg/g.

Pyrogens. Carry out the test as described under "Test for pyrogens" (vol. 1, p. 155) injecting, per kg of the rabbit's mass, 0.5 ml of a solution in sterile water R containing 2.0 mg of the substance to be examined per ml, except that the temperature of 0.6 °C is replaced by 1.1 °C, the temperature of 1.4 °C by 3.0 °C, and the temperature of 3.7 °C by 8.0 °C.

Undue toxicity. Carry out the test as described under "Test for undue toxicity" (vol. 1, p. 154), administering orally 0.4 ml of a solution in acacia (5 g/l) TS containing a quantity equivalent to 50 mg/ml.

ARGENTI NITRAS

Silver nitrate

Molecular formula. $AgNO_3$

Relative molecular mass.   169.9

Chemical name.   Silver(1+) nitrate; CAS Reg. No. 7761-88-8.

Description.   Colourless or white crystals or white cylindrical rods; odourless.

Solubility.   Soluble in 0.5 parts of water; soluble in ethanol ($\sim$750 g/l) TS.

Category.   Antiinfective agent.

Storage.   Silver nitrate should be kept in a tightly closed, non-metallic container, protected from light.

Additional information.   Even in the absence of light, Silver nitrate is gradually degraded on exposure to a humid atmosphere, the decomposition being faster at higher temperatures. On exposure to light and in the presence of organic matter, it becomes grey or greyish black.

REQUIREMENTS

General requirement.   Silver nitrate contains not less than 99.0 % and not more than 100.5 % of $AgNO_3$.

Identity tests

A.   Dissolve 20 mg in 1.0 ml of water, add ammonia ($\sim$100 g/l) TS, drop by drop, until the precipitate first formed just dissolves; add about 0.1 ml of formaldehyde TS and warm the mixture; glossy metallic silver forms on the wall of the test-tube.

B.   Dissolve 20 mg in 1.0 ml of water and add a few drops of potassium iodide ($\sim$80 g/l) TS; a cream-coloured precipitate is produced which is insoluble in ammonia ($\sim$100 g/l) TS and nitric acid ($\sim$1000 g/l) TS.

C.   To 2 ml of a 0.05 g/ml solution add 2 ml of ferrous sulfate (15 g/l) TS; it yields reaction A described under "General identification tests" as characteristic of nitrates (vol. 1, p. 114).

Clarity and colour.   A solution of 0.4 g in 10 ml of water is clear and colourless.

Acidity or alkalinity.   Dissolve 0.4 g in 10 ml of water; to a 2-ml portion add 0.1 ml of bromocresol green/ethanol TS; the colour of the solution is blue. To another 2-ml portion of the test solution add 0.1 ml of phenol red/ethanol TS; the colour of the solution is yellow.

Foreign salts.   Dissolve 1.2 g in 30 ml of water, add 7.5 ml of hydrochloric acid ($\sim$70 g/l) TS, shake vigorously, heat on a water-bath for 5 minutes and filter. Evaporate 20 ml of the filtrate to dryness on a water-bath and dry at 105 °C; the residue weighs not more than 2.0 mg.

Bismuth, copper, and lead.   Dissolve 1.0 g in 5 ml of water, add drop by drop ammonia ($\sim$100 g/l) TS until the precipitate first formed just dissolves; the solution is clear and colourless.

Assay.   Dissolve about 0.3 g, accurately weighed, in 50 ml of water, add 2 ml of nitric acid ($\sim$130 g/l) TS and 4 ml of ferric ammonium sulfate (45 g/l) TS. Titrate with ammonium thiocyanate (0.1 mol/l) VS until a reddish yellow colour is produced. Each ml of ammonium thiocyanate (0.1 mol/l) VS is equivalent to 16.99 mg of $AgNO_3$.

AZATHIOPRINUM

Azathioprine

Molecular formula. $C_9H_7N_7O_2S$

Relative molecular mass.   277.3

Graphic formula.

Chemical name.   6-[(1-Methyl-4-nitroimidazol-5-yl)thio]purine; 6-[(1-methyl-4-nitro-1H-imidazol-5-yl)thio]-1H-purine; CAS Reg. No. 446-86-6.

Description.   A pale yellow powder; odourless.

Solubility.   Practically insoluble in water; very slightly soluble in ethanol ($\sim$750 g/l) TS and chloroform R; sparingly soluble in dilute mineral acids; soluble in dilute solutions of alkali hydroxides.

Category. Immunosuppressive drug.

Storage. Azathioprine should be kept in a well-closed container, protected from light.

Additional information. Azathioprine decomposes in strong solutions of alkali hydroxides. CAUTION: Azathioprine must be handled with care, avoiding contact with the skin and inhalation of airborne particles.

REQUIREMENTS

General requirement. Azathioprine contains not less than 98.0 % and not more than 101.5 % of $C_9H_7N_7O_2S$, calculated with reference to the dried substance.

Identity tests

● Either test A alone or tests B and C may be applied.

A. Carry out the examination as described under "Spectrophotometry in the infrared region" (vol. 1, p. 40). The infrared absorption spectrum is concordant with the spectrum obtained from azathioprine RS or with the *reference spectrum* of azathioprine.

B. See the test described below under "Related substances". The principal spot obtained with solution B corresponds in position, appearance, and intensity with that obtained with solution C.

C. Heat 20 mg with 100 ml of water and filter. To 5 ml of the filtrate add 1 ml of hydrochloric acid (~420 g/l) TS, 10 mg of zinc R powder, and allow to stand for 5 minutes; the solution becomes yellow. Filter, cool in ice, add 0.1 ml of sodium nitrite (100 g/l) TS and 0.1 g of sulfamic acid R, and shake until the bubbles disappear. Add 1 ml of 2-naphthol TS1; a pale pink precipitate is produced.

Sulfated ash. Not more than 1.0 mg/g.

Loss on drying. Dry at 105 °C under reduced pressure (not exceeding 0.6 kPa or about 5 mm of mercury) for 5 hours; it loses not more than 10 mg/g.

Acidity or alkalinity. Shake 0.5 g with 25 ml of water for 15 minutes, and filter; to 20 ml of the filtrate add 0.15 ml of methyl red/ethanol TS; not more than 0.10 ml of hydrochloric acid (0.02 mol/l) VS or 0.10 ml of sodium hydroxide (0.02 mol/l) VS is required to obtain the midpoint of the indicator (orange).

Related substances. Carry out the test as described under "Thin-layer chromatography" (vol. 1, p. 83), using cellulose R3 (a precoated plate from a commercial source is suitable) and 1-butanol R saturated with ammonia (~100 g/l) TS as the mobile phase. Apply separately to the plate 10 µl of each of 3 solutions in ammonia (~100 g/l) TS containing (A) 10 mg of the test substance per ml, (B) 0.15 mg of the test substance per ml, and (C) 0.15 mg of azathioprine RS per ml. After removing the plate from the chromatographic chamber, allow it to dry in air and examine the chromatogram in ultraviolet light (254 nm). Any spot obtained with solution A, other than the principal spot, is not more intense than that obtained with solution B.

Assay.   Dissolve about 0.5 g, accurately weighed, in 50 ml of dimethylformamide R and titrate with tetrabutylammonium hydroxide (0.1 mol/l) VS, determining the endpoint potentiometrically as described under "Non-aqueous titration", Method B (vol. 1, p. 132). Each ml of tetrabutylammonium hydroxide (0.1 mol/l) VS is equivalent to 27.73 mg of $C_9H_7N_7O_2S$.

BACITRACINUM

Bacitracin

Bacitracin (non-injectable)
Bacitracin, sterile

Composition.   Bacitracin is a polypeptide produced by the growth of an organism of the *licheniformis* group of *Bacillus subtilis*. The main components are Bacitracin A, B_1, and B_2. CAS Reg. No. 1405-87-4.

Description.   A white or pale brownish yellow powder; odourless or with a faint characteristic odour.

Solubility.   Freely soluble in water, methanol R and ethanol ($\sim$750 g/l) TS; practically insoluble in acetone R, chloroform R and ether R.

Category.   Antiinfective drug.

Storage.   Bacitracin should be kept in a tightly closed container, protected from light, and stored at a temperature not exceeding 15 °C. If it is intended for parenteral administration, the container should be sterile and sealed so as to exclude microorganisms.

Labelling.   The designation sterile Bacitracin indicates that the substance complies with the additional requirements for sterile Bacitracin and may be used for parenteral administration or for other sterile applications.

Additional information.   Bacitracin is hygroscopic. Its solutions deteriorate rapidly at room temperature. Even in the absence of light, it is gradually degraded on exposure to a humid atmosphere, the decomposition being faster at higher temperatures.

REQUIREMENTS

General requirement. Bacitracin contains not less than 55 International Units per mg, calculated with reference to the dried substance.

Identity test

Carry out the test as described under "Thin-layer chromatography" (vol. 1, p. 83), using silica gel R1 as the coating substance and a mixture of 60 volumes of 1-butanol R, 10 volumes of water, 6 volumes of pyridine R, 15 volumes of glacial acetic acid R, and 5 volumes of ethanol ($\sim$750 g/l) TS as the mobile phase. Apply separately to the plate 1 µl of each of 2 solutions in disodium edetate (10 g/l) TS containing (A) 6.0 mg of the test substance per ml and (B) 6.3 mg of bacitracin zinc RS per ml. A third spot (C) is made by applying 1 µl of each of solutions A and B at the same point of application, allowing to dry between the two loadings. After removing the plate from the chromatographic chamber, allow it to dry in air, spray it with triketohydrindene/pyridine/butanol TS, and heat it at 110 °C for 10 minutes. Allow to cool, and examine the chromatogram in daylight. The spots obtained with solution A correspond in position, appearance, and intensity with that obtained with solution B. A single spot is obtained with solution C.

Sulfated ash. Not more than 20 mg/g.

Loss on drying. Dry at 60 °C under reduced pressure (not exceeding 0.6 kPa or about 5 mm of mercury) for 3 hours; it loses not more than 50 mg/g.

pH value. Shake 1.0 g with 10 ml of carbon-dioxide-free water R; the pH is between 5.5 and 7.5.

Bacitracin F and related substances. Prepare a solution containing 30 mg in 100 ml of sulfuric acid (0.05 mol/l) VS. The ratio of the absorbance at 290 nm to that at 252 nm is not greater than 0.15.

Assay. Dissolve 0.05 g, accurately weighed, in 5 ml of water and add 0.5 ml of hydrochloric acid ($\sim$70 g/l) TS and sufficient water to produce 100 ml. Allow to stand at room temperature for 30 minutes and carry out the assay as described under "Microbiological assay of antibiotics" (vol. 1, p. 145), using *Micrococcus luteus* (NCTC 7743 or ATCC 10240) as the test organism, culture medium Cml with a final pH of either 7.0–7.1 or 6.5–6.6, sterile phosphate buffer TS of pH either 7.0 or 6.0, an appropriate concentration of bacitracin (usually 1–4 IU per ml), and an incubation temperature of either 35–39 °C or 32–35 °C. The precision of the assay is such that the fiducial limits of error of the estimated potency ($P = 0.95$) are not less than 95 % and not more than 105 % of the estimated potency. The upper fiducial limit of error of the estimated potency ($P = 0.95$) is not less than 55 IU per mg, calculated with reference to the dried substance.

Additional Requirements for Sterile Bacitracin

Storage.   Sterile Bacitracin should be kept in a hermetically closed container, protected from light, and stored at a temperature not exceeding 15 °C.

Undue toxicity.   Carry out the test as described under "Test for undue toxicity" (vol. 1, p. 154), injecting intravenously 0.5 ml of a solution in saline TS containing a quantity equivalent to 200 IU per ml.

Pyrogens.   Carry out the test as described under "Test for pyrogens" (vol. 1, p. 155), injecting per kg of the rabbit's mass 1 ml of a solution in saline TS containing 300 IU per ml.

Sterility.   Complies with the "Sterility testing of antibiotics" (vol. 1, p. 152), applying the membrane filtration test procedure.

BACITRACINUM ZINCUM

Bacitracin zinc

Bacitracin zinc (non-injectable)
Bacitracin zinc, sterile

Composition.   Bacitracin zinc is a zinc complex of bacitracin, a polypeptide produced by the growth of an organism of the *licheniformis* group of *Bacillus subtilis*. The main components are Bacitracin A, B_1 and B_2. CAS Reg. No. 1405-89-6.

Description.   A white or pale brownish yellow powder; odourless or with a faint characteristic odour.

Solubility.   Soluble in 900 parts of water and in 500 parts of ethanol (~750 g/l) TS; very slightly soluble in ether R; practically insoluble in chloroform R.

Category.   Antiinfective drug.

Storage.   Bacitracin zinc should be kept in a tightly closed container, protected from light, and stored at a temperature not exceeding 25 °C. If it is intended for parenteral administration, the container should be sterile and sealed so as to exclude microorganisms.

Labelling.   The designation sterile Bacitracin zinc indicates that the substance complies with the additional requirements for sterile Bacitracin zinc and may be used for other sterile applications.

Additional information.   Bacitracin zinc is hygroscopic.

REQUIREMENTS

General requirement. Bacitracin zinc contains not less than 55 International Units of bacitracin per mg, calculated with reference to the dried substance.

Identity tests

A.   Carry out the test as described under "Thin-layer chromatography" (vol. 1, p. 83), using silica gel R1 as the coating substance and a mixture of 60 volumes of 1-butanol R, 10 volumes of water, 6 volumes of pyridine R, 15 volumes of glacial acetic acid R, and 5 volumes of ethanol ($\sim$750 g/l) TS as the mobile phase. Apply separately to the plate 1 µl of each of 2 solutions in disodium edetate (10 g/l) TS containing (A) 6.0 mg of the test substance per ml and (B) 6.0 mg of bacitracin zinc RS per ml. A third spot (C) is made by applying 1 µl of each of solutions A and B at the same point of application, allowing the plate to dry between the two loadings. After removing the plate from the chromatographic chamber, allow it to dry in air, spray it with triketohydrindene/pyridine/butanol TS, and heat it at 110 °C for 10 minutes. Allow to cool, and examine the chromatogram in daylight. The spots obtained with solution A correspond in position, appearance, and intensity with that obtained with solution B. A single spot is obtained with solution C.

B.   Ignite 30 mg; dissolve half of the residue in 1.0 ml of hydrochloric acid ($\sim$70 g/l) TS and add 1.0 ml of potassium ferrocyanide (45 g/l) TS; a white precipitate is produced. Dissolve the remaining residue in 1.0 ml of sulfuric acid ($\sim$100 g/l) TS, add 0.05 ml of copper(II) sulfate (1 g/l) TS and 2.0 ml of ammonium mercurithiocyanate TS; a violet precipitate is produced.

Loss on drying.   Dry at 60 °C under reduced pressure (not exceeding 0.6 kPa or about 5 mm of mercury) for 3 hours; it loses not more than 50 mg/g.

pH value.   Shake 1.0 g with 10 ml of carbon-dioxide-free water R and filter; pH of the filtrate, 6.0–7.5.

Bacitracin F and related substances.   Prepare a solution containing 30 mg in 100 ml of sulfuric acid (0.05 mol/l) VS. The ratio of the absorbance at 290 nm to that at 252 nm is not greater than 0.15.

Zinc.   Dissolve 0.20 g in 5 ml of acetic acid ($\sim$60 g/l) TS and add 50 ml of water, 50 mg of xylenol orange indicator mixture R, and sufficient methenamine R to produce a red solution. Add 2.0 g of methenamine R in excess and titrate with disodium edetate (0.01 mol/l) VS until the colour changes to yellow. Each ml of disodium edetate (0.01 mol/l) VS is equivalent to 0.6537 mg of Zn; the zinc content is not less than 40 mg/g and not more than 60 mg/g, calculated with reference to the dried substance.

Assay. Suspend 0.05 g, accurately weighed, in 5 ml of water and add 0.5 ml of hydrochloric acid ($\sim$70 g/l) TS and sufficient water to produce 100 ml. Allow to stand at room temperature for 30 minutes and carry out the assay as described under "Microbiological assay of antibiotics" (vol. 1, p. 145), using *Micrococcus luteus* (NCTC 7743 or ATCC 10240) as the test organism, culture medium Cm1 with a final pH of either 7.0–7.1 or 6.5–6.6, sterile phosphate buffer TS of pH either 7.0 or 6.0, an appropriate concentration of bacitracin (usually 1–4 IU per ml), and an incubation temperature of either 35–39 °C or 32–35 °C. The precision of the assay is such that the fiducial limits of error of the estimated potency (P = 0.95) are not less than 95 % and not more than 105 % of the estimated potency. The upper fiducial limit of error of the estimated potency (P = 0.95) is not less than 55 IU of bacitracin per mg, calculated with reference to the dried substance.

Additional Requirements for Sterile Bacitracin Zinc

Storage. Sterile Bacitracin zinc should be kept in a hermetically closed container, protected from light, and stored at a temperature not exceeding 25 °C.

Sterility. Complies with the "Sterility testing of antibiotics" (vol. 1, p. 152), applying the membrane filtration test procedure. Dissolve the test substance in peptone (1 g/l) TS1 to which disodium edetate R has been added.

BARII SULFAS

Barium sulfate

Molecular formula. $BaSO_4$

Relative molecular mass. 233.4

Chemical name. Barium sulfate (1 : 1); CAS Reg. No. 7727-43-7.

Description. A white, heavy, fine powder; free from grittiness; odourless.

Solubility. Practically insoluble in water and in organic solvents; very slightly soluble in acids and in solutions of alkali hydroxides.

Category. Radiocontrast medium.

Storage. Barium sulfate should be kept in a well-closed container.

Additional information. Barium sulfate is inclined to caking.

REQUIREMENTS

Identity tests

A.   Boil 0.2 g in a solution of 5.0 g of sodium carbonate R dissolved in 5 ml of water for 5 minutes, then add 10 ml of water and filter (keep the precipitate for test B). To 5 ml of the filtrate add 5 ml of hydrochloric acid ($\sim$70 g/l) TS; this solution yields reaction A described under "General identification tests" as characteristic of sulfates (vol. 1, p. 115).

B.   Wash the precipitate from test A with 3 successive small quantities of water. To the residue add 5 ml of hydrochloric acid ($\sim$70 g/l) TS, filter, and to the filtrate add 0.3 ml of sulfuric acid ($\sim$100 g/l) TS; a white precipitate is produced which is insoluble in sodium hydroxide ($\sim$80 g/l) TS.

Sedimentation.   Place 5.0 g, previously sifted, in a glass-stoppered 50-ml graduated cylinder, having the 50-ml graduation mark 11–14 cm from the base. Add sufficient water to produce 50 ml, shake for 5 minutes and allow to stand for 15 minutes; the barium sulfate does not settle below the 15-ml graduation mark.

Heavy metals.   For the preparation of the test solution boil 4 g with 6 ml of acetic acid ($\sim$60 g/l) PbTS and 44 ml of water for 10 minutes, filter, allow to cool and dilute to 50 ml with water. Determine the heavy metals content in 25 ml of the filtrate as described under "Limit test for heavy metals", according to Method A (vol. 1, p. 119); not more than 10 µg/g.

Arsenic.   Transfer 0.5 g to a long-necked combustion flask, add 30 ml of water and 2 ml of nitric acid ($\sim$1000 g/l) TS, insert a small funnel into the neck of the flasks and heat in an inclined position on a water-bath for 2 hours. Allow to cool, adjust to the original volume with water, and filter. Wash the residue three times with 5 ml of water, combine the filtrate and washings, add 1 ml of sulfuric acid ($\sim$1760 g/l) TS, and evaporate on a water-bath until white fumes are evolved. Dissolve the residue in 10 ml of sulfuric acid ($\sim$100 g/l) TS, add 10 ml of water, and proceed as described under "Limit test for arsenic" (vol. 1, p. 122); the arsenic content is not more than 2 µg/g.

Soluble barium salts.   Boil 10 g with 20 ml of water and 30 ml of acetic acid ($\sim$60 g/l) TS for 5 minutes, filter, allow to cool and dilute to 50 ml with water. To a 10-ml portion of this solution add 1 ml of sulfuric acid ($\sim$100 g/l) TS and to a second 10-ml portion add 1 ml of water. When compared after 1 hour, the two solutions remain equally clear.

Phosphates.   To 1.0 g add 3 ml of nitric acid ($\sim$130 g/l) TS and 7 ml of water and heat on a water-bath for 5 minutes. Filter and dilute the filtrate to 10 ml with water. Add 5 ml of ammonium molybdate/vanadate TS and allow to stand for 5 minutes; any yellow colour produced is not more intense than that of a reference solution prepared similarly using 10 ml of phosphate standard (5 µg/ml) TS.

Oxidizable sulfur compounds.   Shake 1.0 g with 5 ml of water for 30 seconds and filter. To the filtrate add 0.1 ml of starch TS, 0.1 g of potassium iodide R, 1 ml of freshly prepared potassium iodate (3.6 mg/l) TS, and 1 ml of hydrochloric acid (1 mol/l) VS, and shake well; the colour produced is more intense than that of a solution prepared in a similar way, but omitting the potassium iodate.

Acid-soluble substances.   Boil 5 g with 15 ml of acetic acid ($\sim$300 g/l) TS and 10 ml of water for 5 minutes. Filter, evaporate the filtrate to dryness on a water-bath, and dry to constant weight at 105 °C; the residue weighs not more than 15 mg.

Loss on ignition.   Ignite 1.0 g at 600 °C; it loses not more than 20 mg/g.

Acidity or alkalinity.   Heat 5.0 g with 20 ml of carbon-dioxide-free water R on a water-bath for 5 minutes and filter. To 10 ml of the filtrate add 0.05 ml of bromothymol blue/ethanol TS; not more than 0.5 ml of hydrochloric acid (0.01 mol/l) VS or 0.5 ml of carbonate-free sodium hydroxide (0.01 mol/l) VS is required to obtain the midpoint of the indicator (green).

BECLOMETASONI DIPROPIONAS

Beclometasone dipropionate

Molecular formula. $C_{28}H_{37}ClO_7$

Relative molecular mass.   521.0

Graphic formula.

Chemical name.   9-Chloro-11β,17,21-trihydroxy-16β-methylpregna-1,4-diene-3,20-dione 17,21-dipropionate; 9-chloro-11β-hydroxy-16β-methyl-17,21-bis(1-oxopropoxy)pregna-1,4-diene-3,20-dione; CAS Reg. No. 5534-09-8.

Description.   A white to creamy white powder; odourless.

Solubility. Practically insoluble in water; soluble in 60 parts of ethanol (~750 g/l) TS and in 8 parts of chloroform R.

Category. Antiasthmatic drug.

Storage. Beclometasone dipropionate should be kept in a well-closed container, protected from light.

REQUIREMENTS

General requirement. Beclometasone diproprionate contains not less than 96.0 % and not more than 104.0 % of $C_{28}H_{37}ClO_7$, calculated with reference to the dried substance.

Identity tests

● Either test A or test B may be applied.

A.   Carry out the examination as described under "Spectrophotometry in the infrared region" (vol. 1, p. 40). The infrared absorption spectrum is concordant with the spectrum obtained from beclometasone diproprionate RS or with the *reference spectrum* of beclometasone dipropionate.

B.   Carry out the test as described under "Thin-layer chromatography" (vol. 1, p. 83), using kieselguhr R1 as the coating substance and a mixture of 1 volume of propylene glycol R and 9 volumes of acetone R to impregnate the plate, dipping it about 5 mm into the liquid. After the solvent has reached a height of at least 16 cm, remove the plate from the chromatographic chamber and allow it to stand at room temperature until the solvent has completely evaporated. Use the impregnated plate within 2 hours, carrying out the chromatography in the same direction as the impregnation. Use a mixture of 4 volumes of cyclohexane R and 1 volume of toluene R as the mobile phase. Apply separately to the plate 2 µl of each of 2 solutions in a mixture of 9 volumes of chloroform R and 1 volume of methanol R containing (A) 2.5 mg of the test substance per ml and (B) 2.5 mg of beclometasone dipropionate RS per ml. After removing the plate from the chromatographic chamber, allow it to dry in air until the solvents have evaporated, heat it at 120 °C for 15 minutes, spray the hot plate with sulfuric acid/ethanol TS, and then heat at 120 °C for 10 minutes. Allow to cool, and examine the chromatogram in daylight and in ultraviolet light (365 nm). The principal spot obtained with solution A corresponds in position, appearance, and intensity with that obtained with solution B.

Specific optical rotation. Use a 10 mg/ml solution in dioxan R; $[\alpha]_D^{20\,°C} = +88$ to $+94°$.

Sulfated ash. Not more than 1.0 mg/g.

Loss on drying. Dry to constant weight at 105 °C; it loses not more than 5.0 mg/g.

Related substances. Carry out the test as described under "Thin-layer chromatography" (vol. 1, p. 83), using silica gel R1 as the coating substance and a mixture of 95 volumes of dichloroethane R, 5 volumes of methanol R, and 0.2 volumes of water as the mobile phase. Apply separately to the plate 10 µl of each of 2 solutions in a mixture of 9 volumes of chloroform R and 1 volume of methanol R containing (A) 15 mg of the test substance per ml and (B) 0.30 mg of the test substance per ml. After removing the plate from the chromatographic chamber, allow it to dry in air until the solvents have evaporated and heat at 105 °C for 10 minutes; allow it to cool, spray it with blue tetrazolium/sodium hydroxide TS, and examine the chromatogram in daylight. Any spot obtained with solution A, other than the principal spot, is not more intense than that obtained with solution B.

Assay

● The solutions must be protected from light throughout the assay.

Dissolve about 20 mg, accurately weighed, in sufficient aldehyde-free ethanol (~750 g/l) TS to produce 100 ml. Dilute 20 ml of this solution with sufficient aldehyde-free ethanol (~750 g/l) TS to produce 100 ml. Transfer 10.0 ml of the diluted solution to a 25-ml volumetric flask, add 2.0 ml of blue tetrazolium/ethanol TS, and displace the air in the flask with oxygen-free nitrogen R. Immediately add 2.0 ml of tetramethylammonium hydroxide/ethanol TS and again displace the air with oxygen-free nitrogen R. Stopper the flask, mix the contents by gentle swirling, and allow to stand for 1 hour in a water-bath at 30 °C. Cool rapidly, add sufficient aldehyde-free ethanol (~750 g/l) TS to produce 25 ml, and mix. Measure the absorbance of a 1-cm layer at the maximum at about 525 nm against a solvent cell containing a solution prepared by treating 10 ml of aldehyde-free ethanol (~750 g/l) TS in a similar manner. Calculate the amount of $C_{28}H_{37}ClO_7$ in the substance being tested by comparison with beclometasone dipropionate RS, similarly and concurrently examined.

BENZATHINI BENZYLPENICILLINUM

Benzathine benzylpenicillin

Benzathine benzylpenicillin (non-injectable)
Benzathine benzylpenicillin, sterile

Molecular formula. $(C_{16}H_{18}N_2O_4S)_2,C_{16}H_{20}N_2$ (anhydrous)

Relative molecular mass.   909.1 (anhydrous)

Graphic formula.

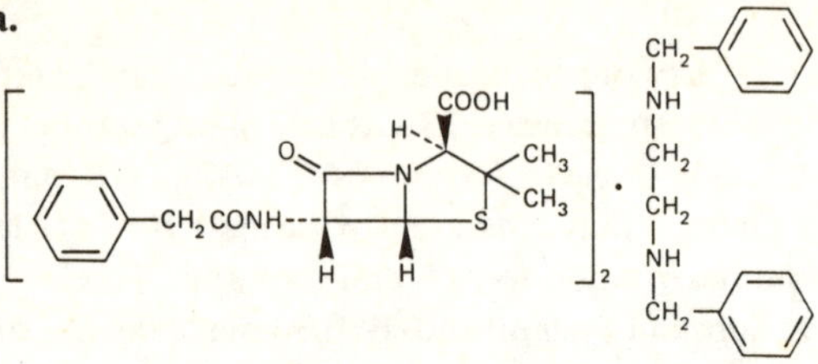

Chemical name. N,N'-Dibenzylethylenediamine compound with $(2S,5R,6R)$-3,3-dimethyl-7-oxo-6-(2-phenylacetamido)-4-thia-1-azabicyclo[3.2.0]heptane-2-carboxylic acid (1:2); N,N'-bis(phenylmethyl)-1,2-ethanediamine compound with [2S-(2α,5α,6β)]-3,3-dimethyl-7-oxo-6-[(phenylacetyl)amino]-4-thia-1-azabicyclo[3.2.0]heptane-2-carboxylic acid (1:2); N,N'-dibenzylethylenediamine salt of benzylpenicillin; CAS Reg. No. 1538-09-6 (anhydrous).

Other name.   Penicillin G benzathine.

Description.   A white powder; odourless or almost odourless.

Solubility.   Very slightly soluble in water; sparingly soluble in ethanol ($\sim$750 g/l) TS; practically insoluble in chloroform R and ether R.

Category.   Antibacterial drug.

Storage.   Benzathine benzylpenicillin should be kept in a tightly closed container, protected from light, and stored at a temperature not exceeding 30 °C.

Labelling.   The designation sterile Benzathine benzylpenicillin indicates that the substance complies with the additional requirements for sterile Benzathine benzylpenicillin and may be used for parenteral administration or for other sterile applications.

Additional information.   Benzathine benzylpenicillin contains a variable amount of water of crystallization.

REQUIREMENTS

General requirement. Benzathine benzylpenicillin contains not less than 96.0% and not more than 100.5% of total penicillins calculated as $(C_{16}H_{18}N_2O_4S)_2,C_{16}H_{20}N_2$, and not less than 24.0% and not more than 27.0% of $C_{16}H_{20}N_2$, both calculated with reference to the anhydrous substance.

Identity tests

A.   To 2 mg in a test-tube add 1 drop of water followed by 2 ml of sulfuric acid ($\sim$1760 g/l) TS and mix; the solution is almost colourless. Immerse the test-tube for 1 minute in a water-bath; the solution remains almost colourless. Place 2 mg in a second test-tube, add 1 drop of water and 2 ml of formaldehyde/sulfuric acid TS and mix; the solution is almost colourless and after a few minutes the colour changes to yellow-brown. Immerse the test-tube for 1 minute in a water-bath; a reddish brown colour is produced.

B.   Shake 0.1 g with 2 ml of sodium hydroxide (1 mol/l) VS for 2 minutes, extract the mixture with 2 quantities, each of 3 ml of ether R, evaporate the combined extracts, and dissolve the residue in 1 ml of ethanol ($\sim$375 g/l) TS. Add 5 ml of trinitrophenol (7 g/l) TS, heat at 90 °C for 5 minutes, and allow to cool slowly. Collect the precipitate and recrystallize it from hot ethanol ($\sim$150 g/l) TS that contains 10 mg/ml of trinitrophenol R; melting temperature, about 214 °C (picrate).

Water.   Determine as described under "Determination of water by the Karl Fischer Method", Method A (vol. 1, p. 135), using about 0.5 g of the substance; the water content is not less than 50 mg/g and not more than 80 mg/g.

pH value.   pH of a saturated solution containing about 0.05 g in 10 ml of carbon-dioxide-free water R, 5.0–7.5.

Assay

A.   *For total penicillins.* Dissolve about 0.065 g, accurately weighed, in 10 ml of dimethylformamide R and dilute with sufficient water to produce 1000 ml. Transfer two 2.0-ml aliquots of this solution into separate stoppered tubes. To one tube add 10.0 ml of imidazole/mercuric chloride TS, mix, stopper the tube and place it in a water-bath at 60 °C for exactly 25 minutes. Cool the tube rapidly to 20 °C (solution A).

To the second tube add 10.0 ml of water and mix (solution B).

Without delay measure the absorbance of a 1-cm layer at the maximum at about 325 nm against a solvent cell containing a mixture of 2.0 ml of water and 10.0 ml of imidazole/mercuric chloride TS for solution A and water for solution B.

From the difference between the absorbance of solution A and that of solution B, calculate the amount of $(C_{16}H_{18}N_2O_4S)_2, C_{16}H_{20}N_2$ in the substance being tested by comparison with 0.050 g of benzylpenicillin sodium RS similarly and concurrently examined, taking into account that each mg of benzylpenicillin sodium RS $(C_{16}H_{17}N_2O_4S)$ is equivalent to 1.275 mg of $(C_{16}H_{18}N_2O_4S)_2, C_{16}H_{20}N_2$. In an adequately calibrated spectrophotometer, the absorbance of the reference solution should be 0.62 ± 0.03.

B.   *For* $C_{16}H_{20}N_2$. To about 1 g, accurately weighed, add 30 ml of sodium chloride (400 g/l) TS and 10 ml of sodium hydroxide ($\sim$150 g/l) TS, shake well, and extract with four quantities, each of 50 ml of ether R. Wash the combined extracts with three quantities, each of 10 ml of water, extract the combined washings with

25 ml of ether R, and add the extract to the main ether solution. Evaporate the ether solution to a low bulk, add 2 ml of dehydrated ethanol R and evaporate to dryness. To the residue add 50 ml of glacial acetic acid R and titrate with perchloric acid (0.1 mol/l) VS, using 1 ml of 1-naphtholbenzein/acetic acid TS as indicator. Repeat the operation without the substance being examined; the difference between the titrations represents the amount of perchloric acid required to neutralize the liberated base. Each ml of perchloric acid (0.1 mol/l) VS is equivalent to 12.02 mg of $C_{16}H_{20}N_2$.

Additional Requirements for Sterile Benzathine Benzylpenicillin

Storage. Sterile Benzathine benzylpenicillin should be kept in a hermetically closed container, protected from light, and stored at a temperature not exceeding 30 °C.

Pyrogens. Carry out the test as described under "Test for pyrogens" (vol. 1, p. 155) injecting, per kg of the rabbit's mass, 5 ml of a solution in sterile water R containing 0.4 mg of the substance to be examined per ml.

Sterility. Complies with the "Sterility testing of antibiotics" (vol. 1, p. 152), applying either the membrane filtration test procedure with added penicillinase TS or the direct test procedure.

BETAMETHASONI VALERAS

Betamethasone valerate

Molecular formula. $C_{27}H_{37}FO_6$

Relative molecular mass.   476.6

Graphic formula.

Chemical name. 9-Fluoro-11β,17,21-trihydroxy-16β-methylpregna-1,4-diene-3,20-dione 17-valerate; 9-fluoro-11β,21-dihydroxy-16β-methyl-17-[(1-oxopentyl)oxyl]pregna-1,4-diene-3,20-dione; CAS Reg. No. 2152-44-5.

Description. A white or creamy white powder; odourless.

Solubility. Practically insoluble in water; soluble in ethanol (~750 g/l) TS; freely soluble in acetone R and chloroform R.

Category. Antiinflammatory drug.

Storage. Betamethasone valerate should be kept in a tightly closed container, protected from light.

REQUIREMENTS

General requirement. Betamethasone valerate contains not less than 96.0 % and not more than 104.0 % of $C_{27}H_{37}FO_6$, calculated with reference to the dried substance.

Identity tests

● Either tests A and B or tests C, D and E may be applied.

A. Carry out the examination as described under "Spectrophotometry in the infrared region" (vol. 1, p. 40). The infrared absorption spectrum is concordant with the spectrum obtained from betamethasone valerate RS or with the *reference spectrum* of betamethasone valerate.

B. Dissolve 20 mg in 20 ml of ethanol (~750 g/l) TS and dilute 2 ml to 20 ml with the same solvent. To 2 ml of this solution placed in a stoppered test-tube add 10 ml of phenylhydrazine/sulfuric acid TS, mix, heat in a water-bath at 60 °C for 20 minutes, and cool immediately. The absorbance of a 1-cm layer at the maximum at about 423 nm is not more than 0.25.

C. See the test described below under "Related steroids". The principal spots obtained with solutions A and C correspond in position with that obtained with solution B. In addition, the principal spot obtained with solution A corresponds in appearance and intensity with that obtained with solution B.

D. Carry out the combustion as described under "Oxygen flask method" (vol. 1, p. 125), using 7 mg of the test substance and a mixture of 0.5 ml of sodium hydroxide (0.01 mol/l) VS and 20 ml of water as the absorbing liquid. When the process is complete, add 0.1 ml of a mixture of 0.1 ml of a freshly prepared sodium alizarinsulfonate (1 g/l) TS and 0.1 ml of zirconyl nitrate TS; the red colour of the solution changes to clear yellow.

E.   Heat 0.05 g with 2.0 ml of potassium hydroxide/ethanol TS1 in a water-bath for 5 minutes. Cool, add 2.0 ml of sulfuric acid ($\sim$100 g/l) TS, and boil gently for 1 minute; a pleasant odour of ethyl valerate is perceptible.

Specific optical rotation.   Use a 10 mg/ml solution in dioxan R; $[\alpha]_D^{20\,°C} = +75$ to $+81°$.

Sulfated ash.   Weigh 0.1 g and ignite on a platinum dish; not more than 2.0 mg/g.

Loss on drying.   Dry to constant weight at 105 °C; it loses not more than 5.0 mg/g.

Related steroids.   Carry out the test as described under "Thin-layer chromatography" (vol. 1, p. 83), using silica gel R1 as the coating substance and a mixture of 95 volumes of dichloroethane R, 5 volumes of methanol R, and 0.2 volumes of water as the mobile phase. Apply separately to the plate 1 µl of each of 2 solutions in a mixture of 9 volumes of chloroform R and 1 volume of methanol R containing (A) 15 mg of the test substance per ml and (B) 15 mg of betamethasone valerate RS per ml; also apply to the plate 2 µl of a third solution (C) composed of a mixture of equal volumes of solutions A and B and 1 µl of a fourth solution (D) containing 0.15 mg of the test substance per ml in the same solvent mixture used for solutions A and B. After removing the plate from the chromatographic chamber, allow it to dry in air until the solvents have evaporated. Then heat it at 105 °C for 10 minutes, allow it to cool, spray it with blue tetrazolium/sodium hydroxide TS, and examine the chromatogram in daylight. Any spot obtained with solution A, other than the principal spot, is not more intense than that obtained with solution D.

Assay

● The solutions must be protected from light throughout the assay.

Dissolve about 20 mg, accurately weighed, in sufficient aldehyde-free ethanol ($\sim$750 g/l) TS to produce 100 ml. Dilute 20 ml of this solution with sufficient aldehyde-free ethanol ($\sim$750 g/l) TS to produce 100 ml. Transfer 10.0 ml of the diluted solution to a 25-ml volumetric flask, add 2.0 ml of blue tetrazolium/ethanol TS, and displace the air in the flask with oxygen-free nitrogen R. Immediately add 2.0 ml of tetramethylammonium hydroxide/ethanol TS and again displace the air with oxygen-free nitrogen R. Stopper the flask, mix the contents by gentle swirling, and allow to stand for 1 hour in a water-bath at 30 °C. Cool rapidly, add sufficient aldehyde-free ethanol ($\sim$750 g/l) TS to produce 25 ml, and mix. Measure the absorbance of a 1-cm layer at the maximum at about 525 nm against a solvent cell containing a solution prepared by treating 10 ml of aldehyde-free ethanol ($\sim$750 g/l) TS in a similar manner. Calculate the amount of $C_{27}H_{37}FO_6$ in the substance being tested by comparison with betamethasone valerate RS, similarly and concurrently examined.

BIPERIDENUM

Biperiden

Molecular formula. $C_{21}H_{29}NO$

Relative molecular mass.   311.5

Graphic formula.

N—CH₂CH₂COH   with a phenyl ring and a piperidine ring and a CH₂ (norbornene) substituent

Chemical name.   α-5-Norbornen-2-yl-α-phenyl-1-piperidinepropanol; α-bicyclo[2.2.1]hept-5-en-2-yl-α-phenyl-1-piperidinepropanol; CAS Reg. No. 514-65-8.

Description.   A white or almost white, crystalline powder; odourless.

Solubility.   Practically insoluble in water; freely soluble in chloroform R; soluble in ether R; sparingly soluble in ethanol ($\sim$750 g/l) TS.

Category.   Antiparkinsonism drug.

Storage.   Biperiden should be kept in a well-closed container, protected from light.

REQUIREMENTS

General requirement.   Biperiden contains not less than 98.0% and not more than 101.0% of $C_{21}H_{29}NO$, calculated with reference to the dried substance.

Identity tests

● Either test A alone or tests B, C and D may be applied.

A.   Carry out the examination as described under "Spectrophotometry in the infrared region" (vol. 1, p. 40).   The infrared absorption spectrum is concordant with the spectrum obtained from biperiden RS or with the *reference spectrum* of biperiden.

B.   Dissolve 20 mg in 5 ml of phosphoric acid ($\sim$1440 g/l) TS and allow to stand; a green colour is produced.

C.   To 0.20 g add 80 ml of water, 0.5 ml of hydrochloric acid ($\sim$70 g/l) TS, and warm until dissolved.   Cool and to 5 ml of this solution add bromine TS1 drop by drop; a yellow precipitate is formed which dissolves on shaking. Upon the addition of more bromine TS1, a permanent precipitate is produced.

D. Melting temperature, about 114 °C.

Sulfated ash. Not more than 1.0 mg/g.

Loss on drying. Dry for 3 hours at 105 °C; it loses not more than 10 mg/g.

Related substances. Carry out the test as described under "Thin-layer chromatography" (vol. 1, p. 83), using a plate coated with a suspension of silica gel R1 in sodium hydroxide (0.5 mol/l) VS, and as the mobile phase a mixture of 96.5 volumes of toluene R and 3.5 volumes of methanol R. Apply separately to the plate 5 µl of each of 2 solutions in chloroform R containing (A) 40 mg of the test substance per ml and (B) 0.20 mg of the test substance per ml. After removing the plate from the chromatographic chamber, allow it to dry in air, spray it with potassium iodobismuthate TS2, and examine the chromatogram in daylight. Any spot obtained with solution A, other than the principal spot, is not more intense than that obtained with solution B.

Assay. Dissolve about 0.4 g, accurately weighed, in 30 ml of glacial acetic acid R1, add 0.15 ml of 1-naphtholbenzein/acetic acid TS as indicator and titrate with perchloric acid (0.1 mol/l) VS, as described under "Non-aqueous titration", Method A (vol. 1, p. 131). Each ml of perchloric acid (0.1 mol/l) VS is equivalent to 31.15 mg of $C_{21}H_{29}NO$.

BIPERIDENI HYDROCHLORIDUM

Biperiden hydrochloride

Molecular formula. $C_{21}H_{29}NO,HCl$

Relative molecular mass. 347.9

Graphic formula.

Chemical name. α-5-Norbornen-2-yl-α-phenyl-1-piperidinepropanol hydrochloride; α-bicyclo[2.2.1]hept-5-en-2-yl-α-phenyl-1-piperidinepropanol hydrochloride; CAS Reg. No. 1235-82-1.

Description.   A white, crystalline powder; odourless.

Solubility.   Slightly soluble in water, chloroform R, ethanol ($\sim$750 g/l) TS and ether R; sparingly soluble in methanol R.

Category.   Antiparkinsonism drug.

Storage.   Biperiden hydrochloride should be kept in a well-closed container, protected from light.

REQUIREMENTS

General requirement.   Biperiden hydrochloride contains not less than 98.0% and not more than 101.0% of $C_{21}H_{29}NO,HCl$, calculated with reference to the dried substance.

Identity tests

• Either tests A and D or tests B, C and D may be applied.

A.   Carry out the examination as described under "Spectrophotometry in the infrared region" (vol. 1, p. 40). The infrared absorption spectrum is concordant with the spectrum obtained from biperiden hydrochloride RS or with the *reference spectrum* of biperiden hydrochloride.

B.   Dissolve 20 mg in 5 ml of phosphoric acid ($\sim$1440 g/l) TS and allow to stand; a green colour is produced.

C.   Dissolve 0.10 g in 50 ml of water and to 5 ml of this solution add bromine TS1 drop by drop; a yellow precipitate is formed which dissolves on shaking. Upon the addition of more bromine TS1, a permanent precipitate is produced.

D.   A 20 mg/ml solution yields reaction B described under "General identification tests" as characteristic of chlorides (vol. 1, p. 113).

Sulfated ash.   Not more than 1.0 mg/g.

Loss on drying.   Dry for 3 hours at 105 °C; it loses not more than 5 mg/g.

Related substances.   Carry out the test as described under "Thin-layer chromatography" (vol. 1, p. 83), using a plate coated with a suspension of silica gel R1 in sodium hydroxide (0.5 mol/l) VS, and as the mobile phase a mixture of 96.5 volumes of toluene R and 3.5 volumes of methanol R. Apply separately to the plate 10 µl of each of 2 solutions in methanol R containing (A) 20 mg of the test substance per ml and (B) 0.10 mg of the test substance per ml. After removing the plate from the chromatographic chamber, allow it to dry in air, spray it with potassium iodobismuthate TS2, and examine the chromatogram in daylight. Any spot obtained with solution A, other than the principal spot, is not more intense than that obtained with solution B.

Assay. Dissolve about 0.4 g, accurately weighed, in 30 ml of glacial acetic acid R1, warming slightly to effect solution, add 10 ml of mercuric acetate/acetic acid TS and 0.15 ml of 1-naphtholbenzein/acetic acid TS as indicator. Titrate with perchloric acid (0.1 mol/l) VS, as described under "Non-aqueous titration", Method A (vol. 1, p. 131). Each ml of perchloric acid (0.1 mol/l) VS is equivalent to 34.79 mg of $C_{21}H_{29}NO,HCl$.

BLEOMYCINI HYDROCHLORIDUM

Bleomycin hydrochloride

Bleomycin hydrochloride (non-injectable)
Bleomycin hydrochloride, sterile

Composition. Bleomycin hydrochloride is the hydrochloride salt of a mixture of substances produced by the growth of *Streptomyces verticillus.* The main components of the mixture are bleomycin A_2 and bleomycin B_2; CAS Reg. No. 67763-87-5.

Molecular formula. Bleomycin A_2 hydrochloride: $C_{55}H_{84}N_{17}O_{21}S_3,Cl$. Bleomycin B_2 hydrochloride: $C_{55}H_{84}N_{20}O_{21}S_2,HCl$.

Relative molecular mass. Bleomycin A_2 hydrochloride: 1452; Bleomycin B_2 hydrochloride: 1461.

Graphic formulas for the bleomycin A_2/B_2 bases.

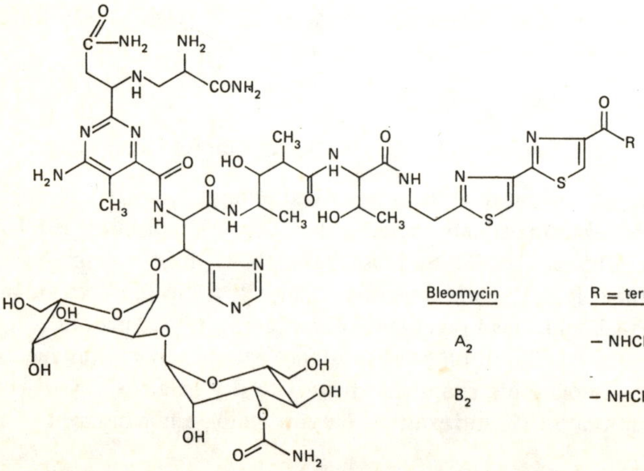

Bleomycin	R = terminal amine
A_2	$-NHCH_2CH_2CH_2S^+(CH_3)_2$
B_2	$-NHCH_2CH_2CH_2CH_2NHC(=NH)NH_2$

Chemical name. Bleomycin A_2 hydrochloride: N^1-[3-(Dimethylsulfonio)-propyl]bleomycinamide chloride; [3-[2′-[2-[(2S,3R)-2-[(2S,3S,4R)-4-[(2S,3R)-2-[6-amino-2-[(1S)-1-[[(2S)-2-amino-2-carbamoylethyl]amino]-2-carbamoylethyl]-5-methyl-4-pyrimidinecarboxamido]-3-[[2-O-(3-O-carbamoyl-α-D-mannopyrano-syl)-α-L-gulopyranosyl]oxy]-3-imidazol-4-ylpropionamido]-3-hydroxy-2-methyl-valeramido]-3-hydroxybutyramido]ethyl][2,4′-bithiazole]-4-carboxamido]pro-pyl]dimethylsulfonium chloride; CAS Reg. No. 49830-49-1.
Bleomycin B_2 hydrochloride: N^1-(Guanidinobutyl)bleomycinamide hydrochlo-ride; (βS)-4-amino-β-[[(2S)-2-amino-2-carbamoylethyl]amino]-6-[[(1S,2R)-2-[[2-O-(3-O-carbamoyl-α-D-mannopyranosyl)-α-L-gulopyranosyl]oxy]-1-[[(1R,2S,3S)-3-[[(1S,2R)-1-[[2-[4-[(4-guanidinobutyl)carbamoyl][2,4′-bithiazol]-2′-yl]ethyl]carbamoyl]-2-hydroxypropyl]carbamoyl]-2-hydroxy-1-methylbutyl]car-bamoyl]-2-imidazol-4-ylethyl]carbamoyl]-5-methyl-2-pyrimidinepropionamide hydrochloride; N^1-[4-[(aminoiminomethyl)amino]butyl]bleomycinamide hydro-chloride; CAS Reg. No. 55658-44-1.

Description.   A white to yellowish white powder.

Solubility.   Freely soluble in water and in methanol R; slightly soluble in ethanol ($\sim$750 g/l) TS; practically insoluble in acetone R and ether R.

Category.   Cytotoxic drug.

Storage.   Bleomycin hydrochloride should be kept in a tightly closed cont-ainer.

Labelling.   The designation sterile Bleomycin hydrochloride indicates that the substance complies with the additional requirements for sterile Bleomycin hydrochloride and may be used for parenteral administration or for other sterile applications. CAUTION: Bleomycin hydrochloride must be handled with care, avoiding contact with the skin and inhalation of airborne particles.

REQUIREMENTS

General requirement.   Bleomycin hydrochloride contains, when tested according to assay A, not less than 1500 and not more than 2000 International Units of bleomycin A_2/B_2 per mg, calculated with reference to the dried substance.

Further, Bleomycin hydrochloride contains, when tested according to assay B, not less than 55.0% and not more than 70.0% of bleomycin A_2 and not less than 25.0% and not more than 32.0% of bleomycin B_2; the total of bleomycin A_2 and bleomycin B_2 is not less than 85%. The content of bleomycin A_5 is not more than 7.0%, of bleomycin B_4 not more than 1.0%, and of demethylbleomycin A_2 not more than 3.0%.

Identity tests

A.   Dissolve about 5 mg in 10 ml of water, add 5 µl of copper(II) sulfate (160 g/l) TS and dilute with water to 100 ml; the absorption spectrum exhibits maxima at about 242 nm and 290 nm, and a minimum at about 268 nm.

B.   A 10 mg/ml solution yields reaction B described under "General identification tests" as characteristic of chlorides (vol. 1, p. 113).

Loss on drying.   Dry at 60 °C under reduced pressure (not exceeding 0.6 kPa or about 5 mm of mercury) for 4 hours; it loses not more than 60 mg/g.

pH value.   pH of a 5.0 mg/ml solution, 4.5–6.0.

Copper content.   Transfer 75 mg, accurately weighed, to a 60-ml separating funnel and dissolve in 10 ml of hydrochloric acid (0.1 mol/l) VS.   Transfer 10 ml of copper standard TS2 to an additional separating funnel.   To both funnels add 10 ml of zinc bis(dibenzyldithiocarbamate) TS and shake vigorously for 1 minute. Allow the layers to separate.   Filter the lower layer through 1 g of anhydrous sodium sulfate R to remove excess water. Measure the absorbances of a 1-cm layer at the maximum at about 435 nm, using a solvent cell containing carbon tetrachloride R.

   Calculate the content of copper in mg/g from the formula $(A_o \times 15)/(A_s \times W)$ where A_o is the absorbance of the substance to be examined, A_s is the absorbance of copper standard TS2, and W is the weight in mg of the substance to be examined; the copper content is not more than 0.2 mg/g.

Assay

A.   *Microbiological assay.*   Carry out the assay as described under "Microbiological assay of antibiotics" (vol. 1, p. 145), using *Mycobacterium smegmatis* (ATCC 607) as the test organism.   Prepare the inoculum as follows: the test organism is grown for 40–48 hours at a temperature of 27 °C on the surface of culture medium Cm8.   Using 3 ml of saline TS wash the growth into a flask containing 100 ml of culture medium Cm9 and 50 g of glass beads, and incubate at 25–27 °C for 5 days with constant mechanical agitation using an orbital shaker.   The resulting suspension should be used for no longer than 14 days, and kept at a temperature below 5 °C.   For the preparation of inoculated plates use 0.5 ml of the suspension or a suitable volume previously determined using test plates with culture medium Cm8 at a temperature of 27 °C.   Prepare the reference solution in phosphate buffer, pH 7.0, TS, diluting the International Reference Preparation of bleomycin A_2/B_2 to an appropriate concentration (usually between 10 and 200 µg per ml). The precision of the assay is such that the fiducial limits of error of the estimated potency ($P = 0.95$) are not less than 95 % and not more than 105 % of the estimated potency.   The upper fiducial limit of error of the estimated potency ($P = 0.95$) is not less than 1500 IU and the lower fiducial limit is not more than 2000 IU of bleomycin A_2/B_2 per mg, calculated with reference to the dried substance.

B. *Content of the bleomycin components.* Carry out the test as described on pp. 373–377 of the Amendments to vol. 1 under "High performance liquid chromatography", using a column 25 cm long and 4.6 mm in internal diameter packed with particles of silica gel, 5–10 μm in diameter, the surface of which has been modified with chemically bonded octadecyl silyl groups. As the mobile phase for a linear gradient development, start with a mixture of 9 volumes of 1-pentanesulfonic acid TS and 1 volume of methanol R, both previously filtered and deaerated, and end with a composition of 6 volumes of 1-pentanesulfonic acid TS and 4 volumes of methanol R, using a suitable linear rate of change of mobile phase so as to reach the final composition in 60 minutes. (If needed, add the following to the mobile phase to obtain satisfactory chromatography: 1.86 g of disodium edetate R per litre.) As detector use an ultraviolet spectrophotometer at a wavelength of about 254 nm, fitted with a low-volume flow cell (8–20 μl is suitable). Inject 5 μl of a solution of the test substance in water containing the equivalent of 5 IU of bleomycin per ml. Proceed with the gradient elution, pumping the mobile phase mixture at the condition mentioned above for about 80 minutes or until the demethylbleomycin A_2 is eluted.

The elution order of the bleomycin components is the following: void volume, bleomycin acid, bleomycin A_2, bleomycin B_2, bleomycin A_5, bleomycin B_4, and demethylbleomycin A_2.

Calculate in % the content of each bleomycin component, comparing the ratios of the individual areas of the peaks with that of the total area of all the bleomycins.

Additional Requirements for Sterile Bleomycin Hydrochloride

Storage. Sterile Bleomycin hydrochloride should be kept in a hermetically closed container.

Histamine-like substances. Carry out the test as described under "Test for histamine-like substances" (vol. 1, p. 157) using 1 ml per kg of body mass of a solution in saline TS containing a quantity equivalent to 500 IU per ml.

Undue toxicity. Carry out the test as described under "Test for undue toxicity" (vol. 1, p. 154), using 0.5 ml of a solution in saline TS containing a quantity equivalent to 5000 IU of bleomycin hydrochloride per ml.

Pyrogens. Carry out the test as described under "Test for pyrogens" (vol. 1, p. 155) injecting per kg of the rabbit's mass, 1 ml of a solution in saline TS containing 500 IU of bleomycin hydrochloride per ml.

Sterility. Complies with the "Sterility testing of antibiotics" (vol. 1, p. 152), applying the membrane filtration test procedure.

————————

BLEOMYCINI SULFAS

Bleomycin sulfate

Bleomycin sulfate (non-injectable)
Bleomycin sulfate, sterile

Composition. Bleomycin sulfate is the sulfate salt of a mixture of substances produced by the growth of *Streptomyces verticillus.* The main components of the mixture are bleomycin A_2 and bleomycin B_2; CAS Reg. No. 9041-93-4.

Molecular formula. Bleomycin A_2 sulfate: $C_{55}H_{84}N_{17}O_{21}S_3,HSO_4$; Bleomycin B_2 sulfate: $C_{55}H_{84}N_{20}O_{21}S_2,H_2SO_4$

Relative molecular mass. Bleomycin A_2 sulfate: 1514; Bleomycin B_2 sulfate: 1524.

Graphic formulas for the bleomycin A_2/B_2 bases.

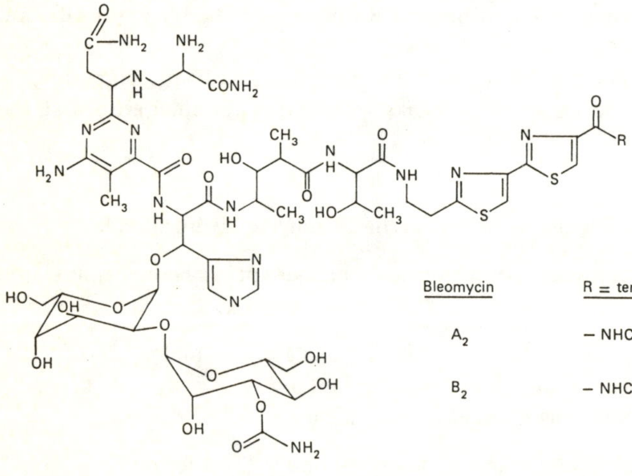

Bleomycin	R = terminal amine
A_2	$-NHCH_2CH_2CH_2S^+(CH_3)_2$
B_2	$-NHCH_2CH_2CH_2CH_2NHC(=NH)NH_2$

Chemical name. Bleomycin A_2 sulfate: N^1-[3-(Dimethylsulfonio)propyl]bleomycinamide hydrogen sulfate; [3-[2′-[2-[(2*S*,3*R*)-2-[(2*S*,3*S*,4*R*)-4-[(2*S*,3*R*)-2-[6-amino-2-[(1*S*)-1-[[(2*S*)-2-amino-2-carbamoylethyl]amino]-2-carbamoylethyl]-5-methyl-4-pyrimidinecarboxamido]-3-[[2-*O*-(3-*O*-carbamoyl-α-D-mannopyranosyl)-α-L-gulopyranosyl]oxy]-3-imidazol-4-ylpropionamido]-3-hydroxy-2-methylvaleramido]-3-hydroxybutyramido]ethyl][2,4′-bithiazole]-4-carboxamido]propyl]dimethylsulfonium hydrogen sulfate.

Bleomycin B_2 sulfate: N^1-(Guanidinobutyl)bleomycinamide; (β*S*)-4-amino-β-[[(2*S*)-2-amino-2-carbamoylethyl]amino]-6-[[(1*S*,2*R*)-2-[[2-*O*-(3-*O*-carbamoyl-α-D-mannopyranosyl)-α-L-gulopyranosyl]oxy]-1-[[(1*R*,2*S*,3*S*)-3-[[(1*S*,2*R*)-1-[[2-[4-

[(4-guanidinobutyl)carbamoyl][2,4′-bithiazol]-2′-yl]ethyl]carbamoyl]-2-hydroxy-propyl]carbamoyl]-2-hydroxy-1-methylbutyl]carbamoyl]-2-imidazol-4-ylethyl]carbamoyl]-5-methyl-2-pyrimidinepropionamide sulfate (salt); N^1-[4-[(amino-iminomethyl)amino]butyl]bleomycinamide sulfate (salt).

Description.   A white or cream-coloured, amorphous powder.

Solubility.   Very soluble in water.

Category.   Cytotoxic drug.

Storage.   Bleomycin sulfate should be kept in a tightly closed container.

Labelling.   The designation sterile Bleomycin sulfate indicates that the substance complies with the additional requirements for sterile Bleomycin sulfate and may be used for parenteral administration or for other sterile applications. CAUTION: Bleomycin sulfate must be handled with care, avoiding contact with the skin and inhalation of airborne particles.

REQUIREMENTS

General requirement.   Bleomycin sulfate contains, when tested according to assay A, not less than 1500 and not more than 2000 International Units of bleomycin A_2/B_2 per mg, calculated with reference to the dried substance.

Further, Bleomycin sulfate contains, when tested according to assay B, not less than 55.0% and not more than 70.0% of bleomycin A_2 and not less than 25.0% and not more than 32.0% of bleomycin B_2; the total of bleomycin A_2 and bleomycin B_2 is not less than 85%. The content of bleomycin A_5 is not more than 7.0%, of bleomycin B_4 not more than 1.0%, and of demethylbleomycin A_2 not more than 3.0%.

Identity tests

A.   Dissolve about 5 mg in 10 ml of water, add 5 µl of copper(II) sulfate (160 g/l) TS, and dilute with water to 100 ml; the absorption spectrum exhibits maxima at about 242 nm and 290 nm, and a minimum at about 268 nm.

B.   A 10 mg/ml solution yields reaction A described under "General identification tests" as characteristic of sulfates (vol. 1, p. 115).

Loss on drying.   Dry at 60 °C under reduced pressure (not exceeding 0.6 kPa or about 5 mm of mercury) for 4 hours; it loses not more than 60 mg/g.

pH value.   pH of a 5.0 mg/ml solution, 4.5–6.0.

Copper content.   Transfer 75 mg, accurately weighed, to a 60-ml separating funnel and dissolve in 10 ml of hydrochloric acid (0.1 mol/l) VS. Transfer 10 ml of copper standard TS2 to an additional separating funnel. To both funnels add

10 ml of zinc bis(dibenzyldithiocarbamate) TS and shake vigorously for 1 minute. Allow the layers to separate. Filter the lower layer through 1 g of anhydrous sodium sulfate R to remove excess water. Measure the absorbances of a 1-cm layer at the maximum at about 435 nm, using a solvent cell containing carbon tetrachloride R.

Calculate the content of copper in mg/g from the formula $(A_o \times 15)/(A_s \times W)$ where A_o is the absorbance of the substance to be examined, A_s is the absorbance of copper standard TS2, and W is the weight in mg of the substance to be examined; the copper content is not more than 0.2 mg/g.

Assay

A. *Microbiological assay.* Carry out the assay as described under "Microbiological assay of antibiotics" (vol. 1, p. 145), using *Mycobacterium smegmatis* (ATCC 607) as the test organism. Prepare the inoculum as follows: the test organism is grown for 40–48 hours at a temperature of 27 °C on the surface of culture medium Cm8. Using 3 ml of saline TS wash the growth into a flask containing 100 ml of culture medium Cm9 and 50 g of glass beads, and incubate at 25–27 °C for 5 days with constant mechanical agitation using an orbital shaker. The resulting suspension should be used for no longer than 14 days, and kept at a temperature below 5 °C. For the preparation of inoculated plates use 0.5 ml of the suspension or a suitable volume previously determined using test plates with culture medium Cm8 at a temperature of 27 °C. Prepare the reference solution in phosphate buffer, pH 7.0, TS, diluting the International Reference Preparation of bleomycin A_2/B_2 to an appropriate concentration (usually between 10 and 200 µg per ml). The precision of the assay is such that the fiducial limits of error of the estimated potency ($P = 0.95$) are not less than 95 % and not more than 105 % of the estimated potency. The upper fiducial limit of error of the estimated potency ($P = 0.95$) is not less than 1500 IU and the lower fiducial limit is not more than 2000 IU of bleomycin A_2/B_2 per mg, calculated with reference to the dried substance.

B. *Content of the bleomycin components.* Carry out the test as described on pp. 373–377 of the Amendments to vol. 1 under "High performance liquid chromatography", using a column 25 cm long and 4.6 mm in internal diameter packed with particles of silica gel, 5–10 µm in diameter, the surface of which has been modified with chemically bonded octadecyl silyl groups. As the mobile phase for a linear gradient development, start with a mixture of 9 volumes of 1-pentanesulfonic acid TS and 1 volume of methanol R, both previously filtered and deaerated, and end with a composition of 6 volumes of 1-pentanesulfonic acid TS and 4 volumes of methanol R, using a suitable linear rate of change of mobile phase so as to reach the final composition in 60 minutes. (If needed, add the following to the mobile phase to obtain satisfactory chromatography: 1.86 g of disodium edetate R per litre.) As detector use an ultraviolet spectrophotometer at a wavelength of about 254 nm, fitted with a low-volume flow cell (8–20 µl is suitable). Inject

5 µl of a solution of the test substance in water containing the equivalent of 5 IU of bleomycin per ml. Proceed with the gradient elution, pumping the mobile phase mixture at the condition mentioned above for about 80 minutes or until the demethylbleomycin A_2 is eluted.

The elution order of the bleomycin components is the following: void volume, bleomycin acid, bleomycin A_2, bleomycin B_2, bleomycin A_5, bleomycin B_4, and demethylbleomycin A_2.

Calculate in % the content of each bleomycin component, comparing the ratios of the individual areas of the peaks with that of the total area of all the bleomycins.

Additional Requirements for Sterile Bleomycin Sulfate

Storage. Sterile Bleomycin sulfate should be kept in a hermetically closed container.

Histamine-like substances. Carry out the test as described under "Test for histamine-like substances" (vol. 1, p. 157) using 1 ml per kg of body mass of a solution in saline TS containing a quantity equivalent to 500 IU per ml.

Undue toxicity. Carry out the test as described under "Test for undue toxicity" (vol. 1, p. 154), using 0.5 ml of a solution in saline TS containing a quantity equivalent to 5000 IU of bleomycin sulfate per ml.

Pyrogens. Carry out the test as described under "Test for pyrogens" (vol. 1, p. 155) injecting, per kg of the rabbit's mass, 1 ml of a solution in saline TS containing 500 IU of bleomycin sulfate per ml.

Sterility. Complies with the "Sterility testing of antibiotics" (vol. 1, p. 152), applying the membrane filtration test procedure.

BUSULFANUM

Busulfan

Molecular formula. $C_6H_{14}O_6S_2$

Relative molecular mass.   246.3

Graphic formula.

$$H-\overset{\displaystyle H}{\underset{\displaystyle H}{C}}-\overset{\displaystyle O}{\underset{\displaystyle O}{S}}-O-(CH_2)_4-O-\overset{\displaystyle O}{\underset{\displaystyle O}{S}}-\overset{\displaystyle H}{\underset{\displaystyle H}{C}}-H$$

Chemical name.   1,4-Butanediol dimethanesulfonate; tetramethylene dimethanesulfonate; CAS Reg. No. 55-98-1.

Other name.   Myelosanum.

Description.   A white, crystalline powder.

Solubility.   Very slightly soluble in water; sparingly soluble in acetone R; slightly soluble in ethanol ($\sim$750 g/l) TS.

Category.   Cytotoxic drug.

Storage.   Busulfan should be kept in a well-closed container, protected from light.

Additional information.   CAUTION: Busulfan must be handled with care, avoiding contact with the skin and inhalation of airborne particles.

REQUIREMENTS

General requirement.   Busulfan contains not less than 98.5% and not more than 100.5% of $C_6H_{14}O_6S_2$, calculated with reference to the dried substance.

Identity tests

A.   Heat 0.1 g with 10 ml of water and 5 ml of sodium hydroxide (1 mol/l) VS until a clear solution is obtained; an intense odour of methanesulfonic acid is perceptible. Cool the solution and divide it into two equal portions for test B.

B.   To one portion of the solution prepared in test A add 0.05 ml of potassium permanganate (10 g/l) TS; the purple colour changes to violet, then to blue, and finally to emerald-green. Acidify the second portion of the solution prepared in test A with 2 ml of sulfuric acid ($\sim$100 g/l) TS, add 0.05 ml of potassium permanganate (10 g/l) TS and shake; the colour of the permanganate is slowly discharged.

C.   To a test-tube transfer 0.10 g of the test substance, suspend it in 1.0 ml of copper edetate TS and 0.5 ml of ammonia ($\sim$260 g/l) TS, then add 0.5 ml of hydrogen peroxide ($\sim$60 g/l) TS; this constitutes solution 1. Similarly, prepare a blank without the test substance; this constitutes solution 2. Place both tubes in a water-bath for 5 minutes, cool and add 1.0 ml of hydrochloric acid ($\sim$70 g/l) TS and 4.0 ml of barium chloride (50 g/l) TS; solution 2 remains clear and an opalescence is produced in solution 1, which changes to a white precipitate after a few minutes.

Melting range.   115–118 °C.

Sulfated ash.   Not more than 1.0 mg/g.

Loss on drying.   Dry to constant weight at 60 °C under reduced pressure (not exceeding 0.6 kPa or about 5 mm of mercury); it loses not more than 20 mg/g.

Assay.   To about 0.25 g, accurately weighed, add 25 ml of water and boil gently under reflux for 30 minutes. Wash the condenser with a small quantity of water, cool, and titrate with carbonate-free sodium hydroxide (0.1 mol/l) VS, using phenolphthalein/ethanol TS as indicator. Repeat the operation without the substance being examined and make any necessary corrections. Each ml of carbonate-free sodium hydroxide (0.1 mol/l) VS is equivalent to 12.32 mg of $C_6H_{14}O_6S_2$.

CALCII CARBONAS

Calcium carbonate

Molecular formula. $CaCO_3$

Relative molecular mass.   100.1

Chemical name.   Calcium carbonate (1:1); CAS Reg. No. 471-34-1.

Description.   A white, fine, microcrystalline powder; odourless.

Solubility.   Practically insoluble in water and ethanol ($\sim$750 g/l) TS. It dissolves with effervescence in acetic acid ($\sim$60 g/l) TS, hydrochloric acid ($\sim$70 g/l) TS, and nitric acid ($\sim$130 g/l) TS.

Category.   Antacid.

Storage.   Calcium carbonate should be kept in a well-closed container.

REQUIREMENTS

General requirement.   Calcium carbonate contains not less than 98.0% and not more than 100.5% of $CaCO_3$, calculated with reference to the dried substance.

Identity tests

A.   Dissolve 20 mg in 0.3 ml of hydrochloric acid ($\sim$70 g/l) TS and 2 ml of water, and filter. The filtrate yields the reactions described under "General identification tests" as characteristic of calcium (vol. 1, p. 112).

B. To 0.10 g add 1.0 ml of acetic acid ($\sim$300 g/l) TS; a gas evolves that is colourless and odourless. Pass the evolved gas into calcium hydroxide TS; a white precipitate is produced immediately.

Heavy metals. Dissolve 5 g in 80 ml of acetic acid ($\sim$60 g/l) TS; when effervescence ceases, boil the solution for 2 minutes, allow to cool, dilute to 100 ml with acetic acid ($\sim$60 g/l) TS and, if necessary, filter through a sintered glass filter (retain the filter for the test of substances insoluble in acetic acid). Determine the heavy metals content in 20 ml of the filtrate (keep the remaining filtrate for the limit test for barium), as described under "Limit test for heavy metals", according to Method A (vol. 1, p. 119); not more than 30 µg/g.

Arsenic. Use a solution of 3.3 g in 35 ml of hydrochloric acid ($\sim$70 g/l) TS and proceed as described under "Limit test for arsenic" (vol. 1, p. 122); the arsenic content is not more than 3 µg/g.

Barium. To 10 ml of the filtrate retained from the limit test for heavy metals add 10 ml of calcium sulfate TS (solution A). Mix a further 10 ml of the filtrate with 10 ml of water (solution B). After not less than 15 minutes, solution A is not more opalescent than solution B.

Iron. Dissolve 0.20 g in 10 ml of hydrochloric acid ($\sim$70 g/l) TS and dilute to 40 ml with water. Proceed with the "Limit test for iron" (vol. 1, p. 121); not more than 200 µg/g.

Magnesium and alkali metals. Dissolve 1.0 g in 10 ml of hydrochloric acid ($\sim$70 g/l) TS, boil for 2 minutes and add 20 ml of water, 1 g of ammonium chloride R, and 0.1 ml of methyl red/ethanol TS. Add ammonia ($\sim$100 g/l) TS drop by drop until the solution changes colour, and then add a further 2 ml. Heat to boiling and add 40 ml of hot ammonium oxalate (50 g/l) TS. Allow to stand for 4 hours, dilute to 100 ml with water and filter. To 50 ml of the filtrate add 0.25 ml of sulfuric acid ($\sim$100 g/l) TS and evaporate to dryness on a water-bath. Ignite the residue to constant weight at 600 °C; not more than 5 mg.

Substances insoluble in acetic acid. Wash the filter retained from the test for heavy metals with 4 successive quantities, each of 5 ml of hot water, and dry at 105 °C for 1 hour; the residue weighs not more than 10 mg.

Loss on drying. Dry to constant weight at 200 °C; it loses not more than 20 mg/g.

Assay. Dissolve about 0.15 g, accurately weighed, in a mixture of 3 ml of hydrochloric acid ($\sim$70 g/l) TS and 20 ml of water, boil for 2 minutes, allow to cool, and dilute to 50 ml with water. Proceed with the titration as described under "Complexometric titrations" for calcium (vol. 1, p. 128). Each ml of disodium edetate (0.05 mol/l) VS is equivalent to 5.004 mg of $CaCO_3$.

CALCII FOLINAS

Calcium folinate

Molecular formula. $C_{20}H_{21}CaN_7O_7,5H_2O$

Relative molecular mass. 601.6

Graphic formula.

Chemical name. Calcium N-[p-[[(2-amino-5-formyl-5,6,7,8-tetrahydro-4-hydroxy-6-pteridinyl)methyl]amino]benzoyl]-L-glutamate (1:1) pentahydrate; calcium N-[4-[[(2-amino-5-formyl-1,4,5,6,7,8-hexahydro-4-oxo-6-pteridinyl)-methyl]amino]benzoyl]-L-glutamate (1:1) pentahydrate; CAS Reg. No. 6035-45-6 (pentahydrate).

Other name. Leucovorin calcium.

Description. A white or creamy white powder; odourless.

Solubility. Very soluble in water; practically insoluble in ethanol ($\sim$750 g/l) TS.

Category. Cytotoxic drug.

Storage. Calcium folinate should be kept in a well-closed container, protected from light.

Additional information. CAUTION: Calcium folinate must be handled with care, avoiding contact with the skin and inhalation of airborne particles.

REQUIREMENTS

General requirement. Calcium folinate contains not less than 95.0% and not more than 105.0% of $C_{20}H_{21}CaN_7O_7$, calculated with reference to the anhydrous substance.

Identity tests

- Either tests A and C or tests B, C and D may be applied.

A. Carry out the examination as described under "Spectrophotometry in the infrared region" (vol. 1, p. 40). The infrared absorption spectrum is concordant with the spectrum obtained from calcium folinate RS or with the *reference spectrum* of calcium folinate.

B. Dissolve 20 mg in 3.0 ml of water, add 0.5 ml of hydrochloric acid ($\sim$70 g/l) TS and 0.5 ml of sodium nitrite (100 g/l) TS. Shake for 2 minutes and add 1.5 ml of 2-naphthol TS1; a yellow-brown precipitate appears and the solution turns green.

C. Dissolve 20 mg in 2.0 ml of water and add 1.0 ml of ammonium oxalate (25 g/l) TS; a white precipitate is produced, which is insoluble in acetic acid ($\sim$300 g/l) TS and ammonia ($\sim$260 g/l) TS, but is soluble in hydrochloric acid ($\sim$70 g/l) TS.

D. Dissolve 20 mg in 5 ml of water and add 1.0 ml of silver nitrate (40 g/l) TS; a white, curdy precipitate is produced. Add a few drops of nitric acid ($\sim$130 g/l) TS; the precipitate dissolves.

Water. Determine as described under "Determination of water by the Karl Fischer method", Method A (vol. 1, p. 135), using about 0.2 g of the substance; the water content is not less than 0.080 g/g and not more than 0.150 g/g.

Assay

● Use freshly deionized water throughout the procedure, and perform the assay in low-actinic glassware or protect the solutions containing calcium folinate from light. Complete the assay without prolonged interruption.

Carry out the test as described on pp. 373–377 of the Amendments to vol. 1 under "High performance liquid chromatography", using a column 30 cm long and 4 mm in internal diameter, packed with particles of porous silica gel or ceramic, 5–10 µm in diameter, the surface of which has been modified with chemically bonded octadecyl silyl groups.

As the mobile phase, use a mixture of 15 ml of tetrabutylammonium hydroxide/methanol TS with 835 ml of water, add 125 ml of acetonitrile R, adjust the pH to 7.5 $\pm$ 0.1 with sodium dihydrogen phosphate (275 g/l) TS, dilute with water to 1000 ml, and filter. Adjust the concentration of acetonitrile, if necessary.

Dilute the following solution for use in the preparation of the test solutions: To 15 ml of tetrabutylammonium hydroxide/methanol TS add 900 ml of water, adjust the pH to 7.5 $\pm$ 0.1 with sodium dihydrogen phosphate (275 g/l) TS, dilute with water to 1000 ml, and mix. Weigh accurately a quantity of calcium folinate RS, dissolve it in the above solution and dilute with the same solution to contain about 175 µg per ml (solution A). Dissolve 20 mg of the substance to be examined in a sufficient volume of the above solution to produce 100 ml, and mix (solution B). For the system suitability test, dissolve a quantity of folic acid RS in the above solution and dilute with the same solution to contain about 175 µg per ml. Mix 1 part of this solution with 4 parts of solution A (solution C).

Operate at a flow rate of $1-2$ ml per minute. As detector use an ultraviolet spectrophotometer at a wavelength of about 254 nm, fitted with a suitable recorder.

Make 6 replicate injections, each of 15 µl of solution C. The resolution factor between calcium folinate and folic acid should be not less than 3.6, with a relative standard deviation for the calcium folinate peak of not more than 2.0%. The relative retention times for calcium folinate and folic acid are 1.0 and about 1.6, respectively.

Then inject 15 µl of each of solutions A and B. Measure the peak responses at the corresponding retention times and calculate the quantity, in %, of $C_{20}H_{21}CaN_7O_7$, using the following formula: $100(0.1C)(r_U/r_S)$ in which C is the concentration in µg per ml of calcium folinate RS in solution A, and r_U and r_S are the peak responses obtained from solutions B and A, respectively.

CARBAMAZEPINUM

Carbamazepine

Molecular formula. $C_{15}H_{12}N_2O$

Relative molecular mass.   236.3

Graphic formula.

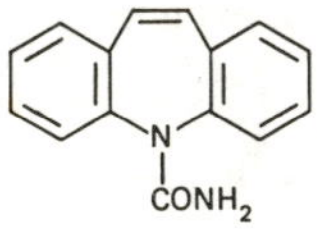

Chemical name.   5*H*-Dibenz[*b,f*]azepine-5-carboxamide; CAS Reg. No. 298-46-4.

Description.   A white to yellowish white, crystalline powder; odourless or almost odourless.

Solubility.   Practically insoluble in water and ether R; soluble in ethanol ($\sim$750 g/l) TS and chloroform R.

Category.   Antiepileptic drug.

Storage.   Carbamazepine should be kept in a tightly closed container.

REQUIREMENTS

General requirement. Carbamazepine contains not less than 98.0% and not more than 102.0% of $C_{15}H_{12}N_2O$, calculated with reference to the dried substance.

Identity tests

- Either test A or tests B, C and D may be applied.

A. Carry out the examination as described under "Spectrophotometry in the infrared region" (vol. 1, p. 40). The infrared absorption spectrum obtained from the test substance without pretreatment is concordant with the spectrum obtained from carbamazepine RS or with the *reference spectrum* of carbamazepine.

B. See the test described below under "Related substances". The principal spot obtained with solution C corresponds in position, appearance, and intensity with that obtained with solution D.

C. Expose a small amount of the test substance to ultraviolet light (365 nm); an intense blue fluorescence is observed.

D. Heat 0.1 g with 2 ml of nitric acid ($\sim$1000 g/l) TS in a water-bath for 3 minutes; an orange-red colour is produced.

Melting range. 189–193 °C.

Heavy metals. Use 1.0 g for the preparation of the test solution as described under "Limit test for heavy metals", Procedure 3 (vol. 1, p. 118); determine the heavy metals content according to Method A (vol. 1, p. 119); not more than 10 µg/g.

Sulfated ash. Not more than 1.0 mg/g.

Loss on drying. Dry to constant weight at 105 °C; it loses not more than 5.0 mg/g.

Acidity or alkalinity. Stir 1.0 g with 20 ml of carbon-dioxide-free water R for 15 minutes and filter. To 10 ml of the filtrate add 0.1 ml of phenolphthalein/ethanol TS and titrate with carbonate-free sodium hydroxide (0.01 mol/l) VS; not more than 0.5 ml is required to obtain a pink colour. Add 0.15 ml of methyl red/ethanol TS and titrate with hydrochloric acid (0.01 mol/l) VS; not more than 1.0 ml is required to obtain a red colour.

Related substances. Carry out the test as described under "Thin-layer chromatography" (vol. 1, p. 83), using silica gel R6 as the coating substance and a mixture of 86 volumes of toluene R and 14 volumes of methanol R as the mobile phase. Apply separately to the plate 2 µl of each of 5 solutions in a mixture of equal volumes of ethanol ($\sim$750 g/l) TS and chloroform R containing (A) 0.050 g of the test substance per ml, (B) 0.050 mg of iminodibenzyl R per ml, (C) 5.0 mg of the test substance per ml, (D) 5.0 mg of carbamazepine RS per ml, and (E) 5.0 µg of carbamazepine RS per ml. After removing the plate from the chromatographic chamber, allow it to dry in air, spray it with potassium dichromate TS3, and examine the chromatogram in daylight. Any spot obtained with solution A, other than the principal spot, is not more intense than that obtained with solution B. Then heat the plate at 140 °C for 15 minutes and examine the chromatogram in ultraviolet light (254 nm). Any additional spot obtained with solution A is not more intense than that obtained with solution E.

Assay. Dissolve about 0.1 g, accurately weighed, in sufficient ethanol ($\sim$750 g/l) TS to produce 100 ml. Dilute 10 ml of this solution to 100 ml with the same solvent, and again dilute 10 ml of this dilution to 100 ml with ethanol ($\sim$750 g/l) TS. Measure the absorbance of a 1-cm layer of the resulting solution at the maximum at about 285 nm. Calculate the amount of $C_{15}H_{12}N_2O$ in the substance being tested by comparison with carbamazepine RS, similarly and concurrently examined. In an adequately calibrated spectrophotometer the absorbance of the reference solution should be 0.49 $\pm$ 0.02.

CARBIDOPUM

Carbidopa

Molecular formula. $C_{10}H_{14}N_2O_4,H_2O$

Relative molecular mass. 244.2

Graphic formula.

$$HO-\text{C}_6H_3(OH)-CH_2-\underset{\underset{NHNH_2}{|}}{\overset{\overset{CH_3}{|}}{C}}-COOH \quad \cdot \quad H_2O$$

Chemical name. (–)-L-α-Hydrazino-3,4-dihydroxy-α-methylhydrocinnamic acid monohydrate; (S)-α-hydrazino-3,4-dihydroxy-α-methylbenzenepropanoic acid monohydrate; CAS Reg. No. 38821-49-7 (monohydrate).

Description. A white to creamy white powder; odourless or almost odourless.

Solubility. Slightly soluble in water; very slightly soluble in ethanol ($\sim$750 g/l) TS; practically insoluble in chloroform R and ether R.

Category. Antiparkinsonism drug.

Storage. Carbidopa should be kept in a well-closed container, protected from light.

REQUIREMENTS

General requirement.   Carbidopa contains not less than 99.0% and not more than 101.0% of $C_{10}H_{14}N_2O_4$, calculated with reference to the anhydrous substance.

Identity tests

A.   Carry out the examination as described under "Spectrophotometry in the infrared region" (vol. 1, p. 40). The infrared absorption spectrum is concordant with the spectrum obtained from carbidopa RS or with the *reference spectrum* of carbidopa.

B.   To 5 mg add 1 ml of water, 1 ml of pyridine R, and 5 mg of 4-nitrobenzoyl chloride R, mix and allow to stand for 3 minutes; the solution remains colourless, but after boiling changes to a pale yellow colour. While shaking, add 0.1 ml of sodium carbonate (200 g/l) TS; an orange colour is produced.

Specific optical rotation.   Use a 10 mg/ml solution in aluminium chloride TS and calculate with reference to the anhydrous substance; $[\alpha]_D^{20\,°C} = -22.5$ to $-26.5°$.

Heavy metals.   Use 1.0 g for the preparation of the test solution as described under "Limit test for heavy metals", Procedure 3 (vol. 1, p. 118); determine the heavy metals content according to Method A (vol. 1, p. 119); not more than 20 µg/g.

Sulfated ash.   Not more than 1.0 mg/g.

Water.   Determine as described under "Determination of water by the Karl Fischer Method", Method A (vol. 1, p. 135), using about 0.5 g of the substance; the water content is not less than 69 mg/g and not more than 79 mg/g.

Methyldopa and 3-*O*-Methylcarbidopa.   Carry out the test as described on pp. 373–377 of the Amendments to vol. 1 under "High performance liquid chromatography", using a stainless steel column 20 cm long and 4 mm in internal diameter packed with particles of silica gel, 10 µm in diameter, the surface of which has been modified with chemically bonded octylsilyl groups (suitable packing or columns are commercially available). As the mobile phase, use a mixture of 98 volumes of potassium dihydrogen phosphate (13.6 g/l) TS and 2 volumes of methanol R at a flow rate of 1.5 ml per minute. As detector use an ultraviolet spectrophotometer at a wavelength of about 282 nm, fitted with a low-volume flow cell (10 µl is suitable).

Prepare the following solutions in hydrochloric acid (0.1 mol/l) VS containing (A) 0.050 mg of methyldopa RS, 0.050 mg of (–)-3-(4-hydroxy-3-methoxyphenyl)-2-hydrazino-2-methylalanine RS and 0.10 mg of (–)-3-(4-hydroxy-3-methoxyphenyl)-2-methylalanine RS per ml, the last serving as an internal standard, (B) 10 mg of the test substance per ml, and (C) 10 mg of the test substance and 0.10 mg of the internal standard per ml.

In the chromatogram obtained with solution A the peaks, excluding the solvent peak, are due to (*a*) methyldopa, (*b*) (–)-3-(4-hydroxy-3-methoxyphenyl)-2-methylalanine and (*c*) (–)-3-(4-hydroxy-3-methoxyphenyl)-2-hydrazino-2-methylalanine in order of their emergence. The ratios of the areas of the peaks (*a*) and (*c*) to the area of the peak due to the internal standard are greater than the corresponding ratios in the chromatogram obtained with solution C.

Assay. Dissolve about 0.3 g, accurately weighed, in 25.0 ml of perchloric acid (0.1 mol/l) VS with the aid of a minimum of heat. Titrate the excess perchloric acid with sodium acetate/glacial acetic acid (0.1 mol/l) VS, determining the endpoint potentiometrically as described under "Non-aqueous titration", Method A (vol. 1, p. 131). Each ml of perchloric acid (0.1 mol/l) VS is equivalent to 22.62 mg of $C_{10}H_{14}N_2O_4$.

CHLORAMBUCILUM

Chlorambucil

Molecular formula. $C_{14}H_{19}Cl_2NO_2$

Relative molecular mass. 304.2

Graphic formula.

$$(ClCH_2CH_2)_2N \text{---} \langle \text{phenyl} \rangle \text{---} CH_2CH_2CH_2COOH$$

Chemical name. 4-[*p*-[Bis(2-chloroethyl)amino]phenyl]butyric acid; 4-[bis(2-chloroethyl)amino]benzenebutanoic acid; CAS Reg. No. 305-03-3.

Description. A white or almost white, crystalline or slightly granular powder.

Solubility. Practically insoluble in water; freely soluble in ethanol (~750 g/l) TS, chloroform R, and acetone R.

Category. Cytotoxic drug.

Storage. Chlorambucil should be kept in a well-closed container, protected from light.

Additional information. CAUTION: Chlorambucil must be handled with care, avoiding contact with the skin and inhalation of airborne particles.

REQUIREMENTS

General requirement. Chlorambucil contains not less than 98.0% and not more than 101.0% of $C_{14}H_{19}Cl_2NO_2$, calculated with reference to the anhydrous substance.

Identity tests

A.   Place 20 mg in a test-tube, add 0.20 ml of potassium dichromate TS2, cover the tube with a piece of filter-paper moistened with sodium nitroprusside (8.5 g/l) TS and 0.05 ml of piperidine R.   Heat the tube over a small flame; a blue spot appears on the filter-paper.

B.   Dissolve 0.05 g in 5 ml of acetone R, and dilute with water to 10 ml.   Add 0.05 ml of sulfuric acid ($\sim$ 100 g/l) TS, then add 0.20 ml of silver nitrate (0.1 mol/l) VS; no opalescence is observed immediately (absence of chloride ion). Warm the solution on a water-bath; an opalescence develops (presence of ionizable chlorine).

C.   Mix 0.4 g with 10 ml of hydrochloric acid ($\sim$ 70 g/l) TS and allow to stand for 30 minutes, shaking occasionally.   Filter, wash the residue with 2 quantities, each of 10 ml of water, and dry at ambient temperature under reduced pressure (not exceeding 0.6 kPa or about 5 mm of mercury) over phosphorus pentoxide R for 3 hours; melting temperature, about 146 °C.

Melting range.   64 – 69 °C.

Sulfated ash.   Not more than 1.0 mg/g.

Water.   Determine as described under "Determination of water by the Karl Fischer method", Method A (vol. 1, p. 135), using about 0.5 g of the substance; the water content is not more than 5.0 mg/g.

Related substance.   Carry out the test as described under "Thin-layer chromatography" (vol. 1, p. 83), using silica gel R2 as the coating substance and allowing the coated plate to dry at room temperature for 24 hours.   Use as the mobile phase a mixture of 8 volumes of toluene R, 5 volumes of methanol R, 4 volumes of heptane R, and 4 volumes of ethylmethylketone R.   Apply separately to the plate 10 µl of each of 2 solutions in acetone R containing (A) 20 mg of the test substance per ml and (B) 0.40 mg of the test substance per ml.   After removing the plate from the chromatographic chamber, allow it to dry in air and examine the chromatogram in ultraviolet light (254 nm).   Any spot obtained with solution A, other than the principal spot, is not more intense than that obtained with solution B.

Assay.   Dissolve about 0.2 g, accurately weighed, in 10 ml of acetone R, add 10 ml of water, and titrate with carbonate-free sodium hydroxide (0.1 mol/l) VS using phenolphthalein/ethanol TS as indicator. Repeat the operation without the substance being examined and make any necessary corrections. Each ml of carbonate-free sodium hydroxide (0.1 mol/l) VS is equivalent to 30.42 mg of $C_{14}H_{19}Cl_2NO_2$.

CHLORAMPHENICOLI PALMITAS

Chloramphenicol palmitate

Molecular formula. $C_{27}H_{42}Cl_2N_2O_6$

Relative molecular mass.   561.5

Graphic formula.

$$O_2N-\text{C}_6H_4-\underset{\underset{H}{|}}{\overset{\overset{HO}{|}}{C}}-\underset{\underset{NHCOCHCl_2}{|}}{\overset{\overset{H}{|}}{C}}-CH_2OCO(CH_2)_{14}CH_3$$

Chemical name.   D-*threo*-(−)-2,2-Dichloro-*N*-[β-hydroxy-α-(hydroxymethyl)-*p*-nitrophenethyl]acetamide α-palmitate; [*R*-(*R**,*R**)]-2-[(dichloroacetyl)amino]-3-hydroxy-3-(4-nitrophenyl)propyl hexadecanoate; CAS Reg. No. 530-43-8.

Description.   A fine, white, unctuous, crystalline powder; odour, faint.

Solubility.   Practically insoluble in water; sparingly soluble in ethanol ($\sim$750 g/l) TS; soluble in chloroform R and ether R.

Category.   Antibacterial drug.

Storage.   Chloramphenicol palmitate should be kept in a tightly closed container, protected from light.

Additional information.   If Chloramphenicol palmitate is to be used to prepare a dosage form in the solid state, it should contain at least 90% of polymorph B. If a liquid dosage form is to be prepared, e.g., a suspension, the method of preparation should be such as to ensure that at least 90% of the chloramphenicol palmitate is present as polymorph B in the final product.

REQUIREMENTS

General requirement.   Chloramphenicol palmitate contains not less than 98.0% and not more than 102.0% of $C_{27}H_{42}Cl_2N_2O_6$, calculated with reference to the dried substance.

Identity tests

A.   Carry out the test as described under "Thin-layer chromatography" (vol. 1, p. 83), using silica gel R4 as the coating substance and a mixture of 9 volumes of chloroform R, 1 volume of methanol R, and 0.1 volume of water as the mobile phase. Apply separately to the plate 10 µl of each of 2 solutions in acetone R containing (A) 10 mg of the test substance per ml and (B) 10 mg of chloramphenicol palmitate RS per ml. After removing the plate from the chromatographic chamber, allow it to dry in air and examine the chromatogram in ultraviolet light (254 nm). The principal spot obtained with solution A corresponds in position, appearance, and intensity with that obtained with solution B.

B.   Dissolve 10 mg in 4 ml of ethanol ($\sim$750 g/l) TS, add 1.0 ml of sulfuric acid ($\sim$100 g/l) TS and 0.05 g of zinc R powder, and allow to stand for 10 minutes. Decant the supernatant liquid or filter if necessary. Cool the resulting solution in ice and add 0.5 ml of sodium nitrite (100 g/l) TS and, after 2 minutes, 1.0 g of urea R, followed by 1.0 ml of 2-naphthol TS1 and 2.0 ml of sodium hydroxide ($\sim$400 g/l) TS; a red colour develops. Repeat the test omitting the zinc R powder; no red colour is produced.

Specific optical rotation.   Use a 50 mg/ml solution in dehydrated ethanol R; $[\alpha]_D^{20\,°C} = +22.5$ to $+25.5°$.

Sulfated ash.   Not more than 1.0 mg/g.

Loss on drying.   Dry to constant weight at ambient temperature under reduced pressure (not exceeding 0.6 kPa or about 5 mm of mercury) over phosphorus pentoxide R; it loses not more than 5.0 mg/g.

Acidity.   Dissolve 1.0 g by warming to 35 °C with 5 ml of a mixture of equal volumes of ethanol ($\sim$750 g/l) TS and ether R, previously neutralized to phenolphthalein/ethanol TS.   Titrate with sodium hydroxide (0.1 mol/l) VS, using phenolphthalein/ethanol TS as indicator, until, on gentle shaking, a pink colour persists for 30 seconds; not more than 0.4 ml is required.

Free chloramphenicol.   Dissolve, with the aid of gentle heat, 1.0 g in 80 ml of xylene R, cool, and extract with 3 quantities, each of 15 ml, of water; discard the xylene and dilute the combined aqueous extracts to 50 ml with water. Extract the solution with 10 ml of carbon tetrachloride R, allow to separate, discard the carbon tetrachloride, and centrifuge a portion of the aqueous solution. Measure the absorbance of the clear supernatant liquid in a 1-cm layer at the maximum at about 278 nm, using as the blank a solution obtained by repeating the procedure without the substance being examined; the absorbance of this blank solution should not exceed 0.05. Calculate the content of free chloramphenicol, using the absorptivity value of 29.8 ($A_{1\,cm}^{1\%} = 298$); not more than 0.45 mg/g.

Assay. Dissolve about 0.03 g, accurately weighed, in sufficient dehydrated ethanol R to produce 100 ml; dilute 10 ml of this solution to 100 ml with the same solvent. Measure the absorbance of the diluted solution in a 1-cm layer at the maximum at about 271 nm and calculate the content of $C_{27}H_{42}Cl_2N_2O_6$ using the absorptivity value of 17.8 ($A_{1\ cm}^{1\%} = 178$).

CHLORHEXIDINI DIACETAS

Chlorhexidine diacetate

Molecular formula. $C_{22}H_{30}Cl_2N_{10},2C_2H_4O_2$

Relative molecular mass. 625.6

Graphic formula.

$$\underset{(CH_2)_6}{\overset{\displaystyle NH\quad\ NH}{NH-CH-NH-CH-NH}}-\!\!\left\langle\ \right\rangle\!-Cl$$

(Hexamethylenebis[5-(4-chlorophenyl)biguanide], with two CH_3CO_2H groups shown as $\cdot\ 2CH_3CO_2H$.)

Chemical name. 1,1'-Hexamethylenebis[5-(p-chlorophenyl)biguanide] diacetate; N,N''-bis(4-chlorophenyl)-3,12-diimino-2,4,11,13-tetraazatetradecanediimidamide diacetate; CAS Reg. No. 56-95-1.

Description. A white or yellowish white, microcrystalline powder; odourless or almost odourless.

Solubility. Soluble in 55 parts of water and in 15 parts of ethanol ($\sim$750 g/l) TS; very slightly soluble in glycerol R.

Category. Disinfectant.

Storage. Chlorhexidine diacetate should be kept in a well-closed container, protected from light.

REQUIREMENTS

General requirement. Chlorhexidine diacetate contains not less than 97.5% and not more than 101.0% of $C_{22}H_{30}Cl_2N_{10},2C_2H_4O_2$, calculated with reference to the dried substance.

Identity tests

A.   Dissolve 0.1 g in 10 ml of methanol R by warming, and add a mixture of 2 ml of sodium hydroxide (~150 g/l) TS and 2 ml of bromine TS1; a deep red colour is produced.

B.   Dissolve 0.1 g in 10 ml of water and add, with shaking, 0.15 ml of copper(II) chloride/ammonia TS; a purple precipitate is produced immediately. Continue to add 0.5 ml of copper(II) chloride/ammonia TS; the colour of the precipitate changes to blue.

C.   Heat gently 0.2 g with 1 ml of ethanol (~750 g/l) TS and 1 ml of sulfuric acid (~1760 g/l) TS; ethyl acetate, perceptible by its odour (proceed with caution), is produced.

Sulfated ash.   Not more than 2.0 mg/g.

Loss on drying.   Dry to constant weight at 105 °C; it loses not more than 35 mg/g.

Chloraniline.   Dissolve 0.20 g in 30 ml of water. Add with mixing 5 ml of hydrochloric acid (1 mol/l) VS, 1 ml of sodium nitrite (35 g/l) TS, 2 ml of ammonium sulfamate (50 g/l) TS, and shake. Then add 5 ml of freshly prepared *N*-(1-naphthyl)ethylenediamine hydrochloride (1 g/l) TS, 1 ml of ethanol (~750 g/l) TS, and sufficient water to produce 50 ml. Allow to stand for 30 minutes. Treat similarly 30 ml of a solution containing 0.10 mg of chloraniline R that has been slightly acidified with hydrochloric acid (~70 g/l) TS. The colour produced in the test solution is not more intense than that of the reference solution when compared as described in "Colour of liquids" (vol. 1, p. 50) (0.5 mg/g).

Related substances.   Carry out the test as described under "Thin-layer chromatography" (vol. 1, p. 83), using silica gel R4 as the coating substance and preparing a slurry as follows: To 8 g of silica gel R4 add 16 ml of water containing 1 g of sodium formate R and coat the plates with a layer 0.5 mm thick. Use a mixture of 50 volumes of chloroform R, 50 volumes of ethanol (~750 g/l) TS and 7 volumes of formic acid (~1080 g/l) TS as the mobile phase. Apply to the plate in the form of a band, 4 cm wide, 20 µl of a solution in acetic acid (~90 g/l) TS containing 72 mg of the test substance per ml (solution A). After removing the plate from the chromatographic chamber, allow it to dry in air and examine the chromatogram in ultraviolet light (254 nm). Score a rectangular area around each group of bands above and below the principal band, quantitatively transfer the enclosed areas of silica gel to a glass-stoppered test-tube, add 5 ml of methanol R, shake for 15 minutes, centrifuge, and measure the absorbance of the clear supernatant liquid in a 1-cm layer at the maximum at about 256 nm. For the blank solution treat in a similar manner equivalent sized areas of silica gel removed from the coating adjacent to the areas previously removed. Prepare solution B in the following manner: Dissolve 0.14 g of the test substance in sufficient acetic acid (~90 g/l) TS to produce 100 ml and dilute 200 µl of this solution to 50 ml with methanol R. The absorbance obtained from the eluted solution A is not greater than the absorbance obtained from solution B.

Assay. Dissolve about 0.45 g, accurately weighed, in 30 ml of glacial acetic acid R1, add 0.15 ml of 1-naphtholbenzein/acetic acid TS as indicator, and titrate with perchloric acid (0.1 mol/l) VS as described under "Non-aqueous titration", Method A (vol. 1, p. 131). Each ml of perchloric acid (0.1 mol/l) VS is equivalent to 15.64 mg of $C_{22}H_{30}Cl_2N_{10},2C_2H_4O_2$.

CHLORHEXIDINI DIHYDROCHLORIDUM

Chlorhexidine dihydrochloride

Molecular formula. $C_{22}H_{30}Cl_2N_{10},2HCl$

Relative molecular mass. 578.4

Graphic formula.

Chemical name. 1,1'-Hexamethylenebis[5-(*p*-chlorophenyl)biguanide] dihydrochloride; *N,N''*-bis(4-chlorophenyl)-3,12-diimino-2,4,11,13-tetraazatetradecanediimidamide dihydrochloride; CAS Reg. No. 3697-42-5.

Description. A white or almost white, crystalline powder; odourless.

Solubility. Sparingly soluble in water; soluble in 450 parts of ethanol (~750 g/l) TS.

Category. Disinfectant.

Storage. Chlorhexidine dihydrochloride should be kept in a well-closed container, protected from light.

REQUIREMENTS

General requirement. Chlorhexidine dihydrochloride contains not less than 98.0% and not more than 101.0% of $C_{22}H_{30}Cl_2N_{10},2HCl$, calculated with reference to the dried substance.

Identity tests

A.   Dissolve 20 mg in 10 ml of methanol R by warming, and add a mixture of 2 ml of sodium hydroxide (~150 g/l) TS and 2 ml of bromine TS1 ; a deep red colour is produced.

B.   Dissolve 0.1 g in 10 ml of water and add, with shaking, 0.15 ml of copper(II) chloride/ammonia TS; a purple precipitate is produced immediately. Continue to add 0.5 ml of copper(II) chloride/ammonia TS; the colour of the precipitate changes to blue.

C.   Dissolve 0.1 g in 50 ml of nitric acid (~130 g/l) TS; the solution yields reaction A described under "General identification tests" as characteristic of chlorides (vol. 1, p. 112).

Sulfated ash.   Not more than 1.0 mg/g.

Loss on drying.   Dry to constant weight at 130 °C; it loses not more than 20 mg/g.

Chloraniline.   Dissolve 0.20 g in 30 ml of water.   Add with mixing 5 ml of hydrochloric acid (1 mol/l) VS, 1 ml of sodium nitrite (35 g/l) TS, 2 ml of ammonium sulfamate (50 g/l) TS and shake.   Then add 5 ml of freshly prepared *N*-(1-naphthyl)ethylenediamine hydrochloride (1 g/l) TS, 1 ml of ethanol (~750 g/l) TS, and sufficient water to produce 50 ml.   Allow to stand for 30 minutes.   Treat similarly 30 ml of a solution containing 0.10 mg of chloraniline R that has been slightly acidified with hydrochloric acid (~70 g/l) TS.   The colour produced in the test solution is not more intense than that of the reference solution when compared as described in "Colour of liquids" (vol. 1, p. 50) (0.5 mg/g).

Related substances.   Carry out the test as described under "Thin-layer chromatography" (vol. 1, p. 83), using silica gel R4 as the coating substance and preparing a slurry as follows: To 8 g of silica gel R4 add 16 ml of water containing 1 g of sodium formate R and coat the plates with a layer, 0.5 mm thick.   Use a mixture of 50 volumes of chloroform R, 50 volumes of ethanol (~750 g/l) TS, and 7 volumes of formic acid (~1080 g/l) TS as the mobile phase.   Prepare solution A by dissolving 1.1 g of the test substance in 35 ml of hydrochloric acid (~330 g/l) TS, add 100 ml of 2-propanol R, cool in ice, make alkaline with sodium hydroxide (~200 g/l) TS, cool in ice, add 200 ml of ice-cooled water, and extract with 100 ml of chloroform R.   Dry the chloroform extract over anhydrous potassium carbonate R, filter, evaporate the chloroform almost to dryness under a stream of nitrogen R, add 50 ml of methanol R, evaporate to dryness under a stream of nitrogen R, and dry the residue at 65 °C for 30 minutes; dissolve 0.56 g of the dried residue in sufficient acetic acid (~90 g/l) TS to produce 100 ml.   Apply to the plate in the form of a band, 4 cm wide, 20 µl of solution A.   After removing the plate from the chromatographic chamber, allow it to dry in air and examine the chromatogram in ultraviolet light (254 nm).   Score a rectangular area around each group of bands above and below the principal band, quantitatively transfer the enclosed areas of silica gel to a glass-stoppered test-tube, add 5 ml of methanol R, shake for 15 minutes, centrifuge, and measure the absorbance of the clear supernatant liquid in a 1-cm layer at the maximum at about 256 nm. For the blank solution treat in a similar manner equivalent-sized areas of silica gel removed from the coating adjacent to the areas previously removed. Prepare solution B in the following manner: Dissolve 0.11 g of the dried residue in sufficient acetic acid (~90 g/l) TS to produce 100 ml and dilute 200 µl of this solution to 50 ml with methanol R. The absorbance obtained from the eluted solution A is not greater than the absorbance obtained from solution B.

Assay. Dissolve about 0.4 g, accurately weighed, in 30 ml of glacial acetic acid R1, add 10 ml of mercuric acetate/acetic acid TS and titrate with perchloric acid (0.1 mol/l) VS, determining the endpoint potentiometrically as described under "Non-aqueous tritration", Method A (vol. 1, p. 131). Each ml of perchloric acid (0.1 mol/l) VS is equivalent to 14.46 mg of $C_{22}H_{30}Cl_2N_{10},2HCl$.

CHLORTETRACYCLINI HYDROCHLORIDUM

Chlortetracycline hydrochloride

Chlortetracycline hydrochloride (non-injectable)
Chlortetracycline hydrochloride, sterile

Molecular formula. $C_{22}H_{23}ClN_2O_8,HCl$

Relative molecular mass. 515.4

Graphic formula.

Chemical name. (4S,4aS,5aS,6S,12aS)-7-Chloro-4-(dimethylamino)-1,4,4a,5,5a,6,11,12a-octahydro-3,6,10,12,12a-pentahydroxy-6-methyl-1,11-dioxo-2-naphthacenecarboxamide monohydrochloride; [4S-(4α,4aα,5aα,6β,12aα)]-7-chloro-4-(dimethylamino)-1,4,4a,5,5a,6,11,12a-octahydro-3,6,10,12,12a-pentahydroxy-6-methyl-1,11-dioxo-2-naphthacenecarboxamide monohydrochloride; CAS Reg. No. 64-72-2.

Description.   Yellow crystals or a yellow, crystalline powder; odourless.

Solubility.   Soluble in about 100 parts of water and in about 250 parts of ethanol (~750 g/l) TS; practically insoluble in acetone R, chloroform R, and ether R.

Category.   Antiinfective drug.

Storage.   Chlortetracycline hydrochloride should be kept in a tightly closed container, protected from light.

Labelling.   The designation sterile Chlortetracycline hydrochloride indicates that the substance complies with the additional requirements for sterile Chlortetracycline hydrochloride and may be used for parenteral administration or for other sterile applications.

Additional information.   Chlortetracycline hydrochloride has a bitter taste. Even in the absence of light, Chlortetracycline hydrochloride is gradually degraded on exposure to a humid atmosphere, the decomposition being faster at higher temperatures.

REQUIREMENTS

General requirement.   Chlortetracycline hydrochloride contains not less than 900 International Units of chlortetracycline per mg, calculated with reference to the dried substance.

Identity tests

A.   Carry out the test as described under "Thin-layer chromatography" (vol. 1, p. 83), using a kieselguhr coating prepared as follows: To 25 g of kieselguhr R1 add 50 ml of a mixture of 2.5 ml of glycerol R and 47.5 ml of disodium edetate (0.1 mol/l) VS previously adjusted to pH 7 with ammonia (~100 g/l) TS. Coat the plates with this mixture, and allow them to dry at room temperature for about 70–90 minutes, or until sufficiently dry to give a satisfactory separation. As the mobile phase, take 200 ml of a mixture of 2 volumes of ethyl acetate R, 2 volumes of chloroform R, and 1 volume of acetone R, shake with 25 ml of disodium edetate (0.1 mol/l) VS previously adjusted to pH 7 with ammonia (~100 g/l) TS, allow to settle, and use the lower layer. Apply separately to the plate 1 µl of each of 3 solutions in methanol R containing (A) 0.50 mg of the test substance per ml, (B) 0.50 mg of chlortetracycline hydrochloride RS per ml, and (C) a mixture of 0.50 mg of chlortetracycline hydrochloride RS per ml, 0.50 mg of oxytetracycline hydrochloride RS per ml, and 0.50 mg of tetracycline hydrochloride RS per ml. After removing the plate from the chromatographic chamber, allow it to dry in air, expose it to the vapour of ammonia (~260 g/l) TS, and examine the chromatogram in ultraviolet light (365 nm). The principal spot obtained with solution A corresponds in position, appearance, and intensity with that obtained with solution B. The test is not valid unless the chromatogram obtained with solution C shows 3 clearly separated spots.

B.   Dissolve 10 mg in 10 ml of phosphate buffer, pH 7.6, TS, heat at 100 °C for 1 minute and examine the solution in ultraviolet light (365 nm); a strong blue fluorescence is observed.

C.   To about 1 mg add 2 ml of sulfuric acid ($\sim$1760 g/l) TS; a blue to bluish green colour is produced, which changes to brown on the addition of about 1 ml of water.

D.   A 0.05 g/ml solution yields reaction B described under "General identification tests" as characteristic of chlorides (vol. 1, p. 113).

Specific optical rotation.   Dissolve 0.125 g in sufficient water to produce 25.0 ml, and allow to stand in the dark for 30 minutes. Measure the rotation at 25 °C and calculate with reference to the dried substance; $[\alpha]_D^{25\,°C} = -235$ to $-250°$.

Heavy metals.   Use 0.5 g for the preparation of the test solution as described under "Limit test for heavy metals", Procedure 3 (vol. 1, p. 118); determine the heavy metals content according to Method A (vol. 1, p. 119); not more than 50 µg/g.

Sulfated ash.   Not more than 5.0 mg/g.

Loss on drying.   Dry at 60 °C under reduced pressure (not exceeding 0.6 kPa or about 5 mm of mercury) over phosphorus pentoxide R for 3 hours; it loses not more than 20 mg/g.

pH value.   pH of a 10 mg/ml solution, 2.3–3.3.

Absorption in the ultraviolet region.   Dissolve 10 mg in sufficient sulfuric acid (0.5 mol/l) VS to produce 100 ml. Dilute 10 ml of this solution to 100 ml with sulfuric acid (0.5 mol/l) VS. Place 10 ml of the resulting solution in a test-tube 25 mm in diameter and 200 mm long and immerse in a water-bath for 8 minutes. Cool, replace the water lost by evaporation, and measure the absorbance of a 1-cm layer at 274 nm; not less than 0.70 and not more than 0.76.

Assay.   Carry out the assay as described under "Microbiological assay of antibiotics" (vol. 1, p. 145), using either (*a*) *Bacillus pumilus* (NCTC 8241 or ATCC 14884) as the test organism, culture medium Cm1 with a final pH of 6.5–6.6, sterile phosphate buffer, pH 4.5 TS, an appropriate concentration of chlortetracycline (usually between 2 and 20 IU per ml), and an incubation temperature of 35–39 °C, or (*b*) *Bacillus cereus* (ATCC 11778) as the test organism, culture medium Cm1 with a final pH of 5.9–6.0, sterile phosphate buffer, pH 4.5 TS, an appropriate concentration of chlortetracycline (usually between 0.05 and 0.2 IU), and an incubation temperature of 29–33 °C. The precision of the assay is such that the fiducial limits of error of the estimated potency ($P = 0.95$) are not less than 95% and not more than 105% of the estimated potency. The upper fiducial limit of error of the estimated potency ($P = 0.95$) is not less than 900 IU of chlortetracycline per mg, calculated with reference to the dried substance.

Additional Requirements for Sterile Chlortetracycline Hydrochloride

Storage.   Sterile Chlortetracycline hydrochloride should be kept in a hermetically closed container, protected from light.

Undue toxicity.   Carry out the test as described under "Test for undue toxicity" (vol. 1, p. 154), using 0.5 ml of a solution in sterile water R containing a quantity equivalent to 2 mg/ml.

Pyrogens.   Carry out the test as described under "Test for pyrogens" (vol. 1, p. 155) injecting, per kg of the rabbit's mass, 1 ml of a solution in sterile water R containing 5 mg of the substance to be examined per ml.

Sterility.   Complies with the "Sterility testing of antibiotics" (vol. 1, p. 152), applying the membrane filtration test procedure.

CIMETIDINUM

Cimetidine

Molecular formula. $C_{10}H_{16}N_6S$

Relative molecular mass.   252.3

Graphic formula.

Chemical name.   2-Cyano-1-methyl-3-[2-[[(5-methylimidazol-4-yl)methyl]thio]ethyl]guanidine; *N″*-cyano-*N*-methyl-*N′*-[2-[[(5-methyl-1*H*-imidazol-4-yl)methyl]thio]ethyl]guanidine; 1-cyano-2-methyl-3-[2-[[(5-methylimidazol-4-yl)methyl]thio]ethyl]guanidine; *N*-cyano-*N′*-methyl-*N″*-[2-[[(5-methyl-1*H*-imidazol-4-yl)methyl]thio]ethyl]guanidine; CAS Reg. No. 51481-61-9.

Description.   A white to off-white powder; odourless or with a faint odour.

Solubility.   Sparingly soluble in water; very soluble in methanol R.

Category.   Antiulcer drug.

Storage.   Cimetidine should be kept in a well-closed container.

Additional information.   Cimetidine exists in three polymorphic forms.   The polymorph specified in the monograph corresponds to the crystal form of cimetidine RS.

REQUIREMENTS

General requirement.   Cimetidine contains not less than 98.5% and not more than 101.0% of $C_{10}H_{16}N_6S$, calculated with reference to the dried substance.

Identity tests

A.   Carry out the examination as described under "Spectrophotometry in the infrared region" (vol. 1, p. 40).   The infrared absorption spectrum obtained from the solid state without prior solvent treatment is concordant with the spectrum similarly obtained from cimetidine RS or with the *reference spectrum* of cimetidine; no shoulder or peak is discernible at 1180 cm $^{-1}$ (confirmation of polymorphic form).

B.   Melting temperature, about 142 °C.

Heavy metals.   Use 1.0 g for the preparation if the test solution as described under "Limit test for heavy metals", Procedure 3 (vol. 1, p. 118); determine the heavy metals content according to Method A (vol. 1, p. 119); not more than 20 µg/g.

Sulfated ash.   Not more than 1.0 mg/g.

Loss on drying.   Dry to constant weight at 105 °C; it loses not more than 10.0 mg/g.

pH value.   pH of a 5.0 mg/ml solution in carbon-dioxide-free water R, 8.0−9.5.

Related substances.   Carry out the test as described on pp. 373−377 of the Amendments to vol. 1 under "High performance liquid chromatography", using a column 25 cm long and 4.6 mm internal diameter, packed with particles of porous silica gel or ceramic, 5−10 µm in diameter, the surface of which has been modified with chemically bonded octadecyl silyl groups.   Prepare the following solvent mixture: Dilute 1 ml of glacial acetic acid R with sufficient water to produce 200 ml. To 190 ml of this solution add 10 ml of ammonium acetate (2 g/l) TS. As the mobile phase use a degassed and filtered mixture of 84 volumes of the above solvent mixture and 16 volumes of acetonitrile R. For the system suitability test prepare a solution containing 18 µg of cimetidine RS and 24 µg of caffeine RS per ml of the above solvent mixture (solution A). Further prepare a solution of the substance to be examined containing 18 µg per ml of solvent mixture (solution B). Operate with a flow rate of about 1 ml per minute. As detector use an ultraviolet spectrophotometer at a wavelength of about 228 nm, fitted with a suitable recorder. Make 6 replicate injections, each of 10 µl of solution A. Measure the peak responses; the relative standard deviation of the ratio of the responses from cimetidine to the sum of all the responses in the chromatogram, excluding any from the solvent mixture, is not more than 2.0%, and the resolution between caffeine and cimetidine is not less than 3.0. The relative retention times are about 1.0 for caffeine and 1.4 for cimetidine. Then inject 10 µl of solution B and measure the peak responses: the ratio of the response from cimetidine to the sum of all the responses in the chromatogram, excluding any from the solvent mixture, is not less than 0.99.

Assay. Dissolve about 0.25 g, accurately weighed, in 30 ml of glacial acetic acid R1, and titrate with perchloric acid (0.1 mol/l) VS, determining the endpoint potentiometrically as described under "Non-aqueous titration", Method A (vol. 1, p. 131). Each ml of perchloric acid (0.1 mol/l) VS is equivalent to 25.23 mg of $C_{10}H_{16}N_6S$.

CLOFAZIMINUM

Clofazimine

Molecular formula. $C_{27}H_{22}Cl_2N_4$

Relative molecular mass. 473.4

Graphic formula.

Chemical name. 3-(p-Chloroanilino)-10-(p-chlorophenyl)-2,10-dihydro-2-(isopropylimino)phenazine; N,5-bis(4-chlorophenyl)-3,5-dihydro-3-[(1-methylethyl)imino]-2-phenazinamine; CAS Reg. No. 2030-63-9.

Description.   A reddish brown, fine powder; odourless or almost odourless.

Solubility.   Practically insoluble in water; soluble in 15 parts of chloroform R; slightly soluble in ethanol ($\sim$750 g/l) TS and in ether R.

Category.   Antileprosy drug.

Storage.   Clofazimine should be kept in a well-closed container.

Additional information.   Clofazimine melts at about 217 °C.

REQUIREMENTS

General requirement.   Clofazimine contains not less than 98.0% and not more than 101.0% of $C_{27}H_{22}Cl_2N_4$, calculated with reference to the dried substance.

Identity tests

● Either test A or tests B and C may be applied.

A.   Carry out the examination as described under "Spectrophotometry in the infrared region" (vol. 1, p. 40). The infrared absorption spectrum is concordant with the spectrum obtained from clofazimine RS or with the *reference spectrum* of clofazimine.

B.   The absorption spectrum of a 5.0 µg/ml solution in hydrochloric acid/methanol (0.01 mol/l) VS, when observed between 230 nm and 600 nm, exhibits 2 maxima at about 283 nm and 487 nm. The absorbances of a 1-cm layer at these wavelengths are about 0.65 and 0.32, respectively.

C.   Dissolve about 2 mg in 3 ml of acetone R and add 0.1 ml of hydrochloric acid ($\sim$420 g/l) TS; an intense violet colour is produced. Add 0.5 ml of sodium hydroxide ($\sim$200 g/l) TS; the colour changes to orange-red.

Heavy metals.   Use 1.0 g for the preparation of the test solution as described under "Limit test for heavy metals", Procedure 3 (vol. 1, p. 118); determine the heavy metals content according to Method A (vol. 1, p. 119); not more than 10 µg/g.

Sulfated ash.   Not more than 1.0 mg/g.

Loss on drying.   Dry to constant weight at 105 °C; it loses not more than 5.0 mg/g.

Related substances.   Carry out the test as described under "Thin-layer chromatography" (vol. 1, p. 83), using silica gel R6 (a precoated plate from a commercial source is suitable), exposed immediately before use to ammonia vapour by suspending the plate for 30 minutes in a chromatographic chamber containing a shallow layer of ammonia ($\sim$17 g/l) TS. As the mobile phase, to be used in a separate chamber, prepare a mixture of 85 volumes of dichloromethane R and 4 volumes of 1-propanol R. Apply separately to the plate 5 µl of each of 3 solutions in chloroform R containing (A) 20 mg of the test substance per ml, (B) 0.16 mg of the test substance per ml, and (C) 0.10 mg of the test substance per ml. Allow the mobile phase to ascend 12 cm above the line of application. After removing the plate from the chromatographic chamber, allow it to dry in air for 5 minutes, and replace it in the chamber. Allow the mobile phase to ascend again 12 cm, remove the plate from the chamber, dry it in air for 5 minutes, and examine the chromatogram in ultraviolet light (254 nm). Any spot obtained with solution A, other than the principal spot, is not more intense than the spot obtained with solution C, except that 2 such spots are not more intense than that obtained with solution B.

Assay. Dissolve about 0.4 g, accurately weighed, in 20 ml of chloroform R, add 50 ml of acetone R, and titrate with perchloric acid (0.1 mol/l) VS as described under "Non-aqueous titration", Method A (vol. 1, p. 131). Each ml of perchloric acid (0.1 mol/l) VS is equivalent to 47.34 mg of $C_{27}H_{22}Cl_2N_4$.

CLOMIFENI CITRAS

Clomifene citrate

Molecular formula. $C_{26}H_{28}ClNO,C_6H_8O_7$

Relative molecular mass. 598.1

Graphic formula.

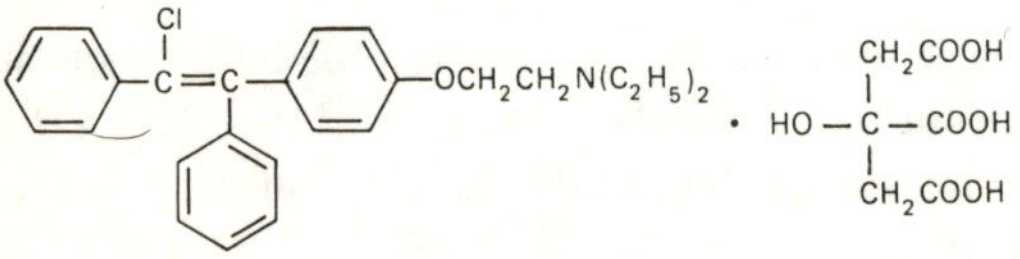

Chemical name. 2-[p-(2-Chloro-1,2-diphenylvinyl)phenoxy]triethylamine citrate (1:1); 2-[2-chloro-1,2-diphenylethenyl)phenoxy]-N,N-diethylethanamine 2-hydroxy-1,2,3-propanetricarboxylate (1:1); CAS Reg. No. 50-41-9.

Description. A white to pale yellow powder; odourless.

Solubility. Slightly soluble in water and chloroform R; freely soluble in methanol R; sparingly soluble in ethanol ($\sim$750 g/l) TS; practically insoluble in ether R.

Category.   Ovulation inducer.

Storage.   Clomifene citrate should be kept in a well-closed container, protected from light.

Additional information.   Clomifene citrate is a mixture of the *E* and *Z* geometric isomers.

REQUIREMENTS

General requirement.   Clomifene citrate contains not less than 97.0% and not more than 101.0% of $C_{26}H_{28}ClNO,C_6H_8O_7$, and not less than 30.0% and not more than 50.0% of the Z-isomer, both calculated with reference to the anhydrous substance.

Identity tests

● Either test A or tests B and C may be applied.

A.   Carry out the examination as described under "Spectrophotometry in the infrared region" (vol. 1, p. 40). The infrared absorption spectrum is concordant with the spectrum obtained from clomifene citrate RS or with the *reference spectrum* of clomifene citrate.

B.   The ultraviolet absorption spectrum of a 25 μg/ml solution in hydrochloric acid (0.1 mol/l) VS, when observed between 220 nm and 350 nm, exhibits maxima at about 235 nm and 292 nm; the absorbances of a 1-cm layer at these wavelengths are about 0.79 and 0.44, respectively.

C.   A 10 mg/ml solution yields reaction B described under "General identification tests" as characteristic of citrates (vol. 1, p. 113).

Heavy metals.   Use 1.0 g for the preparation of the test solution as described under "Limit test for heavy metals", Procedure 3 (vol. 1, p. 118); determine the heavy metals content according to Method A (vol. 1, p. 119); not more than 20 μg/g.

Solution in methanol.   A solution of 1.0 g in 30 ml of methanol R is clear and colourless.

Water.   Determine as described under "Determination of water by the Karl Fischer method", Method A (vol. 1, p. 135), using about 1 g of the substance; the water content is not more than 10 mg/g.

***Z*-isomer.**   Carry out the test as described under "Thin-layer chromatography" (vol. 1, p. 83), using silica gel R2 as the coating substance and a mixture of 90 volumes of chloroform R, 10 volumes of methanol R, and 1 volume of water as the mobile phase. Dissolve 100 mg of the test substance in 50 ml of a mixture of 3 volumes of chloroform R and 1 volume of ethanol ($\sim$750 g/l) TS (solution A), and dissolve 50 mg of clomifene citrate Z-isomer RS in 50 ml of the same solvent mixture (solution B). With a syringe apply 100 µl of solution A to one side and 100 µl of solution B to the other side, keeping the centre of the plate to serve as a blank. After removing the plate from the chromatographic chamber, allow it to dry in air, and examine the chromatogram in ultraviolet light (254 nm). Mark the bands of the Z-isomer with a pencil, scratch off separately the bands of silica gel produced by solutions A and B, as well as a band of a similar size from the centre of the plate for the blank, and transfer them to separate test-tubes. Add 10 ml of ethanol ($\sim$750 g/l) TS to each tube, shake vigorously and then centrifuge or filter. Measure the absorbances of a 1-cm layer of the filtered solutions at 240 nm against a solvent cell containing ethanol ($\sim$750 g/l) TS. Calculate the content of Z-isomer in the following manner: Deduct the absorbance of the blank solution from the absorbances of the test and reference solutions and apply the formula: $(A_1)(W_2)(1000)/(A_2)(W_1)$, where A_1 is the absorbance of the test substance, A_2 the absorbance of clomifene citrate Z-isomer RS, W_1 the weight in mg of the test substance, and W_2 the weight in mg of clomifene citrate Z-isomer RS; the content of the Z-isomer is not less than 300 mg/g and not more than 500 mg/g.

Assay. Dissolve about 1.0 g, accurately weighed, in 30 ml of glacial acetic acid R1, and titrate with perchloric acid (0.1 mol/l) VS as described under "Non-aqueous titration", Method A (vol. 1, p. 131). Each ml of perchloric acid (0.1 mol/l) VS is equivalent to 59.81 mg of $C_{26}H_{28}ClNO,C_6H_8O_7$.

COLCHICINUM

Colchicine

Molecular formula. $C_{22}H_{25}NO_6$

Relative molecular mass.   399.4

Graphic formula.

Chemical name.   (S)-N-(5,6,7,9-Tetrahydro-1,2,3,10-tetramethoxy-9-oxobenzo[a]heptalen-7-yl)acetamide; CAS Reg. No. 64-86-8.

Description.   Pale yellow to pale greenish yellow crystals, amorphous scales or a powder; odourless or almost odourless.

Solubility.   Soluble in water; freely soluble in ethanol ($\sim$750 g/l) TS and chloroform R; slightly soluble in ether R.

Category.   Antigout drug.

Storage.   Colchicine should be kept in a tightly closed container, protected from light.

Additional information.   Colchicine is an alkaloid obtained from *Colchicum autumnale L.* (Fam. Liliaceae).   It darkens on exposure to light.   CAUTION: Colchicine is extremely poisonous and must be handled with care.

REQUIREMENTS

General requirement.   Colchicine contains not less than 97.0% and not more than 103.0% of $C_{22}H_{25}NO_6$, calculated with reference to the anhydrous and solvent-free substance.

Identity tests

● Either test A or tests B, C and D may be applied.

A.   Carry out the examination as described under "Spectrophotometry in the infrared region" (vol. 1, p. 40).   The infrared absorption spectrum is concordant with the spectrum obtained from colchicine RS or with the *reference spectrum* of colchicine.

B.   The absorption spectrum of a 10 µg/ml solution in ethanol ($\sim$750 g/l) TS, when observed between 230 nm and 400 nm, exhibits 2 maxima at about 243 nm and 350 nm.

C.   Dissolve 30 mg in 1 ml of ethanol ($\sim$750 g/l) TS and add 1 drop of ferric chloride (25 g/l) TS; a red colour is immediately produced.

D.   Mix 1 mg with about 0.2 ml of sulfuric acid ($\sim$1760 g/l- TS; a lemon-yellow colour is produced.   Add about 0.1 ml of nitric acid ($\sim$1000 g/l) TS; the colour changes to greenish blue, rapidly becoming reddish and finally yellow or almost colourless.   Then add a few drops of sodium hydroxide ($\sim$80 g/l) TS; the colour changes to red.

Specific optical rotation.   Use a 10 mg/ml solution and calculate with reference to the dried and solvent-free substance; $[\alpha]_D^{20\,°C} = -425$ to $-460°$.

Sulfated ash.   Not more than 1.0 mg/g.

Content of solvent and water. Dry at 130 °C for 4 hours, using about 0.5 g of the substance, and determine the loss of weight. Weigh 0.3 g of the dried material and determine the water content as described under "Determination of water by the Karl Fischer method", Method A (vol. 1, p. 135), using pyridine R as the solvent; the sum of the loss of weight and of the water content, both expressed in mg/g, is not less than 115 mg/g and not more than 145 mg/g.

Colchiceine. Dissolve 0.050 g in 4 ml of water, add 0.2 ml of ferric chloride (25 g/l) TS, dilute to 6 ml with water, and mix; the colour produced in the test solution is not more intense than that of the standard colour solution produced by mixing 2 ml of iron colour TS, 1 ml of cobalt colour TS, 2 ml of copper colour TS and 0.70 ml of hydrochloric acid ($\sim$70 g/l) TS, when compared as described under "Colour of liquids" (vol. 1, p. 50).

Related substances. Carry out the test as described under "Thin-layer chromatography" (vol. 1, p. 83), using a suitable aluminium oxide containing a substance that fluoresces at about 254 nm as the coating substance and a mixture of 25 volumes of chloroform R, 20 volumes of acetone R, and 0.4 volumes of ammonia ($\sim$260 g/l) TS as the mobile phase. Apply separately to the plate 2 µl of each of 2 solutions in ethanol ($\sim$750 g/l) TS containing (A) 50 mg of the test substance per ml and (B) 2.5 mg of the test substance per ml. After removing the plate from the chromatographic chamber, allow it to dry in air, and examine the chromatogram in ultraviolet light (254 nm). Any spot obtained with solution A, other than the principal spot, is not more intense than that obtained with solution B.

Assay. Dissolve about 0.05 g, accurately weighed, in a mixture of 10 ml of acetic anhydride R and 20 ml of toluene R, and titrate with perchloric acid (0.02 mol/l) VS, determining the endpoint potentiometrically as described under "Non-aqueous titration", Method A (vol. 1, p. 131). Each ml of perchloric acid (0.02 mol/l) VS is equivalent to 7.988 mg of $C_{22}H_{25}NO_6$.

CYCLOPHOSPHAMIDUM

Cyclophosphamide

Molecular formula. $C_7H_{15}Cl_2N_2O_2P,H_2O$

Relative molecular mass. 279.1

Graphic formula.

Chemical name.   2-[Bis(2-chloroethyl)amino]tetrahydro-2H-1,3,2-oxazaphos-phorine 2-oxide monohydrate; N,N-bis(2-chloroethyl)tetrahydro-2H-1,3,2-oxa-zaphosphorin-2-amine 2-oxide monohydrate; CAS Reg. No. 6055-19-2 (monohy-drate).

Other name.   Cyclophosphanum.

Description.   A white, crystalline powder.

Solubility.   Soluble in water; freely soluble in ethanol ($\sim$750 g/l) TS; slightly soluble in ether R.

Category.   Cytotoxic drug.

Storage.   Cyclophosphamide should be kept in a tightly closed container and stored at a temperature between 2 and 30 °C.

Additional information.   CAUTION: Cyclophosphamide must be handled with care, avoiding contact with the skin and inhalation of airborne particles.

REQUIREMENTS

General requirement.   Cyclophosphamide contains not less than 98.0% and not more than 101.0% of $C_7H_{15}Cl_2N_2O_2P$, calculated with reference to the anhydrous substance.

Identity tests

A.   Dissolve 0.1 g in 10 ml of water and add 5 ml of silver nitrate (40 g/l) TS; no precipitate is produced. Boil; a white precipitate is produced, which is insoluble in nitric acid ($\sim$130 g/l) TS but soluble in ammonia ($\sim$100 g/l) TS from which it is reprecipitated by the addition of nitric acid ($\sim$130 g/l) TS.

B.   Dissolve 20 mg in 1 ml of sulfuric acid ($\sim$100 g/l) TS and heat until white fumes are evolved. After cooling, add 5 ml of water and shake. Neutralize with ammonia ($\sim$100 g/l) TS, then acidify with nitric acid ($\sim$130 g/l) TS; this test yields reaction A described under "General identification tests" as characteristic of orthophosphates (vol. 1, p. 114).

Melting range.   49-53 °C, determined without previous drying.

Clarity and colour of solution.   A solution of 0.20 g in 10 ml of water is clear and colourless.

Water.   Determine as described under "Determination of water by the Karl Fischer method", Method A (vol. 1, p. 135), using about 0.3 g of the substance; the water content is not less than 55 mg/g and not more than 70 mg/g.

pH value.   pH of a 20 mg/ml solution in carbon-dioxide-free water R, determined 30 minutes after its preparation, 4.0–7.0.

Related substances.   Carry out the test as described under "Thin-layer chromatography" (vol. 1, p. 83), using silica gel R1 as the coating substance and a mixture of 50 volumes of benzene R, 25 volumes of chloroform R, and 25 volumes of methanol R as the mobile phase. Apply separately to the plate 10 µl of each of 2 solutions: (A) 25 mg of the test substance per ml of chloroform R and (B) 0.125 g of the test substance dissolved in 5.0 ml of water, boiled under a reflux condenser for 30 minutes, and then cooled to 20 °C. After removing the plate from the chromatographic chamber, allow it to dry in air and spray it with triketohydrindene/methanol TS. Examine the chromatogram in daylight. With solution B, a pale violet spot is obtained at an R_f value between 0.10 and 0.25; other spots could also appear. With solution A, a brown-violet spot is obtained with an R_r value between 3.50 and 5.50, and no other spot is obtained above this spot.

Assay.   To about 0.2 g, accurately weighed, add 20 ml of potassium hydroxide/ethanol (0.5 mol/l) VS. Boil under a reflux condenser for 1 hour, cool, then add 30 ml of water, 3 ml of nitric acid (~1000 g/l) TS and 20.0 ml of silver nitrate (0.1 mol/l) VS. Shake the flask, add 5 ml of diethyl phthalate R and titrate the excess of silver nitrate with ammonium thiocyanate (0.1 mol/l) VS, using 5 ml of ferric ammonium sulfate (45 g/l) TS as indicator. Repeat the operation without the substance being examined and make any necessary corrections. Each ml of silver nitrate (0.1 mol/l) VS is equivalent to 13.05 mg of $C_7H_{15}Cl_2N_2O_2P$.

CYTARABINUM

Cytarabine

Molecular formula. $C_9H_{13}N_3O_5$

Relative molecular mass.   243.2

Graphic formula.

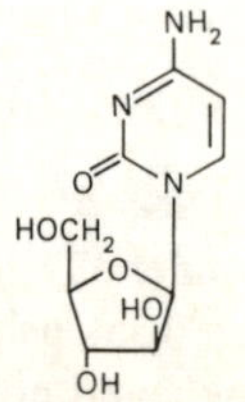

Chemical name.   l-β-D-Arabinofuranosylcytosine; 4-amino-l-β-D-arabinofurano-syl-2(1*H*)-pyrimidone; CAS Reg. No. 147-94-4.

Description.   A white or almost white, crystalline powder; odourless.

Solubility.   Freely soluble in water; slightly soluble in ethanol ($\sim$750 g/l) TS and chloroform R.

Category.   Cytotoxic drug.

Storage.   Cytarabine should be kept in a well-closed container, protected from light, and stored at a temperature not exceeding 15 °C.

Additional information.   CAUTION: Cytarabine must be handled with care, avoiding contact with the skin and inhalation of airborne particles.

REQUIREMENTS

General requirement.   Cytarabine contains not less than 99.0% and not more than 100.5% of $C_9H_{13}N_3O_5$, calculated with reference to the dried substance.

Identity tests

A.   Carry out the examination as described under "Spectrophotometry in the infrared region" (vol. 1, p. 40). The infrared absorption spectrum is concordant with the spectrum obtained from cytarabine RS or with the *reference spectrum* of cytarabine.

B.   The absorption spectrum of a 10 μg/ml solution in hydrochloric acid (0.1 mol/l) VS, when observed between 230 nm and 350 nm, exhibits a maximum at about 280 nm; the absorbance of a 1-cm layer at this wavelength is about 0.55.

Specific optical rotation.   Use a 10 mg/ml solution; $[\alpha]_D^{20\,°C} = +154$ to $+160°$.

Sulfated ash.   Not more 5.0 mg/g.

Loss on drying.   Dry to constant weight at 60 °C under reduced pressure (not exceeding 0.6 kPa or about 5 mm of mercury); it loses not more than 10 mg/g.

Related substances.   Carry out the test as described under "Thin-layer chromatography" (vol. 1, p. 83), using silica gel R4 as the coating substance and a mixture of 13 volumes of ethylmethylketone R, 4 volumes of acetone R, and 3 volumes of water as the mobile phase. Apply separately to the plate 5 μl of each of 3 solutions containing (A) 40 mg of the test substance per ml, (B) 0.20 mg of uridine R per ml, and (C) 0.20 mg of the test substance per ml. After removing the plate from the chromatographic chamber, allow it to dry in air, and examine the chromatogram in ultraviolet light (254 nm). Any spot obtained with solution A with an R_f value of about 1.1, compared with the spot obtained with solution B, is not more intense than that obtained with solution B. Any other spot obtained with solution A, other than the principal spot, is not more intense than that obtained with solution C.

Assay. Dissolve about 0.5 g, accurately weighed, in 30 ml of glacial acetic acid R1, add 0.15 ml of 1-naphtholbenzein/acetic acid TS as indicator and titrate with perchloric acid (0.1 mol/l) VS as described under "Non-aqueous titration", Method A (vol. 1, p. 131). Each ml of perchloric acid (0.1 mol/l) VS is equivalent to 24.32 mg of $C_9H_{13}N_3O_5$.

DEFEROXAMINI MESILAS

Deferoxamine mesilate

Molecular formula. $C_{25}H_{48}N_6O_8,CH_4O_3S$

Relative molecular mass. 656.8

Graphic formula.

$$H_2N(CH_2)_5\underset{\underset{OH}{|}}{N}\overset{\overset{O}{\|}}{C}(CH_2)_2\overset{\overset{O}{\|}}{C}NH(CH_2)_5\underset{\underset{OH}{|}}{N}\overset{\overset{O}{\|}}{C}(CH_2)_2\overset{\overset{O}{\|}}{C}NH(CH_2)_5\underset{\underset{OH}{|}}{N}\overset{\overset{O}{\|}}{C}CH_3 \cdot CH_3SO_3H$$

Chemical name. N-[5-[3-[(5-Aminopentyl)hydroxycarbamoyl]propionamido]pentyl]-3-[[5-(N-hydroxyacetamido)pentyl]carbamoyl]propionohydroxamic acid monomethanesulfonate (salt); N'-[5-[[4-[[5-(acetylhydroxyamino)pentyl]amino]-1,4-dioxobutyl]hydroxyamino]pentyl]-N-(5-aminopentyl)-N-hydroxybutanediamide monomethanesulfonate (salt); CAS Reg. No. 138-14-7.

Other name. Desferrioxamine mesylate.

Description. A white to yellowish white powder; odourless or almost odourless.

Solubility. Soluble in 5 parts of water; soluble in ethanol ($\sim$750 g/l) TS; slightly soluble in methanol R; practically insoluble in chloroform R and ether R.

Category. Antidote to iron poisoning.

Storage. Deferoxamine mesilate should be kept in a well-closed container, protected from light, and stored at a temperature not exceeding 4 °C.

REQUIREMENTS

General requirement.   Deferoxamine mesilate contains not less than 98.0% and not more than 102.0% of $C_{25}H_{48}N_6O_8,CH_4O_3S$, calculated with reference to the anhydrous substance.

Identity tests

A.   Dissolve 5 mg in 5 ml of water, add 2 ml of trisodium orthophosphate (2 g/l) TS, mix, then add 1 ml of sodium 1,2-naphthoquinone-4-sulfonate (5 g/l) TS; a blackish brown colour is produced.

B.   The titrated solution obtained in the assay is reddish brown in colour. To 5 ml of the titrated solution add 2 ml of benzyl alcohol R and shake; the colour is extracted. To a further 5 ml of the titrated solution add 2 ml of ether R and shake; the colour is not extracted.

Heavy metals.   Use 1.0 g for the preparation of the test solution as described under "Limit test for heavy metals", Procedure 3 (vol. 1, p. 118); determine the heavy metals content according to Method A (vol. 1, p. 119); not more than 20 µg/g.

Chlorides.   Dissolve 0.7 g in a mixture of 2 ml of nitric acid ($\sim$130 g/l) TS, and proceed as described under "Limit test for chlorides" (vol. 1, p. 116); the chloride content is not more than 0.35 mg/g.

Sulfates.   Dissolve 0.85 g in 40 ml of water, and proceed as described under "Limit test for sulfates" (vol. 1, p. 116); the sulfate content is not more than 0.6 mg/g.

Clarity and colour of solution.   A solution of 1.0 g in 10 ml of water is clear; measure the absorbance of the solution in a 1-cm layer at 420 nm; not more than 0.10.

Sulfated ash.   Not more than 1.0 mg/g.

Water.   Determine as described under "Determination of water by the Karl Fischer method", Method A (vol. 1, p. 135), using about 1 g of the substance; the water content is not more than 20 mg/g.

pH value.   pH of a 0.10 g/ml solution in carbon-dioxide-free water R, 3.5–6.0.

Assay.   Dissolve about 0.3 g, accurately weighed, in 15 ml of water and add 2 ml of sulfuric acid (0.05 mol/l) VS.   Titrate slowly with ferric ammonium sulfate (0.1 mol/l) VS, determining the endpoint potentiometrically using a platinum electrode and a calomel reference electrode.   Each ml of ferric ammonium sulfate (0.1 mol/l) VS is equivalent to 65.68 mg of $C_{25}H_{48}N_6O_8$, CH_4O_3S.   (Keep the titrated solution for identity test B.)

DEHYDROEMETINI DIHYDROCHLORIDUM

Dehydroemetine dihydrochloride

Molecular formula. $C_{29}H_{38}N_2O_4, 2HCl$

Relative molecular mass.   551.6

Graphic formula.

Chemical name.   ($\pm$)-2,3-Didehydroemetine dihydrochloride; ($\pm$)-2,3-didehydro-6′,7′,10,11-tetramethoxyemetan   dihydrochloride;   ($\pm$)-(11bR*)-3-ethyl-1,6,7,11b-tetrahydro-9,10-dimethoxy-1-[[(1bS*)-1,2,3,4-tetrahydro-6,7-dimethoxy-1-isoquinolyl]methyl]-4H-benzo[a]quinolizine dihydrochloride; CAS Reg. No. 3317-75-7.

Description.   A white to yellowish, crystalline powder; odourless.

Solubility.   Sparingly soluble in water; soluble in methanol R.

Category.   Antiamoebic drug.

Storage.   Dehydroemetine dihydrochloride should be kept in a tightly closed container.

REQUIREMENTS

General requirement.   Dehydroemetine dihydrochloride contains not less than 98.0% and not more than 101.0% of $C_{29}H_{38}N_2O_4, 2HCl$, calculated with reference to the dried substance.

Identity tests

A. The absorption spectrum of a 0.040 mg/ml solution in hydrochloric acid (0.1 mol/l) VS, when observed between 240 nm and 350 nm, exhibits a maximum at about 282 nm. The absorbance of a 1-cm layer at this wavelength is about 0.49.

B.   Sprinkle a small quantity of the powdered substance on the surface of 1 ml of sulfuric acid ($\sim$1760 g/l) TS containing 5 mg of molybdenum trioxide R; a bright green colour is produced.

C.   A 0.1 g/ml solution yields reaction B described under "General identification tests" as characteristic of chlorides (vol. 1, p. 113).

Clarity and colour of solution.   A solution of 0.30 g in 10 ml of water is clear and not more intensely coloured than standard colour solution Yw2 when compared as described under "Colour of liquids" (vol. 1, p. 50).

Sulfated ash.   Not more than 1.0 mg/g.

Loss on drying.   Dry to constant weight at 105 °C; it loses not more than 70 mg/g.

pH value.   pH of a 30 mg/ml solution, 3.5–5.0.

Related substances.   Carry out the test as described under "Thin-layer chromatography" (vol. 1, p. 83), using silica gel R4 as the coating substance and a mixture of 9 volumes of ethyl acetate R and 1 volume of diethylamine R as the mobile phase.   Apply separately to the plate 5 µl of each of 3 solutions in methanol R containing (A) 20 mg of the test substance per ml, (B) 0.10 mg of the test substance per ml, and (C) 0.10 mg of emetine hydrochloride RS per ml.   After removing the plate from the chromatographic chamber, allow it to dry in air, spray it with mercuric acetate/acetic acid TS, heat it at 120 °C for 10 minutes, and examine the chromatogram in ultraviolet light (365 nm).   Any spot obtained with solution A, other than the principal spot, is not more intense than that obtained with solution B or solution C, as appropriate.

Assay.   Dissolve about 0.4 g, accurately weighed, in 75 ml of glacial acetic acid R1, add 10 ml of mercuric acetate/acetic acid TS, and titrate with perchloric acid (0.1 mol/l) VS as described under "Non-aqueous titration", Method A (vol. 1, p. 131).   Each ml of perchloric acid (0.1 mol/l) VS is equivalent to 27.58 mg of $C_{29}H_{38}N_2O_4,2HCl$.

DEXAMETHASONI NATRII PHOSPHAS

Dexamethasone sodium phosphate

Molecular formula. $C_{22}H_{28}FNa_2O_8P$

Relative molecular mass.   516.4

Graphic formula.

Chemical name.   9-Fluoro-11β,17,21-trihydroxy-16α-methylpregna-1,4-diene-3,20-dione 21-(dihydrogen phosphate) disodium salt; 9-fluoro-11β,17-dihydroxy-16α-methyl-21-(phosphonooxy)pregna-1,4-diene-3,20-dione disodium salt; CAS Reg. No. 2392-39-4.

Description.   A white or almost white, crystalline powder; odourless or with a slight odour of ethanol.

Solubility.   Freely soluble in water; slightly soluble in ethanol ($\sim$750 g/l) TS; practically insoluble in chloroform R and ether R.

Category.   Adrenal hormone.

Storage.   Dexamethasone sodium phosphate should be kept in a tightly closed container, protected from light.

Additional information.   Dexamethasone sodium phosphate is very hygroscopic. Even in the absence of light, it is gradually degraded on exposure to a humid atmosphere, the decomposition being faster at higher temperatures.

REQUIREMENTS

General requirement.   Dexamethasone sodium phosphate contains not less than 96.0% and not more than 103.0% of $C_{22}H_{28}FNa_2O_8P$, calculated with reference to the anhydrous and ethanol-free substance.

Identity tests

A.   Carry out the test as described under "Thin-layer chromatography" (vol. 1, p. 83), using silica gel R1 as the coating substance and a freshly prepared mixture of 3 volumes of 1-butanol R, 1 volume of acetic anhydride R, and 1 volume of water as the mobile phase. Apply separately to the plate 2 μl of each of 4 solutions in methanol R containing (A) 2.5 mg of the test substance per ml, (B) 2.5 mg of dexamethasone sodium phosphate RS per ml, (C) a mixture of equal volumes of solutions A and B, and (D) equal volumes of solution A and a solution of 2.5 mg of prednisolone sodium phosphate RS per ml of methanol R. After removing the plate from the chromatographic chamber, allow it to dry in air until the solvents have evaporated, spray it with a mixture of 10 ml of sulfuric acid ($\sim$1760 g/l) TS and 90 ml of ethanol (~750 g/l) TS, heat it at 120 °C for 10 minutes, allow it to cool, and examine the chromatogram in ultraviolet light (365 nm). The principal spot obtained with solution A corresponds in position, appearance, and intensity with that obtained with solution B. The principal spot obtained with solution C appears as a single compact spot, whereas the chromatogram of solution D shows 2 closely running spots.

B. Place 0.5 ml of chromic acid TS in a small test-tube and heat in a water-bath for 5 minutes; the solution wets the sides of the tube but there is no greasiness. Add about 3 mg of the test substance and again heat in a water-bath for 5 minutes; the solution no longer wets the sides of the tube.

C. Heat carefully 0.04 g with 2 ml of sulfuric acid (~1760 g/l) TS until white fumes are evolved, add drop by drop nitric acid (~1000 g/l) TS until oxidation is complete, and cool. Add 2 ml of water, heat until white fumes are again evolved, cool, add 10 ml of water, and neutralize with ammonia (~100 g/l) TS, using pH-indicator paper R. Keep half of the solution for test D. The remaining solution yields reaction A described under "General identification tests" as characteristic of orthophosphates (vol. 1, p. 114).

D. The solution prepared in test C yields reaction B described under "General identification tests" as characteristic of sodium (vol. 1, p. 115).

Specific optical rotation. Use a 10 mg/ml solution and calculate with reference to the anhydrous and ethanol-free substance; $[\alpha]_D^{20\,°C} = +74$ to $+82°$.

Clarity of solution. A solution of 0.10 g in 10 ml of carbon-dioxide-free water R is clear.

Water. Determine as described under "Determination of water by the Karl Fischer Method", method A (vol. 1, p. 135), using about 0.3 g of the substance. The sum of the contents of water and ethanol (described below), both calculated in mg/g, is not more than 160 mg/g.

Ethanol. Carry out the test as described under "Gas chromatography" (vol. 1, p. 94), using 3 solutions in water containing (1) a mixture of 10 μl of 1-propanol R per ml serving as an internal standard and 10 μl of dehydrated ethanol R per ml, (2) 0.10 g of the test substance per ml, and (3) a mixture of 0.10 g of the test substance and 10 μl of the internal standard per ml. It may be necessary to adjust the content of dehydrated ethanol R in solution (1) to produce a peak of similar height to the corresponding peak in the chromatogram obtained with solution (2).

For the procedure use a column 1.5 m long and 4 mm in internal diameter packed with porous polymer beads (particle size 80–100 μm from a commercial source, is suitable). Maintain the column at 135 °C, use nitrogen R as the carrier gas and a flame ionization detector.

Calculate the content of ethanol in mg/g, assuming the weight per ml at 20 °C to be 0.790 g; not more than 80 mg/g.

pH value.   pH of a 10 mg/ml solution in carbon-dioxide-free water R, 7.5–10.5.

Free dexamethasone and other related substances.   Carry out the test as described under "Thin-layer chromatography" (vol. 1, p. 83), using silica gel R1 as the coating substance and methanol R as the mobile phase. Apply separately to the plate 2 µl of each of 2 solutions in methanol R containing (A) 10 mg of the test substance per ml, and (B) 0.20 mg of dexamethasone RS per ml. After removing the plate from the chromatographic chamber, allow it to dry in air for 5 minutes, spray it with a solution of 3 g of zinc chloride R in 10 ml of methanol R, heat it at about 125 °C for 1 hour, and examine the chromatogram in ultraviolet light (365 nm). Any spot obtained with solution A, other than the principal spot, is not more intense than that obtained with solution B.

Assay.   Dissolve about 0.2 g, accurately weighed, in sufficient water to produce 200 ml. Dilute 5 ml to 250 ml with water and measure the absorbance of this solution in a 1-cm layer at the maximum at about 241 nm. Calculate the content of $C_{22}H_{28}FNa_2O_8P$, using the absorptivity value of 29.7 ($A^{1\%}_{1\,cm} = 297$).

DEXTROMETHORPHANI HYDROBROMIDUM

Dextromethorphan hydrobromide

Molecular formula. $C_{18}H_{25}NO,HBr,H_2O$

Relative molecular mass.   370.3

Graphic formula.

Chemical name.   (+)-3-Methoxy-17-methyl-9α,13α-14α-morphinan hydrobromide monohydrate; (+)-cis-1,3,4,9,10,10a-hexahydro-6-methoxy-11-methyl-2H-10,4a-iminoethanophenanthrene hydrobromide monohydrate; CAS Reg. No. 6700-34-1 (monohydrate).

Description.   A white or almost white, crystalline powder; odourless or almost odourless.

Solubility.   Sparingly soluble in water; freely soluble in ethanol ($\sim$750 g/l) TS and chloroform R; practically insoluble in ether R.

Category.   Antitussive drug.

Storage.   Dextromethorphan hydrobromide should be kept in a well-closed container.

REQUIREMENTS

General requirement.   Dextromethorphan hydrobromide contains not less than 98.0% and not more than 101.0% of $C_{18}H_{25}NO,HBr$, calculated with reference to the anhydrous substance.

Identity tests

● Either tests A and E or tests B, C, D and E may be applied.

A.   Dry a small quantity of the test substance for 4 hours under reduced pressure (not exceeding 0.6 kPa or about 5 mm of mercury) over phosphorus pentoxide R, and carry out the examination as described under "Spectrophotometry in the infrared region" (vol. 1, p. 40). The infrared absorption spectrum is concordant with the spectrum obtained from dextromethorphan hydrobromide RS similarly prepared or with the *reference spectrum* of dextromethorphan hydrobromide.

B.   The absorption spectrum of a 0.10 mg/ml solution in sodium hydroxide (0.1 mol/l) VS, when observed between 230 nm and 350 nm, exhibits a maximum at 280 nm; the absorbance of a 1-cm layer at this wavelength is about 0.59.

C.   Dissolve 0.05 g in 2 ml of sulfuric acid ($\sim$100 g/l) TS. Add 1 ml of mercury/nitric acid TS drop by drop while shaking; a white, crystalline precipitate in the form of platelets is produced, and the solution does not immediately turn red. Heat on a water-bath for about 10 minutes; a yellow to red colour develops.

D.   Melting temperature, about 125 °C with decomposition.

E.   To a 5 mg/ml solution add 0.25 ml of nitric acid ($\sim$130 g/l) TS; this test yields reaction B described under "General identification tests" as characteristic of bromides (vol. 1, p. 112).

Specific optical rotation.   Use a 20 mg/ml solution in hydrochloric acid (0.1 mol/l) VS and calculated with reference to the anhydrous substance; $[\alpha]_D^{20\,°C} = +28.0$ to $+30.0°$.

Sulfated ash.   Not more than 1.0 mg/g.

Water.   Determine as described under "Determination of water by the Karl Fischer method", Method A (vol. 1, p. 135), using about 0.2 g of the substance; the water content is not less than 35 mg/g and not more than 55 mg/g.

pH value.   Dissolve 0.4 g in carbon-dioxide-free water R using gentle heat, dilute to 20 ml with the same solvent and measure the pH at 20 °C; the value lies between 5.2 and 6.5.

Dimethylaniline.   Dissolve 0.5 g in 15 ml of water using gentle heat, cool, and add 4 ml of acetic acid (~60 g/l) TS, 1 ml of sodium nitrite (10 g/l) TS, and sufficient water to produce 25 ml. Prepare similarly a reference solution containing 5 µg of *N,N*-dimethylaniline R in 25 ml. The colour produced in the test solution is not more intense than that produced in the reference solution when compared as described under "Colour of liquids" (vol. 1, p. 50); the dimethylaniline content is not more than 10 µg/g.

Phenolic substances.   To 5 mg add 1 drop of hydrochloric acid (~70 g/l) TS, 1 ml of water, and 0.2 ml of ferric chloride (50 g/l) TS. Mix, add 0.2 ml of potassium ferricyanide (50 g/l) TS, dilute to 5 ml with water, shake well, and allow to stand for 15 minutes; the solution is yellowish brown and shows no greenish or blue colour.

Assay.   Dissolve about 0.5 g, accurately weighed, in 40 ml of glacial acetic acid R1, and add 10 ml of mercuric acetate/acetic acid TS, warming slightly if necessary to effect solution. Titrate with perchloric acid (0.1 mol/l) VS as described under "Non-aqueous titration", Method A (vol. 1, p. 131). Each ml of perchloric acid (0.1 mol/l) VS is equivalent to 35.23 mg of $C_{18}H_{25}NO,HBr$.

DICLOXACILLINUM NATRICUM

Dicloxacillin sodium

Molecular formula. $C_{19}H_{16}Cl_2N_3NaO_5S,H_2O$

Relative molecular mass.   510.3

Graphic formula.

Chemical name.   Monosodium (2*S*,5*R*,6*R*)-6-[3-(2,6-dichlorophenyl)-5-methyl-4-isoxazolecarboxamido]-3,3-dimethyl-7-oxo-4-thia-1-azabicyclo[3.2.0]heptane-2-carboxylate monohydrate; monosodium [2*S*-(2α,5α,6β)]-6-[[[3-(2,6-dichlorophenyl)-5-methyl-4-isoxazolyl]carbonyl]amino]-3,3-dimethyl-7-oxo-4-thia-1-azabicyclo[3.2.0]heptane-2-carboxylate monohydrate; monosodium [3-(2,6-dichlorophenyl)-5-methyl-4-isoxazolyl]penicillin monohydrate; CAS Reg. No. 13412-64-1 (monohydrate).

Description.   A white or almost white, crystalline powder.

Solubility.   Freely soluble in water and methanol R; soluble in ethanol ($\sim$750 g/l) TS; sparingly soluble in chloroform R.

Category.   Antibacterial drug.

Storage.   Dicloxacillin sodium should be kept in a tightly closed container, protected from light.

Additional information.   Even in the absence of light, Dicloxacillin sodium is gradually degraded on exposure to a humid atmosphere, the decomposition being faster at higher temperatures.

REQUIREMENTS

General requirement.   Dicloxacillin sodium contains not less than 88.0% of total penicillins calculated as dicloxacillin free acid ($C_{19}H_{17}Cl_2N_3O_5S$) and with reference to the anhydrous substance.

Identity tests

A.   Carry out the examination as described under "Spectrophotometry in the infrared region" (vol. 1, p. 40). The infrared absorption spectrum is concordant with the spectrum obtained from dicloxacillin sodium RS or with the *reference spectrum* of dicloxacillin sodium.

B.   To 10 mg of paraformaldehyde R dissolved in 1 ml of sulfuric acid ($\sim$1760 g/l) TS add about 1 mg of the test substance; a colourless solution is produced. Heat the solution in a water-bath for 2 minutes and cool; the solution remains colourless (distinction from cloxacillin sodium).

C.   Ignite 20 mg and dissolve the residue in acetic acid ($\sim$60 g/l) TS. The solution yields reaction B described under "General identification tests" as characteristic of sodium (vol. 1, p. 115).

Specific optical rotation.   Use a 10 mg/ml solution, and calculate with reference to the anhydrous substance; $[\alpha]_D^{20\,°C} = +128$ to $+143°$.

Water. Determine as described under "Determination of water by the Karl Fischer method", Method A (vol. 1, p. 135), using about 0.25 g of the substance; the water content is not less than 30 mg/g and not more than 50 mg/g.

pH value. pH of a 10 mg/ml solution, 4.5–7.5.

Chlorine. Carry out the combustion as described under "Oxygen flask method" (vol. 1, p. 124), but using 25 mg of the test substance and 10 ml of sodium hydroxide (0.1 mol/l) VS as the absorbing liquid. When the process is complete, transfer the resulting solution to a titration vessel, heat on a water-bath for 30 minutes, cool to room temperature, add 20 ml of nitric acid ($\sim$130 g/l) TS, and titrate with silver nitrate (0.01 mol/l) VS, determining the endpoint potentiometrically using a silver/silver chloride electrode system. Repeat the operation without the substance being tested. Each ml of silver nitrate (0.01 mol/l) VS is equivalent to 0.3546 mg of Cl. Calculate the total content of chlorine in mg/g and subtract from it the content of free chlorides as determined below; the content of chlorine is between 130 mg/g and 142 mg/g.

Free chlorides. Dissolve about 0.12 g, accurately weighed, in 10 ml of sodium hydroxide (0.1 mol/l) VS, add 20 ml of water, and heat on a water-bath for 30 minutes. Cool to room temperature, add 20 ml of nitric acid ($\sim$130 g/l) TS, and titrate with silver nitrate (0.01 mol/l) VS, determining the endpoint potentiometrically using a silver/silver chloride electrode system. Repeat the operation without the substance being tested. Each ml of silver nitrate (0.01 mol/l) VS is equivalent to 0.3546 mg of Cl; the content of free chlorides is not more than 5 mg/g.

Assay. Dissolve about 50 mg, accurately weighed, in sufficient water to produce 1000 ml. Transfer two 2.0-ml aliquots of this solution into separate stoppered tubes. To one tube add 10.0 ml of imidazole/mercuric chloride TS, mix, stopper the tube and place in a water-bath at 60 °C for exactly 25 minutes. Cool the tube rapidly to 20 °C (solution A). To the second tube add 10.0 ml of water and mix (solution B).

Without delay measure the absorbance of a 1-cm layer at the maximum at about 343 nm against a solvent cell containing a mixture of 2.0 ml of water and 10.0 ml of imidazole/mercuric chloride TS for solution A and water for solution B.

From the difference between the absorbance of solution A and that of solution B, calculate the amount of $C_{19}H_{16}Cl_2N_3NaO_5S$ in the substance being tested by comparison with dicloxacillin sodium RS, similarly and concurrently examined.

DILOXANIDI FUROAS

Diloxanide furoate

Molecular formula. $C_{14}H_{11}Cl_2NO_4$

Relative molecular mass.   328.2

Graphic formula.

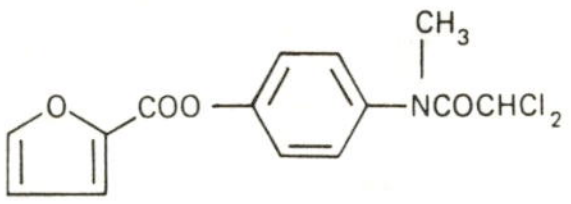

Chemical name.   2,2-Dichloro-4′-hydroxy-*N*-methylacetanilide 2-furoate (ester); 4-[(dichloroacetyl)methylamino]phenyl 2-furancarboxylate; 2,2-dichloro-*N*-(4-hydroxyphenyl)-*N*-methylacetamide 2-furoate; CAS Reg. No. 3736-81-0.

Description.   A white or almost white, crystalline powder; odourless.

Solubility.   Very slightly soluble in water; soluble in 100 parts of ethanol (~750 g/l) TS, in 2.5 parts of chloroform R, and in 130 parts of ether R.

Category.   Antiamoebic drug.

Storage.   Diloxanide furoate should be kept in a well-closed container, protected from light.

REQUIREMENTS

General requirement.   Diloxanide furoate contains not less than 98.0% and not more than 102.0% of $C_{14}H_{11}Cl_2NO_4$, calculated with reference to the dried substance.

Identity tests

● Either test A alone or tests B and C may be applied.

A.   Carry out the examination as described under "Spectrophotometry in the infrared region" (vol. 1, p. 40). The infrared absorption spectrum is concordant with the spectrum obtained from diloxanide furoate RS or with the *reference spectrum* of diloxanide furoate.

B.   The absorption spectrum of a 7.0 µg/ml solution in ethanol (~750 g/l) TS, when observed between 240 nm and 350 nm, exhibits a maximum at about 258 nm; the absorbance of a 1-cm layer at this wavelength is about 0.49.

C.   Carry out the combustion as described under "Oxygen flask method" (vol. 1, p. 125), using 20 mg of the test substance and 10 ml of sodium hydroxide (1 mol/l) VS as the absorbing liquid. When the process is complete, acidify with nitric acid (~130 g/l) TS; the solution yields reaction A, described under "General identification tests" as characteristic of chlorides (vol. 1, p. 112).

Melting range.   114–116 °C.

Sulfated ash.   Not more than 1.0 mg/g.

Loss on drying.   Dry to constant weight at 105 °C; it loses not more than 5.0 mg/g.

Free acidity.   Shake 3.0 g with 50 ml of carbon-dioxide-free water R, filter and wash the residue with 3 quantities, each of 20 ml of carbon-dioxide-free water R. Titrate the combined filtrate and washings with sodium hydroxide (0.1 mol/l) VS, phenolphthalein/ethanol TS being used as indicator; not more than 1.3 ml is required.

Related substances.   Carry out the test as described under "Thin-layer chromatography" (vol. 1, p. 83), using silica gel R2 as the coating substance and a mixture of 24 volumes of dichloromethane R and 1 volume of methanol R as the mobile phase. Apply separately to the plate 5 µl of each of 2 solutions in chloroform R containing (A) 0.10 g of the test substance per ml and (B) 2.5 mg of the test substance per ml. After removing the plate from the chromatographic chamber, allow it to dry in air and examine the chromatogram in ultraviolet light (254 nm). Any spot obtained with solution A, other than the principal spot, is not more intense than that obtained with solution B.

Assay.   Dissolve about 0.3 g, accurately weighed, in 50 ml of anhydrous pyridine R and titrate with tetrabutylammonium hydroxide (0.1 mol/l) VS determining the endpoint potentiometrically as described under "Non-aqueous titration", Method B (vol. 1, p. 132). Each ml of tetrabutylammonium hydroxide (0.1 mol/l) VS is equivalent to 32.82 mg of $C_{14}H_{11}Cl_2NO_4$.

DIMERCAPROLUM

Dimercaprol

Molecular formula. $C_3H_8OS_2$

Relative molecular mass.   124.2

Graphic formula.

$$\underset{\displaystyle \quad SH\ \ SH}{CH_2CHCH_2OH}$$

Chemical name.   2,3-Dimercapto-1-propanol; CAS Reg. No. 59-52-9.

Description.   A clear, colourless or slightly yellow liquid, with an unpleasant, mercaptan-like odour.

Miscibility.   Miscible with 20 parts of water; miscible with ethanol ($\sim$750 g/l) TS and methanol R.

Category.   Antidote for arsenic, gold, and mercury poisoning.

Storage.   Dimercaprol should be kept in a small, well-filled and tightly closed container, protected from light, and stored at a temperature not exceeding 5 °C.

REQUIREMENTS

General requirement.   Dimercaprol contains not less than 98.5% w/w and not more than 101.5% w/w of $C_3H_8OS_2$.

Identity tests

A.   Mix 0.05 ml of cobalt(II) chloride (30 g/l) TS with 5 ml of water and add 0.05 ml of the test liquid; a yellow-brown colour is produced.

B.   Dissolve 0.1 ml in 4 ml of water and add a few drops of lead acetate (80 g/l) TS; a yellow precipitate is formed.

Refractive index. $n_D^{20} = 1.568 - 1.574$.

Relative density. $d_{20}^{20} = 1.239 - 1.259$.

Halides.   Dissolve 2.0 g in 25 ml of potassium hydroxide/ethanol TS1 and heat under a reflux condenser for 2 hours. Evaporate the ethanol in a current of warm air, add 20 ml of water, and cool. Add a mixture of 10 ml of hydrogen peroxide ($\sim$330 g/l) TS and 40 ml of water, boil gently for 10 minutes, cool, and filter rapidly. Add 10 ml of nitric acid ($\sim$130 g/l) TS and 5 ml of silver nitrate (0.1 mol/l) VS and titrate with ammonium thiocyanate (0.1 mol/l) VS, using ferric ammonium sulfate (45 g/l) TS as indicator. Repeat the operation without the test liquid being examined. The difference between the titrations does not exceed 1.0 ml.

pH value.   pH of a 0.5 g/ml solution in carbon-dioxide-free water R, 4.6–6.8.

Assay.   Dissolve about 0.12 g, accurately weighed, in 20 ml of hydrochloric acid (0.1 mol/l) VS and titrate rapidly with iodine (0.05 mol/l) VS, using starch TS as indicator. Repeat the operation without the test liquid being examined and make any necessary corrections. Each ml of iodine (0.05 mol/l) VS is equivalent to 6.211 mg of $C_3H_8OS_2$.

DIPHENOXYLATI HYDROCHLORIDUM

Diphenoxylate hydrochloride

Molecular formula. $C_{30}H_{32}N_2O_2,HCl$

Relative molecular mass.   489.1

Graphic formula.

Chemical name.   Ethyl 1-(3-cyano-3,3-diphenylpropyl)-4-phenylisonipecotate monohydrochloride; ethyl 1-(3-cyano-3,3-diphenylpropyl)-4-phenyl-4-piperidinecarboxylate monohydrochloride; CAS Reg. No. 3810-80-8.

Description.   A white or almost white, crystalline powder; odourless.

Solubility.   Sparingly soluble in water, acetone R and ethanol ($\sim$750 g/l) TS; freely soluble in chloroform R; practically insoluble in ether R.

Category.   Antidiarrhoeal drug.

Storage.   Diphenoxylate hydrochloride should be kept in a well-closed container.

REQUIREMENTS

General requirement.   Diphenoxylate hydrochloride contains not less than 98.0% and not more than 101.0% of $C_{30}H_{32}N_2O_2,HCl$, calculated with reference to the dried substance.

Identity tests

● Either tests A and E or tests B, C, D and E may be applied.

A.   Carry out the examination as described under "Spectrophotometry in the infrared region" (vol. 1, p. 40). The infrared absorption spectrum is concordant with the spectrum obtained from diphenoxylate hydrochloride RS or with the *reference spectrum* of diphenoxylate hydrochloride.

B.   The absorption spectrum of a 0.50 mg/ml solution in a mixture of 1 volume of hydrochloric acid (1 mol/l) VS and 99 volumes of methanol R, when observed between 230 nm and 350 nm, exhibits maxima at about 252 nm, 258 nm, and 265 nm; the absorbances of a 1-cm layer at these wavelengths are about 0.55, 0.65 and 0.50, respectively.

C.   Dissolve 25 mg in 5 ml of water and add 0.1 ml of potassio-mercuric iodide TS; a cream-coloured precipitate is produced.

D.   Melting temperature, about 223 °C.

E.   A 20 mg/ml solution yields reaction B described under "General identification tests" as characteristic of chlorides (vol. 1, p. 113).

Sulfated ash.   Not more than 1.0 mg/g.

Loss on drying.   Dry to constant weight at 105 °C; it loses not more than 5.0 mg/g.

Related substances.   Carry out the test as described under "Thin-layer chromatography" (vol. 1, p. 83), using silica gel R1 as the coating substance and a mixture of 92 volumes of chloroform R, 3 volumes of methanol R, and 5 volumes of glacial acetic acid R as the mobile phase. Apply separately to the plate 10 µl of each of 2 solutions in chloroform R containing (A) 50 mg of the test substance per ml and (B) 0.50 mg of the test substance per ml. After removing the plate from the chromatographic chamber, allow it to dry in air, expose it to the vapour of iodine, and examine the chromatogram in daylight. Any spot obtained with solution A, other than the principal spot, is not more intense than that obtained with solution B.

Assay.   Dissolve about 0.4 g, accurately weighed, in 40 ml of glacial acetic acid R1, add 10 ml of mercuric acetate/acetic acid TS and titrate with perchloric acid (0.1 mol/l) VS as described under "Non-aqueous titration", Method A (vol. 1, p. 131). Each ml of perchloric acid (0.1 mol/l) VS is equivalent to 48.91 mg of $C_{30}H_{32}N_2O_2,HCl$.

DOPAMINI HYDROCHLORIDUM

Dopamine hydrochloride

Molecular formula. $C_8H_{11}NO_2,HCl$

Relative molecular mass.   189.6

Graphic formula.

Chemical name.   4-(2-Aminoethyl)pyrocatechol hydrochloride; 4-(2-amino-ethyl)-1,2-benzenediol hydrochloride; CAS Reg. No. 62-31-7.

Description.   Colourless crystals or a white or almost white, crystalline powder; odourless.

Solubility.   Freely soluble in water; soluble in methanol R; practically insoluble in ether R, chloroform R, and toluene R.

Category.   Cardiovascular drug; sympathomimetic.

Storage.   Dopamine hydrochloride should be kept in a well-closed container, protected from light.

REQUIREMENTS

General requirement.   Dopamine hydrochloride contains not less than 98.0% and not more than 101.0% of $C_8H_{11}NO_2,HCl$, calculated with reference to the dried substance.

Identity tests

● Either tests A and D or tests B, C and D may be applied.

A.   Carry out the examination as described under "Spectrophotometry in the infrared region" (vol. 1, p. 40). The infrared absorption spectrum is concordant with the spectrum obtained from dopamine hydrochloride RS or with the *reference spectrum* of dopamine hydrochloride.

B.   The absorption spectrum of a 0.020 mg/ml solution in hydrochloric acid (0.1 mol/l) VS, when observed between 230 nm and 350 nm, exhibits a maximum at about 280 nm and a minimum at about 249 nm; the absorbance of a 1-cm layer at 280 nm is about 0.54.

C.   Dissolve 0.05 g in 5 ml of water and add while stirring 10 ml of 4-amino-antipyrine TS2; a red colour is produced.

D.   A 20 mg/ml solution yields reaction A described under "General identifica-tion tests" as characteristic of chlorides (vol. 1, p. 113).

Heavy metals.   Use 1.0 g for the preparation of the test solution as described under "Limit test for heavy metals", Procedure 1 (vol. 1, p. 118); determine the heavy metals content according to Method A (vol. 1, p. 119); not more than 20 µg/g.

Clarity and colour of solution.   A solution of 1.0 g in 10 ml of water is clear and colourless.

Sulfated ash.   Not more than 1.0 mg/g.

Loss on drying.   Dry to constant weight at 105 °C; it loses not more than 5.0 mg/g.

Related substances.   Carry out the test as described under "Thin-layer chromatography" (vol. 1, p. 83) using silica gel R1 as the coating substance and a mixture of 13 volumes of chloroform R, 9 volumes of methanol R, and 4 volumes of acetic acid ($\sim$300 g/l) TS as the mobile phase.   Apply separately to the plate 10 µl of each of 2 solutions in methanol R containing (A) 30 mg of the test substance per ml and (B) 0.3 mg of dopamine hydrochloride RS per ml.   After removing the plate from the chromatographic chamber, allow it to dry at room temperature for several minutes, then spray it evenly with a freshly prepared mixture of 2 volumes of ferric chloride (50 g/l) TS and 1 volume of potassium ferricyanide (50 g/l) TS.   Examine the chromatogram in daylight.   Apart from the principal spot, not more than 3 spots are obtained with solution A, and the estimated sum of impurities is not larger than that estimated from the chromatogram obtained with solution B.

Assay.   Dissolve about 0.4 g, accurately weighed, in 140 ml of glacial acetic acid R1, add 10 ml of mercuric acetate/acetic acid TS, and titrate with perchloric acid (0.1 mol/l) VS as described under "Non-aqueous titration", Method A (vol. 1, p. 131).   Each ml of perchloric acid (0.1 mol/l) VS is equivalent to 18.96 mg of $C_8H_{11}NO_2$,HCl.

DOXORUBICINI HYDROCHLORIDUM

Doxorubicin hydrochloride

Molecular formula. $C_{27}H_{29}NO_{11}$,HCl

Relative molecular mass.   580.0

Graphic formula.

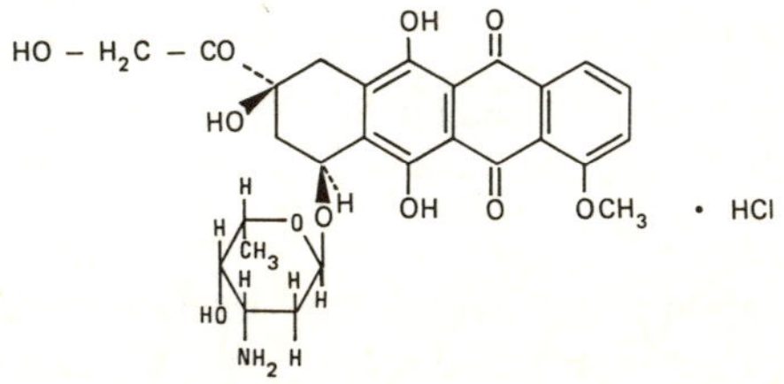

Chemical name.   (8*S*,10*S*)-10-[(3-Amino-2,3,6-trideoxy-α-L-*lyxo*-hexopyrano-syl)oxy]-8-glycoloyl-7,8,9,10-tetrahydro-6,8,11-trihydroxy-1-methoxy-5,12-naphthacenedione hydrochloride; (8*S*-*cis*)-10-[(3-amino-2,3,6-trideoxy-α-L-*lyxo*-hexopyranosyl)oxy]-7,8,9,10-tetrahydro-6,8,11-trihydroxy-8-(hydroxyacetyl)-1-methoxy-5,12-naphthacenedione hydrochloride; CAS Reg. No. 25316-40-9.

Description.   A red-orange, crystalline powder.

Solubility.   Soluble in water and methanol R; practically insoluble in chloroform R and ether R.

Category.   Cytotoxic drug.

Storage.   Doxorubicin hydrochloride should be kept in a tightly closed container.

Additional information.   Doxorubicin hydrochloride is hygroscopic; it is poisonous. CAUTION: Doxorubicin hydrochloride must be handled with care, avoiding contact with the skin and inhalation of airborne particles.

REQUIREMENTS

General requirement.   Doxorubicin hydrochloride contains not less than 97.0% and not more than 102.0% of $C_{27}H_{29}NO_{11}$,HCl, calculated with reference to the anhydrous substance.

Identity tests

A.   The absorption spectrum of a 20 µg/ml solution in methanol R, when observed between 220 nm and 600 nm, is qualitatively similar to that of a 20 µg/ml solution of doxorubicin hydrochloride RS in methanol R (maxima occur at about 233 nm, 253 nm, 290 nm, 477 nm, 495 nm and 530 nm; minima occur at about 245 nm, 280 nm and 350 nm). The absorbances of the solutions at the respective maxima do not differ from each other by more than 3%. The absorbance of a 1-cm layer at the wavelengths of the main maxima are about 1.32, 0.88, 0.30, 0.46, 0.44 and 0.24, respectively.

B.   See the test described below under "Related substances". The principal spot obtained with solution A corresponds in position, appearance and intensity with that obtained with solution B.

C.   Dissolve 2 mg in 2 ml of methanol R, add 2 ml of water and 0.05 ml of sodium hydroxide (~80 g/l) TS; the orange-red colour of the solution turns to blue-violet.

D.   A 0.05 g/ml solution yields reaction B described under "General identification tests" as characteristic of chlorides (vol. 1, p. 113).

Water. Determine as described under "Determination of water by the Karl Fischer method", Method A (vol. 1, p. 135), using about 0.25 g of the substance; the water content is not more than 40 mg/g.

pH value. pH of a 5.0 mg/ml solution, 3.8–6.5.

Related substances. Carry out the test as described under "Thin-layer chromatography" (vol. 1, p. 83), using silica gel R1 as the coating substance and a mixture of 80 volumes of chloroform R, 20 volumes of methanol R and 5 volumes of glacial acetic acid R as the mobile phase. Apply separately to the plate 10 µl of each of 4 solutions in methanol R containing (A) 2.0 mg of the test substance per ml, (B) 2.0 mg of doxorubicin hydrochloride RS per ml, (C) 20 mg of the test substance per ml, and (D) 0.40 mg of the test substance per ml. After removing the plate from the chromatographic chamber, allow it to dry in air and examine the chromatogram in daylight. Any spot obtained with solution C, other than the principal spot, is not more intense than that obtained with solution D.

Assay. Dissolve about 20 mg, accurately weighed, in sufficient methanol R to produce 100 ml; dilute 10 ml of this solution to 100 ml with the same solvent. Measure the absorbance of a 1-cm layer of the diluted solution at the maximum at about 495 nm. Calculate the amount of $C_{27}H_{29}NO_{11}$,HCl in the substance being tested by comparison with doxorubicin hydrochloride RS, similarly and concurrently examined. In an adequately calibrated spectrophotometer the absorbance of the reference solution should be 0.44 ± 0.02.

DOXYCYCLINI HYCLAS

Doxycycline hyclate

Molecular formula. $(C_{22}H_{24}N_2O_8,HCl)_2,C_2H_6O,H_2O$

Relative molecular mass. 1026

Graphic formula.

Chemical name.   (4*S*,4a*R*,5*S*,5a*R*,6*R*,12a*S*)-4-(Dimethylamino)-1,4,4a,5,5a,6, 11,12a-octahydro-3,5,10,12,12a-pentahydroxy-6-methyl-1,11-dioxo-2-naphthacenecarboxamide monohydrochloride, compound with ethyl alcohol (2:1), monohydrate; [4*S*-(4α,4aα,5α,5aα,6α,12aα)]-4-(dimethylamino)-1,4,4a,5,5a,6,11,12a-octahydro-3,5,10,12,12a-pentahydroxy-6-methyl-1,11-dioxo-2-naphthacenecarboxamide monohydrochloride, compound with ethanol (2:1), monohydrate; CAS Reg. No. 24390-14-5.

Description.   A yellow, crystalline powder.

Solubility.   Soluble in 3 parts of water and in 4 parts of methanol R; practically insoluble in chloroform R and ether R.

Category.   Antibacterial drug.

Storage.   Doxycycline hyclate should be kept in a tightly closed container, protected from light.

Additional information.   Even in the absence of light, Doxycycline hyclate is gradually degraded on exposure to a humid atmosphere, the decomposition being faster at higher temperatures.

REQUIREMENTS

General requirement.   Doxycycline hyclate contains not less than 880 International Units of doxycycline per mg, calculated with reference to the anhydrous and ethanol-free substance.

Identity tests

A.   Dissolve 5 mg in 2 ml of sulfuric acid (~1760 g/l) TS; an intense yellow colour is produced.

B.   Dissolve 5 mg in 2.0 ml of water and add 0.05 ml of ferric chloride (~25 g/l) TS; a dark red-brown colour is produced.

C.   Dissolve 5 mg in 2.0 ml of water and add 0.25 ml of alkaline potassiomercuric iodide TS; a fine crystalline, light yellow precipitate is formed.

D.   A 20 mg/ml solution yields reaction B described under "General identification tests" as characteristic of chlorides (vol. 1, p. 113).

Sulfated ash.   Not more than 4.0 mg/g.

Water.   Determine as described under "Determination of water by the Karl Fischer method", Method A (vol. 1, p. 135), using about 1.2 g of the substance; the water content is not less than 14 mg/g and not more than 28 mg/g.

Ethanol.   Carry out the test as described under "Gas chromatography" (vol. 1, p. 94), using 3 solutions in water containing (1) a mixture of 0.50 µl of dehydrated ethanol R per ml, (2) 10 mg of the test substance per ml, and (3) a mixture of 10 mg of the test substance per ml with 0.50 µl of the internal standard.

For the procedure use a column 1.5 m long and 4 mm in internal diameter packed with porous polymer beads (particle size 80–100 µm from a commercial source is suitable). Maintain the column at 135 °C, use nitrogen R as the carrier gas and a flame ionization detector.

Calculate the content of ethanol in mg/g, assuming the weight per ml at 20 °C to be 0.790 g; not less than 43 mg/g and not more than 60 mg/g.

pH value.   pH of a 10 mg/ml solution, 2.0–3.0.

Absorption in the ultraviolet region.   The absorption spectrum of a 10 µg/ml solution in a mixture of 1 volume of hydrochloric acid (1 mol/l) VS and 99 volumes of methanol R exhibits a maximum at about 349 nm. The absorbance of a 1-cm layer at this maximum is not less than 0.28 and not more than 0.31 for the anhydrous and ethanol-free substance.

Light-absorbing impurities.   Prepare a 10 mg/ml solution in a mixture of 1 volume of hydrochloric acid (1 mol/l) VS and 99 volumes of methanol R, and measure the absorbance of a 1-cm layer at 490 nm; the absorbance does not exceed 0.12 for the anhydrous and ethanol-free substance.

Assay.   Carry out the assay as described under "Microbiological assay of antibiotics" (vol. 1, p. 145), using *Bacillus cereus* (NCTC 10320 or ATCC 11778) as the test organism, culture medium Cm10 with a final pH of 6.6, potassium dihydrogen phosphate (13.6 g/l) TS as a buffer, an appropriate concentration of doxycycline (usually between 0.2 and 2.0 IU per ml), and an incubation temperature of 35–39 °C. The precision of the assay is such that the fiducial limits of error of the estimated potency ($P = 0.95$) are not less than 95% and not more than 105% of the estimated potency. The upper fiducial limit of error of the estimated potency ($P = 0.95$) is not less than 880 IU of doxycycline per mg, calculated with reference to the anhydrous and ethanol-free substance.

EDROPHONII CHLORIDUM

Edrophonium chloride

Molecular formula. $C_{10}H_{16}ClNO$

Relative molecular mass.   201.7

Graphic formula.

$$\left[HO-C_6H_4-\overset{\displaystyle\underset{+}{C_2H_5}}{N}(CH_3)_2 \right] Cl^-$$

Chemical name. Ethyl(*m*-hydroxyphenyl)dimethylammonium chloride; *N*-ethyl-3-hydroxy-*N*,*N*-dimethylbenzenaminium chloride; CAS Reg. No. 116-38-1.

Description. A white, crystalline powder; odourless.

Solubility. Soluble in 0.5 parts of water and in 5 parts of ethanol ($\sim$750 g/l) TS; practically insoluble in chloroform R and ether R.

Category. Diagnostic agent.

Storage. Edrophonium chloride should be kept in a well-closed container, protected from light.

REQUIREMENTS

General requirement. Edrophonium chloride contains not less than 98.5% and not more than 101.0% of $C_{10}H_{16}ClNO$, calculated with reference to the dried substance.

Identity tests

A. The absorption spectrum of a 0.050 mg/ml solution in hydrochloric acid (0.1 mol/l) VS, when observed between 230 nm and 350 nm, exhibits a maximum at about 273 nm; the absorbance of a 1-cm layer at this wavelength is about 0.55.

B. The absorption spectrum of a 10 μg/ml solution in sodium hydroxide (0.1 mol/l) VS, when observed between 230 nm and 350 nm, exhibits maxima at about 240 nm and 294 nm; the absorbances of a 1-cm layer at these wavelengths are about 0.55 and 0.17, respectively.

C. Dissolve 0.05 g in 2 ml of water and add 0.05 ml of ferric chloride (25 g/l) TS; a reddish violet colour is produced.

D. Melting temperature, about 168 °C with decomposition.

E. A 20 mg/ml solution yields reaction A described under "General identification tests" as characteristic of chlorides (vol. 1, p. 112).

Sulfated ash. Not more than 1.0 mg/g.

Loss on drying. Dry at ambient temperature under reduced pressure (not exceeding 0.6 kPa or about 5 mm of mercury) over phosphorus pentoxide R for 24 hours; it loses not more than 5.0 mg/g.

pH value. pH of a 0.10 g/ml solution, 4.0–5.0.

Dimethylaminophenol. Dissolve 0.1 g in 10 ml of water, add 5 ml of phosphate buffer, pH 8.0, TS, and extract with 2 quantities, each of 20 ml of chloroform R.

Wash the extracts successively with 2 quantities, each of 10 ml of water, and extract with 10 ml of sodium hydroxide (0.1 mol/l) VS. Measure the absorbance of the sodium hydroxide extract using a 1-cm layer at 293 nm; not greater than 0.25.

Assay. Dissolve about 0.20 g, accurately weighed, in 20 ml of glacial acetic acid R1, add 10 ml of mercuric acetate/acetic acid TS and 0.25 ml of quinaldine red/ethanol TS, and titrate with perchloric acid (0.1 mol/l) VS as described under "Non-aqueous titration", Method A (vol. 1, p. 131). Each ml of perchloric acid (0.1 mol/l) VS is equivalent to 20.17 mg of $C_{10}H_{16}ClNO$.

EMETINI HYDROCHLORIDUM

Emetine hydrochloride

Emetine hydrochloride pentahydrate
Emetine hydrochloride heptahydrate

Molecular formula. $C_{29}H_{40}N_2O_4,2HCl,5H_2O$ (pentahydrate); $C_{29}H_{40}N_2O_4,2HCl,7H_2O$ (heptahydrate).

Relative molecular mass. 643.6 (pentahydrate); 679.7 (heptahydrate).

Graphic formula.

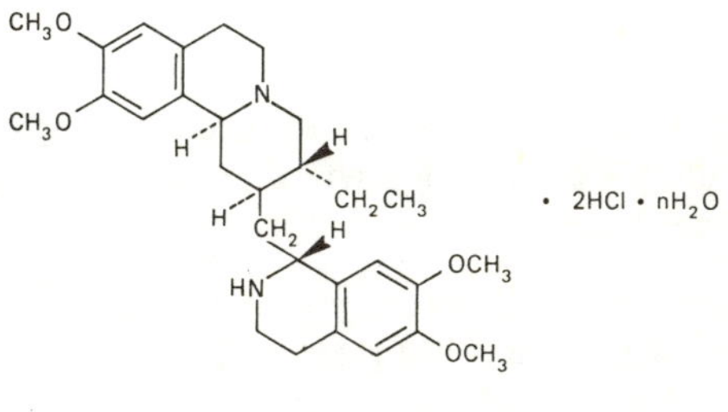

n = 5 (pentahydrate)
n = 7 (heptahydrate)

Chemical name. Emetine dihydrochloride pentahydrate; 6′,7′,10,11-tetramethoxyemetan dihydrochloride pentahydrate; CAS Reg. No. 79300-07-5 (pentahydrate).
Emetine dihydrochloride heptahydrate; 6′,7′,10,11-tetramethoxyemetan dihydrochloride heptahydrate; CAS Reg. No. 79300-08-6 (heptahydrate).

Description. A white or very slightly yellow, crystalline powder; odourless.

Solubility.   Freely soluble in water, ethanol (~750 g/l) TS and chloroform R.

Category.   Antiamoebic drug.

Storage.   Emetine hydrochloride should be kept in a tightly closed container, protected from light.

Labelling.   The designation on the container of Emetine hydrochloride should state whether the substance is the pentahydrate or the heptahydrate.

Additional information.   Emetine hydrochloride is the hydrochloride of an alkaloid obtained from ipecacuanha or prepared by methylation of cephaëline or by synthesis.   Even in the absence of light, Emetine hydrochloride is gradually degraded on exposure to a humid atmosphere, the decomposition being faster at higher temperatures.

REQUIREMENTS

General requirement.   Emetine hydrochloride contains not less than 98.0% and not more than 101.5% of $C_{29}H_{40}N_2O_4,2HCl$, calculated with reference to the dried substance.

Identity tests

● Either tests A and D or tests B, C and D may be applied.

A.   Carry out the examination as described under "Spectrophotometry in the infrared region" (vol. 1, p. 40).   The infrared absorption spectrum is concordant with the spectrum obtained from emetine hydrochloride RS or with the *reference spectrum* of emetine hydrochloride.

B.   See the test described below under "Related alkaloids".   The principal spot obtained with solution A corresponds in position, appearance, and intensity with that obtained with solution D.

C.   Sprinkle 5 mg of the test substance on the surface of 1 ml of ammonium molybdate/sulfuric acid TS; a bright green colour is produced.

D.   A 0.05 g/ml solution yields reaction B described under "General identification tests" as characteristic of chlorides (vol. 1, p. 113).

Specific optical rotation.   Use a 50 mg/ml solution and calculate with reference to the dried substance; $[\alpha]_D^{20\,°C} = +16$ to $+19°$.

Sulfated ash.   Not more than 1.0 mg/g.

Loss on drying.   Dry to constant weight at 105 °C; Emetine hydrochloride pentahydrate loses not less than 110 mg/g and not more than 150 mg/g.   Emetine hydrochloride heptahydrate loses not less than 150 mg/g and not more than 190 mg/g.

Acidity. Dissolve 0.10 g in 10 ml of carbon-dioxide-free water R and titrate with sodium hydroxide (0.02 mol/l) VS, using methyl red/ethanol TS as indicator; not more than 0.5 ml is required to obtain the midpoint of the indicator (orange).

Related alkaloids. Carry out the test as described under "Thin-layer chromatography" (vol. 1, p. 83), using silica gel R1 as the coating substance and a mixture of 100 volumes of chloroform R, 20 volumes of ethylene glycol monomethyl ether R, 5 volumes of methanol R, 2 volumes of water and 0.5 volumes of diethylamine R as the mobile phase. Apply separately to the plate 10 µl of each of 4 solutions in a mixture of 1 volume of ammonia ($\sim$17 g/l) TS and 99 volumes of methanol R containing (A) 0.50 mg of the test substance per ml, (B) 10 µg of cephaëline hydrochloride R per ml, (C) 5.0 µg of the test substance per ml and (D) 0.50 mg of emetine hydrochloride RS per ml. After removing the plate from the chromatographic chamber, allow it to dry in air until the solvents have evaporated, spray it with iodine/chloroform TS, heat it at 60 °C for 15 minutes, and examine the chromatogram in ultraviolet light (365 nm). Any spot obtained with solution A is not more intense than the corresponding spot obtained with solution B. Any other spot obtained with solution A, is not more intense than that obtained with solution C.

Assay. Dissolve about 0.2 g, accurately weighed, in 30 ml of glacial acetic acid R1, add 10 ml of mercuric acetate/acetic acid TS and titrate with perchloric acid (0.1 mol/l) VS as described under "Non-aqueous titration", Method A (vol. 1, p. 131). Each ml of perchloric acid (0.1 mol/l) VS is equivalent to 27.68 mg of $C_{29}H_{40}N_2O_4,2HCl$.

EPHEDRINUM

Ephedrine

Ephedrine, anhydrous
Ephedrine hemihydrate

Molecular formula. $C_{10}H_{15}NO$ (anhydrous); $C_{10}H_{15}NO,\frac{1}{2}H_2O$ (hemihydrate).

Relative molecular mass. 165.2 (anhydrous); 174.2 (hemihydrate).

Graphic formula.

Chemical name.   (–)-Ephedrine; [R-(R*,S*)]-α-[1-(methylamino)ethyl]benzene-methanol; CAS Reg. No. 299-42-3 (anhydrous).
(–)-Ephedrine hemihydrate; [R-(R*,S*)]-α-[1-(methylamino)ethyl]benzene-methanol hemihydrate; CAS Reg. No. 50906-05-3 (hemihydrate).

Description.   Colourless crystals or a white, crystalline powder; odourless or with a slight, aromatic odour.

Solubility.   Soluble in water and chloroform R; very soluble in ethanol (~750 g/l) TS; freely soluble in ether R.

Category.   Antiasthmatic drug.

Storage.   Ephedrine should be kept in a well-closed container, protected from light.

Labelling.   The designation on the container should state whether the substance is the hemihydrate or is in the anhydrous form.

Additional information.   Solutions of Ephedrine in chloroform R may become turbid, especially when the substance contains more than 10 mg of water per g. Even in the absence of light, Ephedrine is gradually degraded on exposure to a humid atmosphere, the decomposition being faster at higher temperatures. Anhydrous Ephedrine melts at about 38 °C, whereas Ephedrine hemihydrate melts at about 42 °C.

REQUIREMENTS

General requirement.   Ephedrine contains not less than 98.5% and not more than 101.0% of $C_{10}H_{15}NO$, calculated with reference to the anhydrous substance.

Identity tests

A.   The absorption spectrum of a 0.50 mg/ml solution in hydrochloric acid (0.1 mol/l) VS, when observed between 230 nm and 350 nm, exhibits 3 maxima at about 251 nm, 257 nm, and 263 nm.

B.   Dissolve 10 mg in 1 ml of water and add 0.1 ml of copper(II) sulfate (80 g/l) TS, followed by 2 ml of sodium hydroxide (~80 g/l) TS; a violet colour is produced. Add 1 ml of ether R and shake; a purple colour is produced in the ethereal layer and a blue colour in the aqueous layer.

C.   Dissolve 0.05 g in 5 ml of water. Add a few drops of sodium hydroxide (~80 g/l) TS and 4 ml of potassium ferricyanide (50 g/l) TS, and heat; an odour of benzaldehyde is perceptible.

Specific optical rotation. Dissolve about 2.25 g, accurately weighed, in 15 ml of hydrochloric acid (~70 g/l) TS and dilute to 50 ml with water. Calculate the result with reference to the anhydrous substance; $[\alpha]_D^{20\,°C} = -41$ to $-43°$.

Chlorides. Dissolve 0.70 g in a mixture of 2 ml of nitric acid (~130 g/l) TS and 20 ml of water, and proceed as described under "Limit test for chlorides" (vol. 1, p. 116); the chloride content is not more than 0.35 mg/g.

Sulfates. Dissolve 1.2 g in 20 ml of water and proceed as described under "Limit test for sulfates" (vol. 1, p. 116); the sulfate content is not more than 0.4 mg/g.

Sulfated ash. Not more than 1.0 mg/g.

Water. Determine as described under "Determination of water by the Karl Fischer method", Method A (vol. 1, p. 135). For the anhydrous form use about 2 g of the substance; the water content is not more than 10 mg/g. For the hemihydrate use about 1 g of the substance; the water content is not less than 45 mg/g and not more than 55 mg/g.

Assay. Dissolve about 0.5 g, accurately weighed, in 5 ml of ethanol (~750 g/l) TS, add 50.0 ml of hydrochloric acid (0.1 mol/l) VS and titrate with sodium hydroxide (0.1 mol/l) VS, using methyl red/ethanol TS as indicator. Each ml of hydrochloric acid (0.1 mol/l) VS is equivalent to 16.52 mg of $C_{10}H_{15}NO$.

EPHEDRINI HYDROCHLORIDUM

Ephedrine hydrochloride

Molecular formula. $C_{10}H_{15}NO,HCl$

Relative molecular mass. 201.7

Graphic formula.

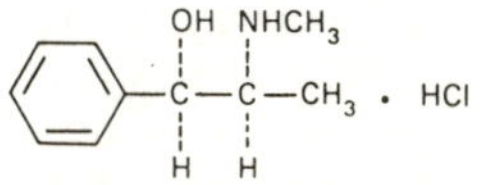
OH NHCH3
C—C—CH3 . HCl
H H

Chemical name. (–)-Ephedrine hydrochloride; [*R*-(*R**,*S**)]-α-[1-(methylamino)ethyl]benzenemethanol hydrochloride; CAS Reg. No. 50-98-6.

Description. Colourless crystals or a white, crystalline powder; odourless.

Solubility. Soluble in 4 parts of water; soluble in ethanol (~750 g/l) TS; very slightly soluble in chloroform R; practically insoluble in ether R.

Category. Antiasthmatic drug.

Storage. Ephedrine hydrochloride should be kept in a well-closed container, protected from light.

Additional information. Ephedrine hydrochloride darkens on exposure to light.

REQUIREMENTS

General requirement. Ephedrine hydrochloride contains not less than 99.0% and not more than 101.0% of $C_{10}H_{15}NO,HCl$, calculated with reference to the dried substance.

Identity tests

A. The absorption spectrum of a 0.50 mg/ml solution, when observed between 230 nm and 350 nm, exhibits maxima at about 251 nm, 257 nm, and 263 nm; the absorbances of a 1-cm layer at these wavelengths are about 0.37, 0.48, and 0.36, respectively.

B. Dissolve 10 mg in 1 ml of water and add 0.1 ml of copper(II) sulfate (80 g/l) TS, followed by 2 ml of sodium hydroxide (~80 g/l) TS; a violet colour is produced. Add 1 ml of ether R and shake; a purple colour is produced in the ethereal layer and a blue colour in the aqueous layer.

C. Dissolve 0.05 g in 5 ml of water. Add a few drops of sodium hydroxide (~80 g/l) TS and 4 ml of potassium ferricyanide (50 g/l) TS, and heat; an odour of benzaldehyde is perceptible.

D. A 0.05 g/ml solution yields reaction A described under "General identification tests" as characteristic of chlorides (vol. 1, p. 112).

Melting range. 217–220 °C.

Specific optical rotation. Use a 50 mg/ml solution; $[\alpha]_D^{20\,°C} = -33.0$ to $-35.5°$.

Sulfates. Dissolve 0.050 g in 40 ml of water and add 1.5 ml of hydrochloric acid (~70 g/l) TS and 1 ml of barium chloride (50 g/l) TS; no turbidity develops within 10 minutes.

Clarity and colour of solution. A solution of 1.0 g in 10 ml of water is clear, or not more opalescent than opalescence standard TS2, and colourless.

Sulfated ash. Not more than 1.0 mg/g.

Loss on drying. Dry to constant weight at 105 °C; it loses not more than 5.0 mg/g.

Acidity and alkalinity. Dissolve 1.0 g in 10 ml of water and add 0.1 ml of methyl red/ethanol TS; not more than 0.1 ml of sodium hydroxide (0.1 mol/l) VS or 0.1 ml of hydrochloric acid (0.1 mol/l) VS is required to obtain the midpoint of the indicator (orange).

Assay. Dissolve about 0.2 g, accurately weighed, in 10 ml of warm mercuric acetate/acetic acid TS, add 50 ml of acetone R and 1 ml of methyl orange/acetone TS as indicator, and titrate with perchloric acid (0.1 mol/l) VS as described under "Non-aqueous titration", Method A (vol. 1, p. 131). Each ml of perchloric acid (0.1 mol/l) VS is equivalent to 20.17 mg of $C_{10}H_{15}NO,HCl$.

EPHEDRINI SULFAS

Ephedrine sulfate

Molecular formula. $(C_{10}H_{15}NO)_2,H_2SO_4$

Relative molecular mass. 428.5

Graphic formula.

$$\left[\underset{\underset{H}{|}}{\overset{\overset{OH}{|}}{C}}-\underset{\underset{H}{|}}{\overset{\overset{NHCH_3}{|}}{C}}-CH_3\right]_2 \cdot H_2SO_4$$

Chemical name. (–)-Ephedrine sulfate (2:1) (salt); [R-(R^*,S^*)]-α-[1-(methyl-amino)ethyl]benzenemethanol sulfate (2:1) (salt); CAS Reg. No. 134-72-5.

Description. Colourless crystals or a white, crystalline powder; odourless.

Solubility. Freely soluble in water; sparingly soluble in ethanol (~750 g/l) TS.

Category. Antiasthmatic drug.

Storage. Ephedrine sulfate should be kept in a well-closed container, protected from light.

Additional information. Ephedrine sulfate darkens on exposure to light. Even in the absence of light, it is gradually degraded on exposure to a humid atmosphere, the decomposition being faster at higher temperatures.

REQUIREMENTS

General requirement. Ephedrine sulfate contains not less than 98.0% and not more than 101.0% of $(C_{10}H_{15}NO)_2,H_2SO_4$, calculated with reference to the dried substance.

Identity tests

A. The absorption spectrum of a 1.0 mg/ml solution, when observed between 230 nm and 350 nm, exhibits maxima at about 251 nm, 257 nm, and 262 nm; the absorbances of a 1-cm layer at these wavelengths are about 0.61, 0.76, and 0.61, respectively.

B. Dissolve 10 mg in 1 ml of water and add 0.1 ml of copper(II) sulfate (80 g/l) TS, followed by 2 ml of sodium hydroxide ($\sim$80 g/l) TS; a violet colour is produced. Add 1 ml of ether R and shake; a purple colour is produced in the ethereal layer and a blue colour in the aqueous layer.

C. Dissolve 0.05 g in 5 ml of water. Add a few drops of sodium hydroxide ($\sim$80 g/l) TS and 4 ml of potassium ferricyanide (50 g/l) TS, and heat; an odour of benzaldehyde is perceptible.

D. A 20 mg/ml solution yields reaction A described under "General identification tests" as characteristic of sulfates (vol. 1, p. 115).

E. Melting temperature, about 245 °C with decomposition.

Specific optical rotation. Use a 50 mg/ml solution and calculate with reference to the dried substance; $[\alpha]_D^{20\,°C} = -30.5$ to -32.5^0.

Chlorides. A quantity of 0.20 g of the test substance shows no more turbidity than 0.40 ml of hydrochloric acid (0.02 mol/l) VS when subjected to the procedure described under "Limit test for chlorides" (vol. 1, p. 116); the chloride content is not more than 1.4 mg/g.

Clarity and colour of solution. A solution of 1.0 g in 10 ml of water is clear, or not more opalescent than opalescence standard TS2, and colourless.

Sulfated ash. Not more than 1.0 mg/g.

Loss on drying. Dry to constant weight at 105 °C; it loses not more than 20 mg/g.

Acidity and alkalinity. Dissolve 1.0 g in 10 ml of water and add 0.1 ml of methyl red/ethanol TS; not more than 0.1 ml of sodium hydroxide (0.1 mol/l) VS or 0.1 ml of hydrochloric acid (0.1 mol/l) VS is required to obtain the midpoint of the indicator (orange).

Assay.   Dissolve about 0.3 g, accurately weighed, in 10 ml of water, add about 3 g of sodium chloride R to saturate the solution, then add 5 ml of sodium hydroxide (1 mol/l) VS and extract with 4 volumes, each of 25 ml, of chloroform R. Wash the combined chloroform extracts with 10 ml of a saturated solution of sodium chloride R, and filter through purified cotton saturated with chloroform R. Shake the aqueous wash solution with 10 ml of chloroform R and add it to the main chloroform extract. Add 0.25 ml of methyl red/ethanol TS and titrate with perchloric acid/dioxan (0.1 mol/l) VS, as described under "Non-aqueous titration", Method A (vol. 1, p. 131). Each ml of perchloric acid/dioxan (0.1 mol/l) VS is equivalent to 21.43 mg of $(C_{10}H_{15}NO)_2,H_2SO_4$.

ERGOCALCIFEROLUM

Ergocalciferol

Molecular formula. $C_{28}H_{44}O$

Relative molecular mass.   396.7

Graphic formula.

Chemical name.   (5Z,7E,22E)-9,10-Secoergosta-5,7,10(19),22-tetraene-3β-ol; 24-methyl-9,10-secocholesta-5,7,10(19),22-tetraene-3β-ol; CAS Reg. No. 50-14-6.

Other name.   Vitamin D_2.

Description.   Colourless or slightly yellowish crystals or a white or slightly yellowish, crystalline powder; odourless or almost odourless.

Solubility.   Practically insoluble in water; freely soluble in ethanol ($\sim$750 g/l) TS, chloroform R, acetone R and ether R.

Category.   Vitamin, antirachitic.

Storage.   Ergocalciferol should be kept in a hermetically closed container, preferably in an inert atmosphere, such as nitrogen, protected from light and stored at a temperature between 2 and 8 °C.

Additional information.   Ergocalciferol is affected by air and by light. Even in the absence of light, it is gradually degraded on exposure to a humid atmosphere, the decomposition being faster at higher temperatures.

REQUIREMENTS

Identity tests

A. Carry out the examination as described under "Spectrophotometry in the infrared region" (vol. 1, p. 40). The infrared absorption spectrum is concordant with the spectrum obtained from ergocalciferol RS or with the *reference spectrum* of ergocalciferol.

B. Dissolve about 2 mg in 10 ml of ethanol (~750 g/l) TS. To 1.0 ml add carefully 5 ml of sulfuric acid (~1760 g/l) TS and mix; a red colour is produced (distinction from colecalciferol, which gives a yellow colour).

C. Dissolve 5 mg in 5 ml of chloroform R, add about 0.5 ml of acetic anhydride R and about 0.1 ml of sulfuric acid (~1760 g/l) TS, shake well; the colour of the solution changes immediately from red to violet, then to blue, and finally to dark green.

D. Dissolve about 1 mg in 40 ml of dichloroethane R. To 1 ml of this solution add 4 ml of antimony trichloride TS; an orange colour is produced, which gradually becomes pink.

Melting range. 112–117 °C, determined without previous grinding or drying.

Specific optical rotation. Dissolve 0.2 g rapidly and without heating in sufficient aldehyde-free ethanol (~750 g/l) TS to produce 25 ml. Determine the rotation within 30 minutes of preparation; $[\alpha]_D^{20\,^\circ C} = +103$ to $+107^\circ$.

Ultraviolet absorbance range. Dissolve 0.05 g rapidly and without heating in sufficient aldehyde-free ethanol (~750 g/l) TS to produce 100 ml; dilute 5.0 ml of this solution to 250 ml with the same solvent. Measure within 30 minutes of preparation the absorbance of a 1-cm layer of the diluted solution at the maximum at about 265 nm; not less than 0.45 and not more than 0.50. The absorbance of a solution of ergocalciferol RS, similarly and concurrently examined, does not differ from that of the test solution by more than 3%.

Ergosterol. Carry out the test as described under "Thin-layer chromatography" (vol. 1, p. 83), using silica gel R1 as the coating substance, and as the mobile phase use a mixture of equal volumes of cyclohexane R and peroxide-free ether R, the mixture containing 0.10 mg of butylated hydroxytoluene R per ml. Apply separately to the plate 10 µl of the following solutions prepared immediately before use in a mixture of dichloroethane R containing 10 mg of squalane R and 0.10 mg of butylated hydroxytoluene R per ml: (A) 0.050 g of the test substance per ml, (B) 0.050 g of ergocalciferol RS per ml, (C) 0.10 mg of ergosterol R per ml; also apply to the plate 20 µl of solution (D) consisting of a mixture of equal volumes of solutions B and C. Develop the plate at once in the dark. After removing the plate from the chromatographic chamber, allow it to dry in air and spray it three times with antimony trichloride TS. Wait after spraying 3–4 minutes, then examine the chromatogram in daylight. The principal spot obtained with solution A is initially orange-yellow and then becomes brown; it corresponds in position, appearance and intensity with that obtained with solution B. Any violet spot obtained with solution A with an R_f value slightly less than that of the principal spot is not more intense than the spot obtained with solution C. The chromatogram obtained with solution A shows no additional spots compared with the chromatograms obtained with solutions B and C. The test is not valid unless the chromatogram obtained with solution D shows two clearly separated spots.

Reducing substances. Dissolve 0.10 g in 10 ml of aldehyde-free ethanol ($\sim$750 g/l) TS, add 0.5 ml of blue tetrazolium/ethanol TS and 0.5 ml of tetramethylammonium hydroxide/ethanol TS. Allow to stand for exactly 5 minutes and then add 1 ml of glacial acetic acid R. Measure the absorbance of a 1-cm layer at the maximum at about 525 nm against a solvent cell containing a solution prepared by treating 10 ml of aldehyde-free ethanol ($\sim$750 g/l) TS in a similar manner. The absorbance is not greater than that obtained by repeating the operation with 10 ml of a solution containing 0.2 µg/ml of hydroquinone R in aldehyde-free ethanol ($\sim$750 g/l) TS.

ERYTHROMYCINUM

Erythromycin

Composition. Erythromycin is a mixture of substances produced by the growth of certain strains of *Streptomyces erythreus*. The main component of the mixture is erythromycin A with lesser amounts of erythromycins B and C.

● *The molecular formula, the relative molecular mass, and the chemical name given below relate to erythromycin A only.*

Molecular formula. $C_{37}H_{67}NO_{13}$

Relative molecular mass. 733.9

Graphic formula.

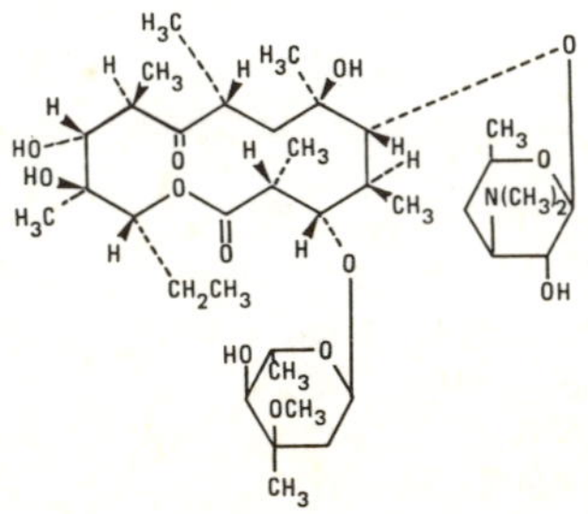

Chemical name.   [3R-(3R*,4S*,5S*,6R*,7R*,9R*,11R*,12R*,13S*,14R*)]-4-[(2,6-Dideoxy-3-C-methyl-3-O-methyl-α-L-*ribo*-hexopyranosyl)oxyl]-14-ethyl-7,12,13-trihydroxy-3,5,7,9,11,13-hexamethyl-6-[[3,4,6-trideoxy-3-(dimethyl-amino)-β-D-*xylo*-hexopyranosyl]oxy]oxacyclotetradecane-2,10-dione; CAS Reg. No. 114-07-8.

Description.   White or slightly yellow crystals or powder; odourless or almost odourless.

Solubility.   Soluble in 1000 parts of water but less soluble in hot water; freely soluble in ethanol (~750 g/l) TS, ether R and chloroform R.

Category.   Antibacterial drug.

Storage.   Erythromycin should be kept in a tightly closed container, protected from light.

Additional information.   Erythromycin is slightly hygroscopic.

REQUIREMENTS

General requirement.   Erythromycin contains not less than 870 International Units per mg, calculated with reference to the anhydrous substance.

Identity tests

● Either test A alone or tests B, C and D may be applied.

A.   Carry out the examination as described under "Spectrophotometry in the infrared region" (vol. 1, p. 40). The infrared absorption is concordant with the spectrum obtained from erythromycin RS or with the *reference spectrum* of erythromycin.

B.   To 5 mg add 2 ml of sulfuric acid (~1760 g/l) TS and shake gently; a reddish brown colour is produced.

C.   Dissolve 3 mg in 2 ml of acetone R and add 2 ml of hydrochloric acid (~420 g/l) TS; an orange colour is produced, which changes to red and then to deep purplish red. Add 2 ml of chloroform R and shake; the chloroform layer becomes purple.

D.   To 5 mg add 5 ml of xanthydrol TS and heat on a water-bath; a red colour is produced.

Specific optical rotation.   Use a 20 mg/ml solution in dehydrated ethanol R, allow to stand for 30 minutes, measure the angle of rotation, and calculate with reference to the anhydrous substance; $[\alpha]_D^{20\,^\circ C} = -71$ to -78°.

Sulfated ash.   Not more than 2.0 mg/g.

Water.   Determine as described under "Determination of water by the Karl Fischer Method", method A (vol. 1, p. 135), using about 1 g of the substance; the water content is not more than 100 mg/g.

pH value.   Dissolve 0.1 g in 50 ml of a mixture composed of 1 volume of methanol R and 19 volumes of carbon-dioxide-free water R; the pH is between 8.0 and 10.5.

Assay.   Carry out the assay as described under "Microbiological assay of antibiotics" (vol. 1, p. 145), using *Bacillus pumilus* (NCTC 8241 or ATCC 14884) as the test organism, culture medium Cml with a final pH of 8.0–8.1, sterile phosphate buffer, pH 8.0 TS or TS2, an appropriate concentration of erythromycin (usually between 5 and 25 IU per ml), and an incubation temperature of 35–39 °C. The precision of the assay is such that the fiducial limits of error of the estimated potency ($P = 0.95$) are not less than 95% and not more than 105% of the estimated potency. The upper fiducial limit of error of the estimated potency ($P = 0.95$) is not less than 870 IU per mg, calculated with reference to the anhydrous substance.

ERYTHROMYCINI ETHYLSUCCINAS

Erythromycin ethylsuccinate

Erythromycin ethylsuccinate for parenteral use

Molecular formula. $C_{43}H_{75}NO_{16}$

Relative molecular mass.   862.1

Graphic formula.

Chemical name.   Erythromycin 2′-(ethylsuccinate); erythromycin 2′(ethyl butanedioate); [3*R*-(3*R**,4*S**,5*S**,6*R**,7*R**,9*R**,11*R**,12*R**,13*S**,14*R**)]-4-[(2,6-dideoxy-3-*C*-methyl-3-*O*-methyl-α-L-*ribo*-hexopyranosyl)oxy]-14-ethyl-7,12,13-trihydroxy-3,5,7,9,11,13-hexamethyl-6-[[3,4,6-trideoxy-3-(dimethylamino)-β-D-*xylo*-hexopyranosyl]oxy]oxacyclotetradecane-2,10-dione 2′-(ethyl butanedioate); CAS Reg. No. 1264-62-6.

Description.   A white or slightly yellow, crystalline powder; odourless or almost odourless.

Solubility.   Very slightly soluble in water; freely soluble in chloroform R; soluble in ethanol (∼750 g/l) TS and macrogol 400 R.

Labelling.   The designation Erythromycin ethylsuccinate for parenteral use indicates that the substance complies with the additional requirement for Erythromycin ethylsuccinate and may be used for parenteral administration.

Category.   Antibacterial drug.

Storage.   Erythromycin ethylsuccinate should be kept in a tightly closed container, protected from light.

REQUIREMENTS

General requirement.   Erythromycin ethylsuccinate contains not less than 740 International Units of erythromycin per mg, calculated with reference to the anhydrous substance.

Identity tests

● Either test A alone or tests B, C and D may be applied.

A.   Carry out the examination as described under "Spectrophotometry in the infrared region" (vol. 1, p. 40).   The infrared absorption spectrum is concordant with the spectrum obtained from erythromycin ethylsuccinate RS or with the *reference spectrum* of erythromycin ethylsuccinate.

B.   To 5 mg add 2 ml of sulfuric acid (∼1760 g/l) TS and shake gently; a reddish brown colour is produced.

C.   Dissolve 3 mg in 2 ml of acetone R and add 2 ml of hydrochloric acid (∼420 g/l) TS; an orange colour is produced, which changes to orange-red and finally to purplish red.   Add 2 ml of chloroform R and shake; the chloroform layer becomes blue.

D.   To 5 mg add 5 ml of xanthydrol TS and heat on a water-bath; a red colour is produced.

Sulfated ash.   Not more than 10 mg/g.

Water.   Determine as described under "Determination of water by the Karl Fischer method", Method A (vol. 1, p. 135), using about 0.5 g of the substance; the water content is not more than 30 mg/g.

pH value.   Shake 0.5 g with 50 ml of carbon-dioxide-free water R; pH of the suspension, 6.0–8.5.

Assay.   Dissolve 50 mg in sufficient methanol R to produce 100 ml and carry out the assay as described under "Microbiological assay of antibiotics" (vol. 1, p. 145), using *Bacillus pumilus* (NCTC 8241 or ATCC 14884) as the test organism, culture medium Cm1 with a final pH of 8.0–8.1, sterile phosphate buffer, pH 8.0 TS1 or TS2, an appropriate concentration of erythromycin (usually between 5 and 25 IU per ml), and an incubation temperature of 35–39 °C. The precision of the assay is such that the fiducial limits of error of the estimated potency ($P = 0.95$) are not less than 95% and not more than 105% of the estimated potency. The upper fiducial limit of error of the estimated potency ($P = 0.95$) is not less than 740 IU of erythromycin per mg, calculated with reference to the anhydrous substance.

Additional Requirement for Erythromycin Ethylsuccinate for Parenteral Use

Undue toxicity.   Carry out the test as described under "Test for undue toxicity" (vol. 1, p. 154), administering orally 0.5 ml of a solution in sterile water R containing a quantity equivalent to 80 mg per ml.

ERYTHROMYCINI STEARAS

Erythromycin stearate

Molecular formula. $C_{37}H_{67}NO_{13}, C_{18}H_{36}O_2$

Relative molecular mass.   1018

Graphic formula.

Chemical name. Erythromycin stearate (salt); erythromycin octadecanoate (salt); [3R-(3R*,4S*,5S*,6R*,7R*,9R*,11R*,12R*,13S*,14R*)]-4-[(2,6-dideoxy-3-C-methyl-3-O-methyl-α-L-*ribo*-hexopyranosyl)oxy]-14-ethyl-7,12,13-trihydroxy-3,5,7,9,11,13-hexamethyl-6-[[3,4,6-trideoxy-3-(dimethylamino)-β-D-*xylo*-hexopyranosyl]oxy]oxacyclotetradecane-2,10-dione octadecanoate (salt); CAS Reg. No. 643-22-1.

Description. Colourless or slightly yellow crystals or a white or slightly yellow powder; odourless or almost odourless.

Solubility. Practically insoluble in water; soluble in ethanol (~750 g/l) TS; soluble in chloroform R, methanol R, and ether R; these solutions may be opalescent.

Category. Antibacterial drug.

Storage. Erythromycin stearate should be kept in a tightly closed container, protected from light.

REQUIREMENTS

General requirement. Erythromycin stearate contains not less than 550 International Units of erythromycin per mg or not less than 77.0% of $C_{37}H_{67}NO_{13}$, $C_{18}H_{36}O_2$, both calculated with reference to the anhydrous substance.

Identity tests

● Either test A or tests B, C and D may be applied.

A. Carry out the examination as described under "Spectrophotometry in the infrared region" (vol. 1, p. 40). The infrared absorption spectrum is concordant with the spectrum obtained from erythromycin stearate RS or with the *reference spectrum* of erythromycin stearate.

B. Dissolve 3 mg in 2 ml of acetone R and add 2 ml of hydrochloric acid (~420 g/l) TS; an orange colour is produced, which changes to red and then to deep purplish red. Add 2 ml of chloroform R and shake; the chloroform layer becomes purple.

C. To 5 mg add 5 ml of xanthydrol TS and heat on a water-bath; a red colour is produced.

D. Heat gently 0.1 g with 5 ml of hydrochloric acid (~70 g/l) TS and 10 ml of water until the solution boils; oily globules rise to the surface. Cool, remove the fatty layer and heat it with 3 ml of sodium hydroxide (0.1 mol/l) VS; allow to cool; the solution sets to a gel. Add 10 ml of hot water and shake; the solution froths. To 1 ml add 1 ml of calcium chloride (~55 g/l) TS; a granular precipitate, insoluble in hydrochloric acid (~250 g/l) TS, is produced.

Erythromycin stearate. Shake 0.5 g with 30 ml of chloroform R. If the solution is clear, add 50 ml of glacial acetic acid R1, previously neutralized with perchloric acid (0.1 mol/l) VS, and continue with the titration as described below.

If the solution is opalescent, shake with an additional 2 quantities, each of 25 ml of chloroform R, filter each extract, wash the filter with chloroform R, and evaporate the combined filtrate and washings on a water-bath to about 30 ml. Add 50 ml of glacial acetic acid R1, previously neutralized with perchloric acid (0.1 mol/l) VS, and titrate with perchloric acid (0.1 mol/l) VS, determining the endpoint potentiometrically. Each ml of perchloric acid (0.1 mol/l) VS is equivalent to 101.8 mg of $C_{37}H_{67}NO_{13},C_{18}H_{36}O_2$; the erythromycin stearate content is not less than 0.770 g/g.

Water. Determine as described under "Determination of water by the Karl Fischer method", Method A (vol. 1, p. 135), using about 0.6 g of the substance; the water content is not more than 40 mg/g.

Free stearic acid. Dissolve 0.4 g in 50 ml of neutralized ethanol TS and titrate with sodium hydroxide (0.1 mol/l) VS, determining the endpoint potentiometrically. Calculate the volume of sodium hydroxide (0.1 mol/l) VS required for each g of the substance and subtract the volume of perchloric acid (0.1 mol/l) VS required for each g of the substance in the test for erythromycin stearate. Each ml of the difference is equivalent to 28.45 mg of $C_{18}H_{36}O_2$; not more than 185 mg/g.

Sodium stearate. Moisten 2.0 g in a platinum dish with a small quantity of sulfuric acid ($\sim$1760 g/l) TS, ignite gently, again moisten with sulfuric acid ($\sim$1760 g/l) TS, ignite at about 800 °C, cool, and weigh. Each g of residue is equivalent to 4.317 g of $C_{18}H_{35}NaO_2$; not more than 60 mg/g.

Total stearic acid, stearates and water. Using the results of the above four determinations, add together the percentages of free stearic acid, erythromycin stearate, sodium stearate (all calculated with reference to the undried substance) and the water content; the total is not less than 98.0% and not more than 103.0%.

Assay. Dissolve 50 mg in sufficient methanol R to produce 100 ml and carry out the assay as described under "Microbiological assay of antibiotics" (vol. 1, p. 145), using *Bacillus pumilus* (NCTC 8241 or ATCC 14884) as the test organism, culture medium Cm1 with a final pH of 8.0–8.1, sterile phosphate buffer, pH 8.0 TS1 or TS2, an appropriate concentration of erythromycin (usually between 5 and 25 IU per ml), and an incubation temperature of 35–39 °C. The precision of the assay is such that the fiducial limits of error of the estimated potency ($P = 0.95$) are not less than 95% and not more than 105% of the estimated potency. The upper fiducial limit of error of the estimated potency ($P = 0.95$) is not less than 550 IU of erythromycin per mg, calculated with reference to the anhydrous substance.

ETHER ANAESTHESICUS

Anaesthetic Ether

Molecular formula. $C_4H_{10}O$

Relative molecular mass.   74.12

Graphic formula. $C_2H_5-.O-C_2H_5$

Chemical name.   Ethyl ether; 1,1'-oxybis[ethane]; diethyl ether; CAS Reg. No. 60-29-7.

Description.   A clear, colourless, volatile, very mobile liquid; odour, characteristic.

Miscibility.   Miscible with 10 parts of water; miscible with ethanol ($\sim$750 g/l) TS and chloroform R.

Category.   General anaesthetic.

Storage.   Anaesthetic Ether should be kept in a securely closed, dry container, protected from light, at a temperature not exceeding 15 °C, and in quantities of not more than 1 kg.

Labelling.   The designation on the container of anaesthetic Ether must state: "Highly flammable. Do not use near an open flame or other sources of heat that may cause ignition." The name and quantity of any antioxidant added must be stated.

Additional information.   Anaesthetic Ether may contain a suitable antioxidant. It must not be used for anaesthesia if it has been removed from its original container for longer than 24 hours. Ether remaining in partially used containers may deteriorate rapidly. CAUTION: Vapours of ether mixed with air, oxygen, or nitrous oxide in certain concentrations are explosive. Do not use an open flame at any time during the testing procedure.

REQUIREMENTS

Distillation range

• It is dangerous to determine the distillation range of the test liquid if it does not comply with the test for Peroxides.

Use a suitable heating device, and take precautions to avoid superheating the distillation flask above the level of the test liquid; it distils completely between 34.0 and 35.0 °C.

Relative density. d_{20}^{20}= 0.713–0.716.

Non-volatile residue

● It is dangerous to determine the non-volatile residue of the test liquid if it does not comply with the test for Peroxides.

Allow 50 ml to evaporate, dry the residue at 105 °C for 1 hour and weigh; it leaves not more than 20 µg/ml.

Acidity. Place 10 ml of ethanol (~750 g/l) TS in a 50-ml glass-stoppered flask, add 0.5 ml of phenolphthalein/ethanol TS and just sufficient carbonate-free sodium hydroxide (0.02 mol/l) VS to produce a pink colour that persists after shaking the mixture for 30 seconds; add 25 ml of the test liquid, mix gently, and add carbonate-free sodium hydroxide (0.02 mol/l) VS until the pink colour persists after shaking the mixture for 30 seconds; not more than 0.4 ml of additional carbonate-free sodium hydroxide is required.

Peroxides. To 10 ml of the test liquid add 2.0 ml of vanadium/sulfuric acid TS and shake. Separately prepare a reference solution by diluting 1.0 ml of hydrogen peroxide (~60 g/l) TS to 100 ml with water. To 0.10 ml of this reference solution add 2.0 ml of vanadium/sulfuric acid TS. The colour produced in the aqueous layer in the tube containing the test liquid, when viewed transversely against a white background, is not more intense than that of the reference solution when compared as described under "Colour of liquids" (vol. 1, p. 50).

Acetone and aldehydes. Transfer 2 ml of alkaline potassio-mercuric iodide TS to a glass-stoppered test-tube of about 12 ml capacity and about 1.5 cm diameter, and add 10 ml of the test liquid. Shake the tube vigorously for 10 seconds and allow to stand in the dark for 5 minutes; no turbidity is produced. If the test liquid does not comply with this requirement, distil 40 ml, previously ensuring that it complies with the test for Peroxides, until only 5 ml remains; repeat the test on the distillate.

Foreign odour. Moisten a section of filter-paper with 10 ml of the test liquid and allow to evaporate; no odour other than that characteristic of ether is perceptible during or after the evaporation.

ETHIONAMIDUM

Ethionamide

Molecular formula. $C_8H_{10}N_2S$

Relative molecular mass. 166.2

Graphic formula.

Chemical name.   2-Ethylthioisonicotinamide; 2-ethyl-4-pyridinecarbothioamide; CAS Reg. No. 536-33-4.

Description.   Small yellow crystals or a yellow, crystalline powder; odour, slight.

Solubility.   Practically insoluble in water; soluble in methanol R; sparingly soluble in ethanol ($\sim$750 g/l) TS; slightly soluble in chloroform R and ether R.

Category.   Antileprosy drug.

Storage.   Ethionamide should be kept in a tightly closed container, protected from light, and stored in a cool place.

Additional information.   Ethionamide darkens on exposure to light.

REQUIREMENTS

General requirement.   Ethionamide contains not less than 98.0% and not more than 101.0% of $C_8H_{10}N_2S$, calculated with reference to the dried substance.

Identity tests

● Either tests A and D or tests B, C and D may be applied.

A.   Carry out the examination as described under "Spectrophotometry in the infrared region" (vol. 1, p. 40). The infrared absorption spectrum is concordant with the spectrum obtained from ethionamide RS or with the *reference spectrum* of ethionamide.

B.   Mix 0.05 g with 0.10 g of 2,4-dinitrochlorobenzene R, then transfer 10 mg of this mixture to a test-tube and heat until melted. Cool and add 3 ml of potassium hydroxide/ethanol TS1; a red to orange-red colour is produced.

C.   Heat 0.1 g with 5 ml of hydrochloric acid (1 mol/l) VS; the vapours evolved blacken lead acetate paper R.

D.   Melting temperature, about 162 °C.

Heavy metals.   Use 1.0 g for the preparation of the test solution as described under "Limit test for heavy metals", Procedure 3 (vol. 1, p. 118); determine the heavy metals content according to Method A (vol. 1, p. 119); not more than 20 µg/g.

Sulfated ash.   Not more than 1.0 mg/g.

Loss on drying.   Dry to constant weight at 105 °C; it loses not more than 5.0 mg/g.

Related substances.   Carry out the test as described under "Thin-layer chromatography" (vol. 1, p. 83), using silica gel R4 as the coating substance and a mixture
of 9 volumes of chloroform R and 1 volume of methanol R as the mobile phase.
Apply separately to the plate 10 µl of each of 3 solutions in acetone R containing
(A) 20 mg of the test substance per ml, (B) 0.10 mg of the test substance per ml, and
(C) 0.04 mg of the test substance per ml.   After removing the plate from the
chromatographic chamber, allow it to dry in air and examine the chromatogram in
ultraviolet light (254 nm).   Any spot obtained with solution A, other than the
principal spot, is not more intense than that obtained with solution B.   Not more
than one of any such spots is more intense than that obtained with solution C.

Assay.   Dissolve about 0.15 g, accurately weighed, in 50 ml of glacial acetic acid
R1, and titrate with perchloric acid (0.1 mol/l) VS as described under "Nonaqueous titration", Method A (vol. 1, p. 131).   Each ml of perchloric acid
(0.1 mol/l) VS is equivalent to 16.62 mg of $C_8H_{10}N_2S$.

FERROSI FUMARAS

Ferrous fumarate

Molecular formula. $C_4H_2FeO_4$

Relative molecular mass.   169.9

Graphic formula.

Chemical name.   Iron(2+) fumarate (1:1); iron(2+) (*E*)-2-butenedioate (1:1);
CAS Reg. No. 141-01-5.

Description.   A fine, reddish orange or reddish brown powder.

Solubility.   Slightly soluble in water; very slightly soluble in ethanol
(~750 g/l) TS.

Category.   Iron supplement.

Storage.   Ferrous fumarate should be kept in a well-closed container.

REQUIREMENTS

General requirement. Ferrous fumarate contains not less than 93.0% and not more than 101.0% of $C_4H_2FeO_4$, calculated with reference to the dried substance.

Identity tests

A. Dissolve with heating 0.4 g in 10 ml of hydrochloric acid (1 mol/l) VS and cool. (Keep 1.0 ml of this solution for test B.) To the remaining solution add 15 ml of sodium hydroxide (1 mol/l) VS. Separate the dark precipitate by filtration. To the filtrate add 0.2 ml of phenolphthalein/ethanol TS and sufficient hydrochloric acid (1 mol/l) VS until the pink colour disappears. To 2.0 ml of the resulting solution add 2.0 ml of copper(II) acetate (45 g/l) TS; a white, crystalline precipitate is produced.

B. The solution prepared in test A yields reaction A described under "General identification tests" as characteristic of ferrous salts (vol. 1, p. 113).

C. Mix 0.5 g with 1 g of resorcinol R. Transfer 0.5 g of the mixture to a crucible, add about 0.15 ml of sulfuric acid ($\sim$1760 g/l) TS and heat gently; a deep red, semi-solid mass is produced. Add the mass to a large volume of water; an orange-yellow solution is obtained which exhibits no fluorescence.

Heavy metals. Ignite 1.0 g gently until free from carbon, dissolve in 5 ml of hydrochloric acid ($\sim$420 g/l) TS by heating on a water-bath, and evaporate to dryness. Dissolve the residue in a mixture of 15 ml of hydrochloric acid ($\sim$420 g/l) TS, 4 ml of nitric acid ($\sim$1000 g/l) TS, and 6 ml of water, boil gently for 1 minute, cool, and extract the iron with 3 portions of ether R, each of 20 ml. Make a fourth extraction with a further 20 ml of ether R if the acid layer is more than slightly yellow and reject the extracts. Heat the acid solution gently to remove the ether, add 1 g of citric acid PbR, make alkaline with ammonia ($\sim$100 g/l) PbTS, add 1 ml of potassium cyanide PbTS and dilute to 40 ml with water; proceed to determine the heavy metals content as described under "Limit test for heavy metals", according to Method A (vol. 1, p. 119); not more than 100 µg/g.

Arsenic. Mix 0.2 g with 1.5 g of anhydrous sodium carbonate R, add 10 ml of bromine AsTS and mix thoroughly. Evaporate to dryness on a water-bath, gently ignite, and dissolve the cooled residue in 20 ml of brominated hydrochloric acid AsTS and 10 ml of water. Transfer to a small flask, add sufficient stannous chloride AsTS to remove the yellow colour, connect to a condenser and distil 22 ml; proceed with the distillate as described under "Limit test for arsenic" (vol. 1, p. 122); the arsenic content is not more than 5 µg/g.

Ferric iron. Dissolve about 3 g, accurately weighed, in a mixture of 100 ml of water and 10 ml of hydrochloric acid ($\sim$420 g/l) TS by heating to boiling until dissolved. Cool rapidly and add 3 g of potassium iodide R, stopper the flask, swirl to mix, and allow to stand in the dark for 15 minutes. Titrate the liberated iodine with sodium thiosulfate (0.1 mol/l) VS, using starch TS as indicator, added towards the end of the titration. Repeat the operation without the substance being examined and determine the difference in the volume of sodium thiosulfate (0.1 mol/l) VS required for the titration. Each ml of sodium thiosulfate (0.1 mol/l) VS is equivalent to 5.585 mg of ferric iron; the ferric iron content is not more than 20 mg/g.

Sulfates. Boil 0.15 g with 8 ml of hydrochloric acid ($\sim$70 g/l) TS and 20 ml of water, cool in ice and filter; proceed with the filtrate as described under "Limit test for sulfates" (vol. 1, p. 116); the sulfate content is not more than 2 mg/g.

Loss on drying. Dry to constant weight at 105 °C; it loses not more than 10 mg/g.

Assay. Dissolve about 0.3 g, accurately weighed, in 7.5 ml of sulfuric acid ($\sim$100 g/l) TS, heating gently. Cool, add 25 ml of water, and immediately titrate with ceric ammonium sulfate (0.1 mol/l) VS, using 0.1 ml of *o*-phenanthroline TS as indicator. Each ml of ceric ammonium sulfate (0.1 mol/l) VS is equivalent to 16.99 mg of $C_4H_2FeO_4$.

FLUCYTOSINUM

Flucytosine

Molecular formula. $C_4H_4FN_3O$

Relative molecular mass. 129.1

Graphic formula.

Chemical name. 5-Fluorocytosine; 4-amino-5-fluoro-2(1*H*)-pyrimidinone; CAS Reg. No. 2022-85-7.

Description. A white or almost white, crystalline powder; odourless or almost odourless.

Solubility. Sparingly soluble in water; slightly soluble in ethanol ($\sim$750 g/l) TS; practically insoluble in chloroform R and ether R.

Category. Antifungal drug.

Storage.   Flucytosine should be kept in a tightly closed container, protected from light.

Additional information.   Flucytosine melts at about 295 °C.

REQUIREMENTS

General requirement.   Flucytosine contains not less than 98.5% and not more than 101.0% of $C_4H_4FN_3O$, calculated with reference to the dried substance.

Identity tests

● Either tests A and C or tests B, C and D may be applied.

A.   Carry out the examination as described under "Spectrophotometry in the infrared region" (vol. 1, p. 40). The infrared absorption spectrum is concordant with the spectrum obtained from flucytosine RS or with the *reference spectrum* of flucytosine.

B.   The absorption spectrum of a 5.0 µg/ml solution in hydrochloric acid (0.1 mol/l) VS, when observed between 230 nm and 350 nm, exhibits a maximum at about 286 nm; the absorbance of a 1-cm layer at this wavelength is about 0.36.

C.   See the test described below under "Fluorouracil". The principal spot obtained with solution A corresponds in position, appearance, and intensity with that obtained with solution B.

D.   Dissolve 0.05 g in 5 ml of water and add 0.15 ml of bromine TS1; the colour is discharged or almost discharged.

Heavy metals.   Use 1.0 g for the preparation of the test solution as described under "Limit test for heavy metals", Procedure 3 (vol. 1, p. 118); determine the heavy metals content according to Method A (vol. 1, p. 119); not more than 20 µg/g.

Sulfated ash.   Not more than 1 mg/g.

Loss on drying.   Dry to constant weight at 105 °C; it loses not more than 15 mg/g.

Fluorouracil.   Carry out the test as described under "Thin-layer chromatography" (vol. 1, p. 83), using silica gel R6 as the coating substance (a precoated plate from a commercial source is suitable) and a mixture of 70 volumes of nitromethane R, 20 volumes of ethanol (~750 g/l) TS, and 10 volumes of lithium chloride (10 g/l) TS as the mobile phase. Apply separately to the plate 1 µl of each of 2 solutions in a solvent mixture composed of 15 volumes of methanol R and

10 volumes of water, containing (A) 10 mg of the test substance per ml and (B) 10 mg of flucytosine RS per ml; then apply also 10 µl of each of the 2 following solutions in the above solvent mixture containing (C) 20 mg of the test substance per ml and (D) 20 µg of fluorouracil RS per ml. Develop the plate in an unsaturated chromatographic chamber. After removing the plate from the chromatographic chamber, allow it to dry in a current of air and examine the chromatogram in ultraviolet light (254 nm). The spot obtained with solution D is more intense than any corresponding spot obtained with solution C.

Assay. Dissolve about 0.3 g, accurately weighed, in a mixture of 50 ml of acetic anhydride R and 100 ml of glacial acetic acid R1 with warming, if necessary, and titrate with perchloric acid (0.1 mol/l) VS, determining the endpoint potentiometrically as described under "Non-aqueous titration", Method A (vol. 1, p. 131). Each ml of perchloric acid (0.1 mol/l) VS is equivalent to 12.91 mg of $C_4H_4FN_3O$.

FLUDROCORTISONI ACETAS

Fludrocortisone acetate

Molecular formula. $C_{23}H_{31}FO_6$

Relative molecular mass. 422.5

Graphic formula.

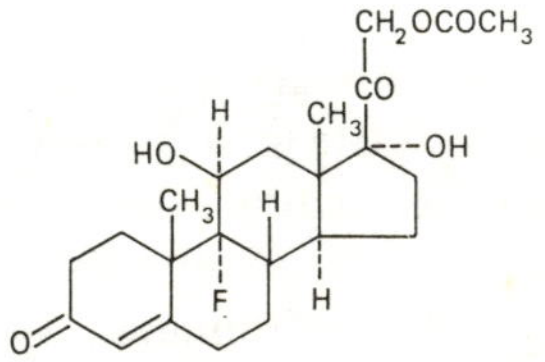

Chemical name. 9-Fluoro-11β,17,21-trihydroxypregn-4-ene-3,20-dione 21-acetate; 21-(acetyloxy)-9-fluoro-11β,17-dihydroxypregn-4-ene-3,20-dione; CAS Reg. No. 514-36-3.

Description. A white or almost white, crystalline powder; odourless or almost odourless.

Solubility. Practically insoluble in water; sparingly soluble in ethanol (~750 g/l) TS and chloroform R; slightly soluble in ether R.

Category. Adrenal hormone.

Storage.   Fludrocortisone acetate should be kept in a well-closed container, protected from light.

Additional information.   Fludrocortisone acetate is hygroscopic.

REQUIREMENTS

General requirement.   Fludrocortisone acetate contains not less than 96.0% and not more than 104.0% of $C_{23}H_{31}FO_6$, calculated with reference to the dried substance.

Identity tests

● Either test A alone or tests B and C may be applied.

A.   Carry out the examination as described under "Spectrophotometry in the infrared region" (vol. 1, p. 40). The infrared absorption spectrum is concordant with the spectrum obtained from fludrocortisone acetate RS or with the *reference spectrum* of fludrocortisone acetate.

B.   Carry out the test as described under "Thin-layer chromatography" (vol. 1, p. 83), using kieselguhr R1 as the coating substance and a mixture of 10 volumes of formamide R and 90 volumes of acetone R to impregnate the plate, dipping it about 5 mm into the liquid. After the solvent has reached a height of at least 16 cm, remove the plate from the chromatographic chamber and allow it to stand at room temperature until the solvent has completely evaporated. Use the impregnated plate within 2 hours and carry out the chromatography in the same direction as the impregnation. As the mobile phase, use a mixture of 75 volumes of toluene R and 25 volumes of chloroform R. Apply separately to the plate 2 µl of each of 2 solutions in a mixture of 9 volumes of chloroform R and 1 volume of methanol R containing (A) 2.5 mg of the test substance per ml and (B) 2.5 mg of fludrocortisone acetate RS per ml. Develop the plate for a distance of 15 cm. After removing the plate from the chromatographic chamber, allow it to dry in air until the solvents have evaporated, heat it at 120 °C for 15 minutes, spray it with sulfuric acid/ethanol TS, and then heat it at 120 °C for 10 minutes. Allow it to cool, and examine the chromatogram in daylight and in ultraviolet light (365 nm). The principal spot obtained with solution A corresponds in position, appearance, and intensity with that obtained with solution B.

C.   Heat 0.5 ml of chromic acid TS in a small test-tube in a water-bath for 5 minutes; the solution wets the sides of the tube but there is no greasiness. Add about 3 mg of the test substance and again heat in a water-bath for 5 minutes; the solution no longer wets the sides of the tube.

Specific optical rotation.   Use a 10 mg/ml solution in dioxan R; $[\alpha]_D^{20\,°C} = +148$ to $+156°$.

Sulfated ash.   Not more than 1.0 mg/g.

Loss on drying.   Dry to constant weight at 105 °C; it loses not more than 10 mg/g.

Ultraviolet absorption.   Absorbance of a 1-cm layer of a 10 μg/ml solution in dehydrated ethanol R at about 240 nm; 0.39–0.42.

Related substances.   Carry out the test as described under "Thin-layer chromatography" (vol. 1, p. 83) using silica gel R2 as the coating substance and a mixture of 95 volumes of dichloroethane R, 5 volumes of methanol R, and 0.2 volumes of water as the mobile phase. Apply separately to the plate 1 μl of each of 2 solutions in a mixture of 9 volumes of chloroform R and 1 volume of methanol R containing (A) 15 mg of the test substance per ml and (B) 0.30 mg of the test substance per ml. After removing the plate from the chromatographic chamber allow it to dry in air until the solvents have evaporated; then heat it at 105 °C for 10 minutes, allow it to cool, and examine the chromatogram in ultraviolet light (254 nm). Any spot obtained with solution A, other than the principal spot, is not more intense than that obtained with solution B.

Assay

● The solutions must be protected from light throughout the assay.

Dissolve about 25 mg, accurately weighed, in sufficient aldehyde-free ethanol (~750 g/l) TS to produce 250 ml. Dilute 10 ml of this solution with sufficient aldehyde-free ethanol (~750 g/l) TS to produce 50 ml. Transfer 10.0 ml of the diluted solution to a 25-ml volumetric flask, add 2.0 ml of blue tetrazolium/ethanol TS, and displace the air in the flask with oxygen-free nitrogen R. Immediately add 2.0 ml of tetramethylammonium hydroxide/ethanol TS and again displace the air with oxygen-free nitrogen R. Stopper the flask, mix the contents by gentle swirling, and allow to stand for 1 hour in a water-bath at 30 °C. Cool rapidly, add sufficient aldehyde-free ethanol (~750 g/l) TS to produce 25 ml and mix. Measure the absorbance of a 1-cm layer at the maximum at about 525 nm against a solvent cell containing a solution prepared by treating 10 ml of aldehyde-free ethanol (~750 g/l) TS in a similar manner. Calculate the amount of $C_{23}H_{31}FO_6$ in the substance being tested by comparison with fludrocortisone acetate RS, similarly and concurrently examined.

FLUORESCEINUM NATRICUM

Fluorescein sodium

Molecular formula. $C_{20}H_{10}Na_2O_5$

Relative molecular mass.   376.3

Graphic formula.

Chemical name.   Fluorescein disodium salt; 2-(6-hydroxy-3-oxo-3H-xanthen-9-yl)benzoic acid disodium salt; 3′,6′-dihydroxyspiro[isobenzofuran-1(3H),9′-[9H]xanthene]-3-one disodium salt; CAS Reg. No. 518-47-8.

Description.   An orange-red powder; odourless.

Solubility.   Soluble in 1.5 parts of water; soluble in ethanol (~750 g/l) TS; practically insoluble in chloroform R.

Category.   Diagnostic agent in ophthalmology.

Storage.   Fluorescein sodium should be kept in a well-closed container, protected from light.

Additional information.   Fluorescein sodium is hygroscopic.

REQUIREMENTS

General requirement.   Fluorescein sodium contains not less than 98.0% and not more than 100.5% of $C_{20}H_{10}Na_2O_5$, calculated with reference to the dried substance.

Identity tests

A.   A solution in water is strongly fluorescent, even in extreme dilution; the fluorescence disappears when the solution is made acid and reappears when it is made alkaline.

B.   Ignite 20 mg and dissolve the residue in acetic acid (~60 g/l) TS. The solution yields reaction B described under "General identification tests" as characteristic of sodium (vol. 1, p. 115).

C.   Dissolve 1 mg in 2 ml of water, place 0.05 ml of this solution on a piece of filter-paper; a yellow spot is produced. Expose the moist paper to the vapour of bromine R for 1 minute and then to the vapour of ammonia (~260 g/l) TS; the yellow colour of the spot changes to deep pink.

Chlorides.   Dissolve 0.07 g in a mixture of 2 ml of nitric acid (~130 g/l) TS and 20 ml of water, and proceed as described under "Limit test for chlorides" (vol. 1, p. 116); the chloride content is not more than 3.5 mg/g.

Sulfates.   Dissolve 0.05 g in 20 ml of water and proceed as described under "Limit test for sulfates" (vol. 1, p. 116); the sulfate content is not more than 10 mg/g.

Zinc.   Dissolve 0.10 g in 10 ml of water, add 2 ml of hydrochloric acid (~420 g/l) TS, filter, and add 0.1 ml of potassium ferrocyanide (45 g/l) TS; no turbidity or precipitate is produced immediately.

Chloroform-soluble matter.   Dissolve 0.20 g in 10 ml of sodium hydroxide (0.1 mol/l) VS and extract with 10 ml of chloroform R. Allow to separate, dry the chloroform layer over anhydrous sodium sulfate R, and filter. Measure the absorbance of the filtrate in a 1-cm cell at a maximum of 480 nm against a solvent cell containing chloroform R; the absorbance does not exceed 0.10.

Ethanol-insoluble matter.   Boil 0.2 g with 20 ml of ethanol (~750 g/l) TS for 1 minute, filter through a sintered glass filter, wash the filter with ethanol (~750 g/l) TS until the filtrate is almost colourless, dry the filter at 105 °C for 1 hour and weigh; the residue is not more than 2.0 mg.

Loss on drying.   Dry to constant weight at 105 °C; it loses not more than 100 mg/g.

pH value.   pH of a 20 mg/ml solution in carbon-dioxide-free water R, 7.0–9.0.

Dimethylformamide.   Carry out the test as described under "Gas chromatography" (vol. 1, p. 94). Prepare an internal standard consisting of a mixture of 20 µl of dimethylacetamide R in 100 ml of water. Inject the following 3 solutions: (1) a mixture of 2 µl of dimethylformamide R in 10 ml of water and containing 10 ml of the solution of the internal standard; (2) for the determination of the retention time of the substance being examined, dissolve 1.0 g of the test substance in 10 ml of water, add with stirring 10 ml of hydrochloric acid (0.5 mol/l) VS, allow to stand for 15 minutes, centrifuge, and then dissolve 0.10 g of trisodium orthophosphate R in 5 ml of the supernatant liquid; (3) dissolve 1.0 g of the test substance in 10 ml of the solution of the internal standard, add with stirring 10 ml of hydrochloric acid (0.5 mol/l) VS, allow to stand for 15 minutes, centrifuge, and then dissolve 0.10 g of trisodium orthophosphate R in 5 ml of the supernatant liquid.

For the procedure, use a glass column 1.5 m long and 4 mm in internal diameter packed with an adequate quantity of an adsorbent composed of 1 g of macrogol 1000 R supported on 9 g of acid-washed, silanized diatomaceous support R and maintained at 120 °C. Use nitrogen R as the carrier gas and a flame ionization detector.

In the chromatogram obtained with solution 3, the ratio of the area of any peak due to dimethylformamide to the area of the peak due to the internal standard is not greater than the corresponding ratio for the chromatogram obtained with solution 1.

Resorcinol.   Carry out the test as described under "Thin-layer chromatography" (vol. 1, p. 83), using silica gel R1 as the coating substance (a precoated plate from a commercial source is suitable) and a mixture of 6 volumes of hexane R and 4 volumes of ethyl acetate R as the mobile phase. Apply separately to the plate 5 µl of each of the 2 following solutions: (A) dissolve 1.0 g of the test substance in 10 ml of water, add slowly with constant stirring 10 ml of hydrochloric acid (0.5 mol/l) VS, allow to stand for 15 minutes, centrifuge, and use the supernatant liquid; (B) dissolve 2.5 mg of resorcinol R in 10 ml of water. After removing the plate from the chromatographic chamber, allow it to dry in air, and expose it to the vapour of iodine R for 30 minutes. Examine the chromatogram in daylight. The spot obtained with solution B is more intense than any corresponding spot obtained with solution A.

Related substances.   Carry out the test as described under "Thin-layer chromatography" (vol. 1, p. 83), using silica gel R1 as the coating substance (a precoated plate from a commercial source is suitable) and a mixture of 8 volumes of chloroform R and 2 volumes of methanol R as the mobile phase. Apply separately to the plate 5 µl of each of 2 solutions in hydrochloric acid/methanol (0.1 mol/l) VS containing (A) 10 mg of the test substance per ml and (B) 20 µg of the test substance per ml. After removing the plate from the chromatographic chamber, allow it to dry in air, and expose the plate to the vapour of iodine R for 30 minutes. Examine the chromatogram in daylight. Any spot obtained with solution A, other than the principal spot, is not more intense than that obtained with solution B.

Assay.   Dissolve about 0.5 g, accurately weighed, in 20 ml of water, add 5 ml of hydrochloric acid (~70 g/l) TS, and extract with 4 volumes, each of 20 ml, of a solvent mixture composed of equal volumes of 2-butanol R and chloroform R. Separate and combine the extracts, wash with 10 ml of water, extract the washings with 5 ml of the above solvent mixture, and add to the combined extracts. Evaporate the mixed extracts to dryness on a water-bath in a current of air, dissolve the residue in 10 ml of ethanol (~750 g/l) TS, evaporate to dryness on a water-bath and dry to constant weight at 105 °C. Each g of residue is equivalent to 1.132 g of $C_{20}H_{10}Na_2O_5$.

———————

FLUOROURACILUM

Fluorouracil

Molecular formula. $C_4H_3FN_2O_2$

Relative molecular mass.   130.1

Graphic formula.

Chemical name.   5-Fluorouracil; 5-fluoro-2,4(1H,3H)-pyrimidinedione; CAS Reg. No. 51-21-8.

Description.   A white or almost white, crystalline powder.

Solubility.   Sparingly soluble in water; slightly soluble in ethanol (∼750 g/l) TS; practically insoluble in chloroform R and ether R.

Category.   Cytotoxic drug.

Storage.   Fluorouracil should be kept in a tightly closed container, protected from light.

Additional information.   Fluorouracil melts at about 282 °C with decomposition. CAUTION: Fluorouracil must be handled with care, avoiding contact with the skin and inhalation of airborne particles.

REQUIREMENTS

General requirement.   Fluorouracil contains not less than 98.5% and not more than 101.0% of $C_4H_3FN_2O_2$, calculated with reference to the dried substance.

Identity tests

● Either test A alone or tests B, C and D may be applied.

A.   Carry out the examination as described under "Spectrophotometry in the infrared region" (vol. 1, p. 40). The infrared absorption spectrum is concordant with the spectrum obtained from fluorouracil RS or with the *reference spectrum* of fluorouracil.

B.   The absorption spectrum of a 10 µg/ml solution in acetate buffer, pH 4.7, TS, when observed between 220 nm and 350 nm, is qualitatively similar to that of a

10.0 µg/ml solution of fluorouracil RS in acetate buffer, pH 4.7, TS (a maximum occurs at about 266 nm and a minimum occurs at about 232 nm). The absorbances of the solutions at the maximum do not differ from each other by more than 3%. The absorbance of a 1-cm layer at 266 nm is about 0.54.

C.   Heat 0.5 ml of chromic acid TS in a small test-tube in a water-bath for 5 minutes; the solution wets the sides of the tube but there is no greasiness. Add about 3 mg of the test substance and again heat in a water-bath for 5 minutes; the solution no longer wets the sides of the tube.

D.   Dissolve 0.05 g in 5 ml of water, add 1 ml of bromine TS1; the colour of the bromine is discharged.

Heavy metals.   Use 1.0 g for the preparation of the test solution as described under "Limit test for heavy metals", Procedure 3 (vol. 1, p. 118); determine the heavy metals content according to Method A (vol. 1, p. 119); not more than 20 µg/g.

Sulfated ash.   Not more than 1.0 mg/g.

Loss on drying.   Dry at 80 °C under reduced pressure (not exceeding 0.6 kPa or about 5 mm of mercury) over phosphorus pentoxide R for 4 hours; it loses not more than 5.0 mg/g.

Related substances.   Carry out the test as described under "Thin-layer chromatography" (vol. 1, p. 83), using silica gel R6 as the coating substance (a precoated plate from a commercial source is suitable) and a mixture of 70 volumes of ethyl acetate R, 15 volumes of methanol R, and 15 volumes of water as the mobile phase. Apply separately to the plate 5 µl of each of 2 solutions in a mixture of equal volumes of water and methanol R containing (A) 20 mg of the test substance per ml and (B) 0.050 mg of fluorouracil RS per ml. After removing the plate from the chromatographic chamber, allow it to dry in air and examine the chromatogram in ultraviolet light (254 nm). Any spot obtained with solution A, other than the principal spot, is not more intense than that obtained with solution B.

Fluorine content.   Carry out the combustion as described under "Oxygen flask method" (vol. 1, p. 124), using 7 mg of the test substance, and adding about 15 mg of sodium peroxide R and 15 ml of sodium hydroxide (0.1 mol/l) VS as the absorbing liquid. When the process is complete, allow the flask to stand for not less than 10 minutes with intermittent shaking, then dilute the contents to 100 ml with water. Proceed with 5.0 ml as described under "Oxygen flask method" for the determination of fluorine (vol. 1, p. 125); not more than 55 µg of F.

Assay.   Dissolve about 0.4 g, accurately weighed, in 80 ml of dimethylformamide R, add 0.25 ml of thymol blue/dimethylformamide TS and titrate with tetrabutylammonium hydroxide (0.1 mol/l) VS to a blue endpoint as described under "Non-aqueous titration", Method B (vol. 1, p. 132). Each ml of tetrabutylammonium hydroxide (0.1 mol/l) VS is equivalent to 13.01 mg of $C_4H_3FN_2O_2$.

GALLAMINI TRIETHIODIDUM

Gallamine triethiodide

Molecular formula. $C_{30}H_{60}I_3N_3O_3$

Relative molecular mass.   891.5

Graphic formula.

$$\left[\begin{array}{c} OCH_2CH_2N^+(C_2H_5)_3 \\ OCH_2CH_2N^+(C_2H_5)_3 \\ OCH_2CH_2N^+(C_2H_5)_3 \end{array}\right] 3I^-$$

Chemical name.   [v-Phenenyltris(oxyethylene)]tris[triethylammonium] triiodide; 2,2′,2″-[1,2,3-benzenetriyltris(oxy)]tris[N,N,N-triethylethanaminium triiodide; 1,2,3-tris(2-diethylaminoethoxy)benzene triethiodide; CAS Reg. No. 65-29-2.

Description.   A white or almost white powder; odourless.

Solubility.   Very soluble in water; sparingly soluble in ethanol ($\sim$750 g/l) TS; very slightly soluble in chloroform R; practically insoluble in ether R.

Category.   Muscle relaxant.

Storage.   Gallamine triethiodide should be kept in a tightly closed container, protected from light.

Additional information.   Gallamine triethiodide is hygroscopic.

REQUIREMENTS

General requirement.   Gallamine triethiodide contains not less than 98.0% and not more than 101.0% of $C_{30}H_{60}I_3N_3O_3$, calculated with reference to the dried substance.

Identity tests

● Either tests A and D or tests B, C and D may be applied.

A.   Carry out the examination as described under "Spectrophotometry in the infrared region" (vol. 1, p. 40). The infrared absorption spectrum is concordant with the spectrum obtained from gallamine triethiodide RS or with the *reference spectrum* of gallamine triethiodide.

B.   The absorption spectrum of a 10 μg/ml solution in hydrochloric acid (0.01 mol/l) VS, when observed between 220 nm and 350 nm exhibits a maximum at about 225 nm; the absorbance of a 1-cm layer at this wavelength is between 0.50 and 0.55.

C.   Dissolve 0.05 g in 5 ml of water and add 1 ml of potassio-mercuric iodide TS; a yellow precipitate is produced.

D.   A 0.01 g/ml solution yields reaction A described under "General identification tests" as characteristic of iodides (vol. 1, p. 113).

Clarity and colour of solution.   A freshly prepared solution of 0.20 g in 10 ml of carbon-dioxide free water R is clear and not more intensely coloured than standard colour solution Yw1 when compared as described under "Colour of liquids" (vol. 1, p. 50).

Sulfated ash.   Not more than 1.0 mg/g.

Loss on drying.   Dry to constant weight at 105 °C; it loses not more than 15 mg/g.

Acidity or alkalinity.   To 50 ml of water add 0.2 ml of methyl red/ethanol TS and adjust to pH 6 by adding either sulfuric acid (0.01 mol/l) VS or sodium hydroxide (0.02 mol/l) VS until the colour is orange-yellow. Add 1.0 g of the substance being examined and shake to dissolve; not more than 0.2 ml of either sulfuric acid (0.01 mol/l) VS or sodium hydroxide (0.02 mol/l) VS is required to restore the original orange-yellow colour.

Related substances.   Carry out the test as described under "Thin-layer chromatography" (vol. 1, p. 83), using cellulose R1 as the coating substance and a mixture of 17 volumes of glacial acetic acid R, 17 volumes of water and 66 volumes of 1-butanol R as the mobile phase. Apply separately to the plate 10 µl of each of 2 solutions in ethanol ($\sim$750 g/l) TS containing (A) 5.0 mg of the test substance per ml and (B) 0.05 mg of the test substance per ml. Allow the mobile phase to ascend 10 cm. After removing the plate from the chromatographic chamber, dry it in a current of warm air and spray it with potassium iodoplatinate TS. An elongated blue spot, which may appear to be double, is obtained on the chromatogram from test solution A. Any spot above the principal spot obtained with solution A is not more intense than the principal spot obtained with solution B.

Assay.   Dissolve about 0.5 g, accurately weighed, in 40 ml of acetone R, and add 15 ml of mercuric acetate/acetic acid TS. Titrate with perchloric acid (0.1 mol/l) VS, determining the endpoint potentiometrically as described under "Non-aqueous titration", Method A (vol. 1, p. 131). Each ml of perchloric acid (0.1 mol/l) VS is equivalent to 29.72 mg of $C_{30}H_{60}I_3N_3O_3$.

GENTAMICINI SULFAS

Gentamicin sulfate

Gentamicin sulfate (non-injectable)
Gentamicin sulfate, sterile

Composition.   Gentamicin sulfate is the sulfate salt of gentamicin fractions C_1, C_2, and C_{1a} produced by the growth of *Micromonospora purpurea;* CAS Reg. No. 1405-41-0.

Graphic formula.

Gentamicin	R
C_1	$H_3C-HN-\overset{CH_3}{\underset{H}{C}}-H$
C_2	$H_2N-\overset{CH_3}{\underset{H}{C}}-H$
C_{1a}	CH_2NH_2

Description.   A white to cream-coloured powder; odourless.

Solubility.   Soluble in water; practically insoluble in ethanol ($\sim$750 g/l) TS, ether R, and chloroform R.

Category.   Antibacterial drug.

Storage.   Gentamicin sulfate should be kept in a tightly closed container, protected from light.

Labelling.   The designation sterile Gentamicin sulfate indicates that the substance complies with the additional requirements for sterile Gentamicin sulfate and may be used for parenteral administration or for other sterile applications.

Additional information.   Gentamicin sulfate is hygroscopic. Even in the absence of light, it is gradually degraded on exposure to a humid atmosphere, the decomposition being faster at higher temperatures.

REQUIREMENTS

General requirement. Gentamicin sulfate contains not less than 590 International Units of gentamicin per mg, calculated with reference to the anhydrous substance.

Identity tests

A.   Carry out the test as described under "Thin-layer chromatography" (vol. 1, p. 83), using silica gel R5 as the coating substance (a precoated plate from a commercial source is suitable); shake together 1 volume of chloroform R, 1 volume of methanol R, and 1 volume of ammonia (~260 g/l) TS, allow to separate and use the lower layer as the mobile phase. Apply separately to the plate 1 µl of each of 2 solutions containing (A) 20 mg of the test substance per ml and (B) 20 mg of gentamicin sulfate RS per ml. After removing the plate from the chromatographic chamber, allow it to dry in air, spray it with triketohydrindene/pyridine/acetone TS, and heat it at 105 °C for 2 minutes. Examine the chromatogram in daylight.   The 3 principal spots obtained with solution A correspond with the 3 principal spots obtained with solution B.

B.   A 10 mg/ml solution yields reaction A described under "General identification tests" as characteristic of sulfates (vol. 1, p. 115).

Specific optical rotation.   Use a 0.10 g/ml solution, and calculate with reference to the anhydrous substance: $[\alpha]_D^{20\,^{\circ}C} = +107$ to $+121^{\circ}$.

Sulfated ash.   Not more than 10 mg/g.

Water.   Determine as described under "Determination of water by the Karl Fischer method", Method A (vol. 1, p. 135), using about 0.2 g of the substance; the water content is not more than 150 mg/g.

pH value.   pH of a 40 mg/ml solution, 3.5–5.5.

Assay.   Carry out the assay as described under "Microbiological assay of antibiotics" (vol. 1, p. 145), using either *Bacillus pumilus* (NCTC 8241; ATCC 14884), *Bacillus subtilis* (ATCC 6633), or *Staphylococcus aureus* (ATCC 6538P) as the test organism, culture medium Cml with a final pH of 7.8, sterile phosphate buffer pH 8.0 TS1 or TS2, an appropriate concentration of gentamicin (usually between 2 and 20 IU per ml), and an incubation temperature of 35–39 °C. The precision of the assay is such that the fiducial limits of error of the estimated potency ($P = 0.95$) are not less than 95% and not more than 105% of the estimated potency. The upper fiducial limit of error of the estimated potency ($P = 0.95$) is not less than 590 IU per mg, calculated with reference to the anhydrous substance.

Additional Requirements for Sterile Gentamicin Sulfate

Undue toxicity.   Carry out the test as described under "Test for undue toxicity" (vol. 1, p. 154), using 0.5 ml of a solution in saline TS containing a quantity equivalent to 1 mg of gentamicin base per ml.

Pyrogens.   Carry out the test as described under "Test for pyrogens" (vol. 1, p. 155), injecting a solution containing, per kg of the rabbit's mass, not less than 10 000 IU of gentamicin in not more than 5 ml of sterile water R.

Sterility.   Complies with the "Sterility testing of antibiotics" (vol. 1, p. 152), applying the membrane filtration test procedure.

GLIBENCLAMIDUM

Glibenclamide

Molecular formula. $C_{23}H_{28}ClN_3O_5S$

Relative molecular mass.   494.0

Graphic formula.

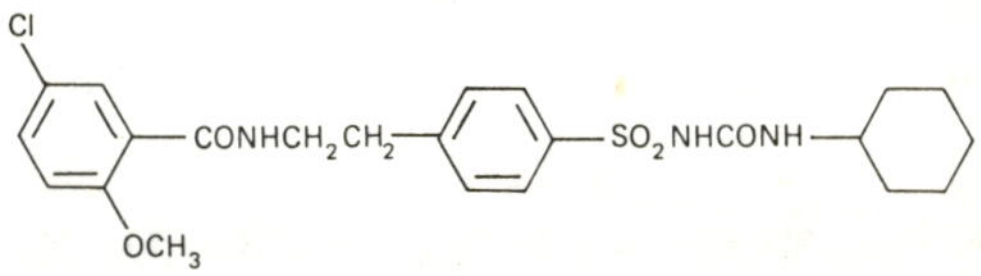

Chemical name.   1-[[p-[2-(5-Chloro-o-anisamido)ethyl]phenyl]sulfonyl]-3-cyclo-hexylurea; 5-chloro-N-[4-[[[(cyclohexylamino)carbonyl]amino]sulfonyl]-phenyl]-ethyl]-2-methoxybenzamide; 1-[4-[2-(5-chloro-2-methoxybenzamido)ethyl]phenylsulfonyl]-3-cyclohexylurea; CAS Reg. No. 10238-21-8.

Other name.   Glyburide.

Description.   A white or almost white, crystalline powder; odourless or almost odourless.

Solubility.   Practically insoluble in water and ether R; slightly soluble in ethanol ($\sim$750 g/l) TS and methanol R; sparingly soluble in chloroform R.

Category.   Antidiabetic agent.

Storage.   Glibenclamide should be kept in a well-closed container.

REQUIREMENTS

General requirement.   Glibenclamide contains not less than 98.5% and not more than 101.0% of $C_{23}H_{28}ClN_3O_5S$, calculated with reference to the dried substance.

Identity tests

- Either test A alone or tests B and C may be applied.

A. Carry out the examination as described under "Spectrophotometry in the infrared region" (vol. 1, p. 40). The infrared absorption spectrum is concordant with the spectrum obtained from glibenclamide RS or with the *reference spectrum* of glibenclamide.

B. The absorption spectrum of a 0.10 mg/ml solution in hydrochloric acid/methanol (0.01 mol/l) VS, when observed between 230 nm and 350 nm, exhibits a maximum at about 300 nm and a less intense maximum at about 275 nm; the absorbance of a 1-cm layer at 300 nm is about 0.63.

C. Melting temperature, about 172 °C.

Heavy metals. Use 1.0 g for the preparation of the test solution as described under "Limit test for heavy metals", Procedure 3 (vol. 1, p. 118); not more than 20 µg/g.

Sulfated ash. Not more than 1.0 mg/g.

Loss on drying. Dry to constant weight at 105 °C; it loses not more than 10 mg/g.

Related substances. Carry out the test as described under "Thin-layer chromatography" (vol. 1, p. 83), using silica gel R4 as the coating substance and a mixture of 45 volumes of chloroform R, 45 volumes of cyclohexane R, 5 volumes of ethanol (~750 g/l) TS, and 5 volumes of glacial acetic acid R as the mobile phase. Apply separately to the plate 10 µl of each of 2 solutions in chloroform R containing (A) 10 mg of the test substance per ml and (B) 0.05 mg of the test substance per ml. After removing the plate from the chromatographic chamber, allow it to dry in air and examine the chromatogram in ultraviolet light (254 nm). Any spot obtained with solution A, other than the principal spot, is not more intense than that obtained with solution B.

Assay. Dissolve about 0.5 g, accurately weighed, in 100 ml of hot neutralized ethanol TS, and titrate with carbonate-free sodium hydroxide (0.1 mol/l) VS, using phenolphthalein/ethanol TS as indicator. Repeat the operation without the substance being examined and make any necessary correction. Each ml of carbonate-free sodium hydroxide (0.1 mol/l) VS is equivalent to 49.40 mg of $C_{23}H_{28}ClN_3O_5S$.

HOMATROPINI HYDROBROMIDUM

Homatropine hydrobromide

Molecular formula. $C_{16}H_{21}NO_3,HBr$

Relative molecular mass.   356.3

Graphic formula.

Chemical name. $1\alpha H,5\alpha H$-Tropan-3α-ol mandelate (ester) hydrobromide; (±)-*endo*-8-methyl-8-azabicyclo[3.2.1]oct-3-yl α-hydroxybenzeneacetate hydrobromide; CAS Reg. No. 51-56-9.

Description.   Colourless crystals or a white, crystalline powder; odourless.

Solubility.   Freely soluble in water; sparingly soluble in ethanol (~750 g/l) TS; slightly soluble in chloroform R; practically insoluble in ether R.

Category.   Mydriatic.

Storage.   Homatropine hydrobromide should be kept in a tightly closed container, protected from light.

REQUIREMENTS

General requirement.   Homatropine hydrobromide contains not less than 98.5% and not more than 101.0% of $C_{16}H_{21}NO_3,HBr$, calculated with reference to the dried substance.

Identity tests

A.   Dissolve 10 mg in 1 ml of water, add ammonia (~100 g/l) TS to render the solution slightly alkaline, and shake with 5 ml of chloroform R. Evaporate the chloroform layer to dryness on a water-bath and add 1.5 ml of mercuric chloride/ethanol TS to the residue; a yellow colour is produced, which turns red on heating.

B.   A 20 mg/ml solution yields reaction A described under "General identification tests" as characteristic of bromides (vol. 1, p. 112).

C. Melting temperature, about 215 °C with decomposition.

Sulfated ash. Not more than 1.0 mg/g.

Loss on drying. Dry to constant weight at 105 °C; it loses not more than 15 mg/g.

pH value. pH of a 20 mg/ml solution, 5.5 – 7.0.

Foreign alkaloids. Dissolve 10 mg in 2 ml of water and add 0.25 ml of tannic acid (50 g/l) TS; no precipitate is produced.

Related alkaloids. Dissolve 5 mg in 0.25 ml of fuming nitric acid R and evaporate to dryness on a water-bath. Allow to cool, add 0.1 ml of acetone R and 0.1 ml of a mixture of 1 volume of potassium hydroxide/ethanol (0.5 mol/l) VS and 4 volumes of aldehyde-free ethanol (~750 g/l) TS; no violet or reddish violet colour is produced.

Assay. Dissolve about 0.3 g, accurately weighed, in 30 ml of glacial acetic acid R1, add 10 ml of mercuric acetate/acetic acid TS, and titrate with perchloric acid (0.1 mol/l) VS, determining the endpoint potentiometrically as described under "Non-aqueous titration", Method A (vol. 1, p. 131). Each ml of perchloric acid (0.1 mol/l) VS is equivalent to 35.63 mg of $C_{16}H_{21}NO_3,HBr$.

HYDRALAZINI HYDROCHLORIDUM

Hydralazine hydrochloride

Molecular formula. $C_8H_8N_4,HCl$

Relative molecular mass. 196.6

Graphic formula.

Chemical name. 1-Hydrazinophthalazine monohydrochloride; 1(2H)-phthalazinone hydrazone monohydrochloride; CAS Reg. No. 304-20-1.

Other name. Apressinum.

Description. A white or almost white, crystalline powder; odourless.

Solubility. Soluble in 25 parts of water; slightly soluble in ethanol (~750 g/l) TS; very slightly soluble in ether R.

Category. Antihypertensive drug.

Storage. Hydralazine hydrochloride should be kept in a well-closed container, protected from light.

Additional information. Hydralazine hydrochloride melts at about 275 °C with decomposition. Even in the absence of light, it is gradually degraded on exposure to a humid atmosphere, the decomposition being faster at higher temperatures.

REQUIREMENTS

General requirement. Hydralazine hydrochloride contains not less than 98.0% and not more than 101.0% of $C_8H_8N_4,HCl$, calculated with reference to the dried substance.

Identity tests

A. The absorption spectrum of a 10 µg/ml solution, when observed between 220 nm and 350 nm, exhibits maxima at 240 nm, 260 nm, 303 nm, and 315 nm; the absorbances of a 1-cm layer at these wavelenghts are about 0.58, 0.54, 0.27, and 0.21, respectively.

B. Dissolve 0.5 g in a mixture of 100 ml of water and 8 ml of hydrochloric acid ($\sim$70 g/l) TS, add 20 ml of sodium nitrite (10 g/l) TS, allow to stand for 10 minutes and filter. Wash the residue with water and dry at 105 °C; melting temperature, about 210 °C.

C. A 20 mg/ml solution yields reaction A described under "General identification tests" as characteristic of chlorides (vol. 1, p. 112).

Water-insoluble substances. Transfer 2.0 g to a 250-ml conical flask, add 100 ml of water, and shake by mechanical means for 30 minutes. Filter the solution through a tared sintered glass crucible, rinse the flask, and wash any undissolved residue into the crucible. Wash the residue with three 10-ml portions of water, dry at 105 °C for 3 hours, cool and weigh; the residue weighs not more than 10 mg (5 mg/g).

Sulfated ash. Not more than 1.0 mg/g.

Loss on drying. Dry at ambient temperature under reduced pressure (not exceeding 0.6 kPa or about 5 mm of mercury) over phosphorus pentoxide R for 8 hours; it loses not more than 5.0 mg/g.

Related substances. Carry out the test as described under "Thin-layer chromatography" (vol. 1, p. 83), using silica gel R1 as the coating substance. For the mobile phase, shake a mixture of 2 volumes of ethyl acetate R, 2 volumes of ammonia ($\sim$260 g/l)TS and 8 volumes of hexane R, allow to separate and use the upper layer. For the preparation of the test solution dissolve 0.10 g of the test substance in a mixture of 100 volumes of methanol R and 1 volume of hydrochloric acid ($\sim$420 g/l)TS, and dilute to 20 ml with the same solvent mixture; to 2.0 ml of this solution add 1.0 ml of salicylaldehyde TS, centrifuge and decant the supernatant liquid (solution A). For the reference solution, dissolve 25.0 mg of hydrazine sulfate R in 10 ml of water and dilute to 100 ml using a mixture of 1 volume of hydrochloric acid ($\sim$420 g/l)TS and 100 volumes of methanol R; dilute 1.0 ml to 100 ml with the same solvent mixture. To 2.0 ml of this solution add 1.0 ml of salicylaldehyde TS, centrifuge and decant the supernatant liquid (solution B). Apply separately to the plate 40 µl of each of solutions A and B. After removing the plate from the chromatographic chamber, allow it to dry in air and spray with 4-dimethylaminobenzaldehyde TS6. Examine the chromatogram in ultraviolet light (254 nm). Any spot obtained with solution A, other than the principal spot, is not more intense than that obtained with solution B.

Assay. Dissolve about 0.15 g, accurately weighed, in 25 ml of water, add 25 ml of hydrochloric acid ($\sim$420 g/l) TS, cool to room temperature, add 5 ml of chloroform R, and titrate with potassium iodate (0.05 mol/l) VS, shaking continuously, until the purple colour of iodine in the chloroform layer disappears. The endpoint is reached when the chloroform layer remains colourless for at least 5 minutes. Each ml of potassium iodate (0.05 mol/l) VS is equivalent to 9.832 mg of $C_8H_8N_4,HCl$.

HYDROCORTISONI NATRII SUCCINAS

Hydrocortisone sodium succinate

Molecular formula. $C_{25}H_{33}NaO_8$

Relative molecular mass. 484.5

Graphic formula.

Chemical name. Cortisol 21-(sodium succinate); 21-(3-carboxy-1-oxopropoxy)-11β,17-dihydroxypregn-4-ene-3,20-dione monosodium salt; CAS Reg. No. 125-04-2.

Description. A white or almost white, crystalline powder or amorphous solid; odourless.

Solubility.   Freely soluble in water; soluble in 34 parts of ethanol ($\sim$750 g/l) TS and in 200 parts of dehydrated ethanol R; practically insoluble in chloroform R and ether R.

Category.   Adrenal hormone.

Storage.   Hydrocortisone sodium succinate should be kept in a tightly closed container, protected from light.

Additional information.   Hydrocortisone sodium succinate is hygroscopic. Even in the absence of light, it is gradually degraded on exposure to a humid atmosphere, the decomposition being faster at higher temperatures.

REQUIREMENTS

General requirement.   Hydrocortisone sodium succinate contains not less than 97.0% and not more than 103.0% of $C_{25}H_{33}NaO_8$, calculated with reference to the dried substance.

Identity tests

A.   Carry out the examination as described under "Spectrophotometry in the infrared region" (vol. 1, p. 40). The infrared absorption spectrum is concordant with the spectrum obtained from hydrocortisone sodium succinate RS or with the *reference spectrum* of hydrocortisone sodium succinate.

B.   Carry out the test as described under "Thin-layer chromatography" (vol. 1, p. 83), using silica gel R1 as the coating substance and a freshly prepared mixture of 3 volumes of 1-butanol R, 1 volume of acetic anhydride R, and 1 volume of water as the mobile phase. Apply separately to the plate 2 µl of each of 2 solutions in methanol R containing (A) 2.5 mg of the test substance per ml and (B) 2.5 mg of hydrocortisone sodium succinate RS per ml. After removing the plate from the chromatographic chamber, allow it to dry in air until the solvents have evaporated, spray it with a mixture of 10 ml of sulfuric acid ($\sim$1760 g/l) TS and 90 ml of ethanol ($\sim$750 g/l) TS, heat it at 120 °C for 10 minutes, allow it to cool, and examine the chromatogram in ultraviolet light (365 nm). The principal spot obtained with solution A corresponds in position, appearance, and intensity with that obtained with solution B.

C.   When tested for sodium as described under "General identification tests" (vol. 1, p. 115), it yields the characteristic reactions. If reaction B is to be used, prepare a 20 mg/ml solution.

Specific optical rotation.   Use a 10 mg/ml solution in ethanol ($\sim$750 g/l) TS and calculate with reference to the dried substance; $[\alpha]_D^{20\,°C} = +135$ to $+145°$.

Loss on drying. Dry to constant weight at 105 °C; it loses not more than 30 mg/g.

Related steroids. Carry out the test as described under "Thin-layer chromatography" (vol. 1, p. 83), using silica gel R1 as the coating substance and a mixture of 77 volumes of dichloromethane R, 15 volumes of ether R, 8 volumes of methanol R, and 1.2 volumes of water as the mobile phase. Apply separately to the plate 1 µl of each of 2 solutions in a mixture of equal volumes of chloroform R and methanol R containing (A) 15 mg of the test substance per ml and (B) 0.15 mg of the test substance per ml. After removing the plate from the chromatographic chamber, allow it to dry in air until the solvents have evaporated, then heat it at 105 °C for 10 minutes; allow it to cool, spray it with blue tetrazolium/sodium hydroxide TS, and examine the chromatogram in daylight. Any spot obtained with solution A, other than the principal spot, is not more intense than that obtained with solution B.

Sodium. Dissolve with gentle heating about 1 g, accurately weighed, in 75 ml of glacial acetic acid R. Add 20 ml of dioxan R, 0.15 ml of crystal violet/acetic acid TS, and titrate with perchloric acid (0.1 mol/l) VS. Each ml of perchloric acid (0.1 mol/l) VS is equivalent to 2.299 mg of Na; the content is not less than 46.0 mg and not more than 48.4 mg of Na per g, calculated with reference to the dried substance.

Assay. Dissolve about 20 mg, accurately weighed, in sufficient water to produce 100 ml; dilute 5 ml to 100 ml with water. Measure the absorbance of a 1-cm layer of the diluted solution at the maximum at about 248 nm. Calculate the amount of $C_{25}H_{33}NaO_8$ in the substance being tested by comparison with hydrocortisone sodium succinate RS, similarly and concurrently examined. In an adequately calibrated spectrophotometer the absorbance of the reference solution should be 0.34 ± 0.02.

HYDROXOCOBALAMINUM

Hydroxocobalamin

Hydroxocobalamin anhydrous
Hydroxocobalamin hydrate

Molecular formula. $C_{62}H_{89}CoN_{13}O_{15}P$ (anhydrous); $C_{62}H_{89}CoN_{13}O_{15}P,H_2O$ (monohydrate).

Relative molecular mass.   1346 (anhydrous); 1365 (monohydrate).

Graphic formula.

n = 0 (anhydrous)
n = 1 (monohydrate)

Chemical name. Cobinamide dihydroxide dihydrogen phosphate (ester),
mono(inner salt), 3′-ester with 5,6-dimethyl-1-α-D-ribofuranosylbenzimidazole;
cobinamide dihydrogen phosphate (ester)-mono(inner salt), 3′-ester with 5,6-
dimethyl-1-α-D-ribofuranosyl-1H-benzimidazole; Coα-[α-(5,6-dimethylbenzimi-
dazolyl)]-Coβ-hydroxocobamide; CAS Reg. No. 13422-51-0 (anhydrous).
Cobinamide dihydroxide monohydrate, dihydrogen phosphate (ester), mono(inner salt), 3′-ester with 5,6-dimethyl-1-α-D-ribofuranosylbenzimidazole; cobinamide dihydroxide monohydrate, dihydrogen phosphate (ester), mono(inner salt)
3′-ester with 5,6-dimethyl-1-α-D-ribofuranosyl-1H-benzimidazole; Coα-[α-(5,6-
dimethylbenzimidazolyl)]-Coβ-hydroxocobamide monohydrate; CAS Reg. No.
13422-52-1 (monohydrate).

Other names.   Vitamin B_{12a} for anhydrous Hydroxocobalamin and Vitamin B_{12b}
for Hydroxocobalamin hydrate.

Description.   Dark red crystals or a red, crystalline powder; odourless.

Solubility.   Sparingly soluble in water and ethanol (~750 g/l) TS; practically
insoluble in acetone R and chloroform R.

Category.   Antianaemia drug.

Storage.   Hydroxocobalamin should be kept in a tightly closed container, protected from light, and stored in a cool place.

Labelling.   The designation on the container should state whether the substance
is in the anhydrous or hydrated form.

Additional information.   In aqueous solution, Hydroxocobalamin exists as hy-
droxocobamide in equilibrium with the hydrated ionic form. The anhydrous form

of Hydroxocobalamin is very hygroscopic. Even in the absence of light, it is gradually degraded on exposure to a humid atmosphere, the decomposition being faster at higher temperatures.

REQUIREMENTS

General requirement. Hydroxocobalamin contains not less than 96.0% and not more than 102.0% of $C_{62}H_{89}CoN_{13}O_{15}P$, calculated with reference to the dried substance.

Identity tests

A. The absorption spectrum of a 40 µg/ml solution in pH 4.5 acetate buffer TS, when observed between 230 nm and 550 nm, exhibits 3 maxima at about 274 nm, 351 nm, and 525 nm; the ratio of the absorbance of a 1-cm layer at 525 nm to that at 351 nm is about 0.34, and the ratio of the absorbance at 274 nm to that at 351 nm is about 0.80.

B. Heat cautiously about 2 mg in a porcelain crucible with a few drops of sulfuric acid ($\sim$1760 g/l) TS until a faintly bluish residue is produced. Cool, add 0.05 ml of water and then a few drops of a saturated solution of ammonium thiocyanate R; a blue-green colour is produced.

C. Place about 2 mg in a 100-ml glass-stoppered flask, dissolve in 2 ml of water and add 5 ml of phosphoric acid ($\sim$1440 g/l) TS. Insert in the flask a flat-bottomed glass tube 1 cm in diameter and 2 cm long, containing 1 ml of lithium carbonate/trinitrophenol TS. Close the flask and expose it for 4 hours to a bright light; the colour of the reagent in the glass tube remains unchanged (distinction from cyanocobalamin).

Loss on drying. Dry Hydroxocobalamin hydrate at 100 °C under reduced pressure (not exceeding 0.6 kPa or about 5 mm of mercury) for 2 hours; it loses between 140 mg/g and 180 mg/g.

pH value. pH of a 20 mg/ml solution in carbon-dioxide-free water R, 8.0–10.0.

Other cobalamins. Carry out the test as described under "Column chromatography" (vol. 1, p. 86), shaking 20 g of diethylaminoethylcellulose R with 200 ml of sodium hydroxide (0.5 mol/l) VS, dilute with water to obtain a homogeneous suspension, allow to settle, and discard the supernatant liquid. Using a suitable filter, wash with water until the washings are free from alkali, then transfer the adsorbent to a tube, length 22 cm, diameter 1.2 cm, and provided with a stopcock. Allow to settle and tap the tube until the height of the adsorbent is about 14 cm. Wash with water until the pH of the eluate is the same as that of the water.

Similarly prepare a second column, slurrying carboxymethylcellulose R with hydrochloric acid (0.5 mol/l) VS, dilute with water, allow to settle, and discard the supernatant liquid. Using a suitable filter, wash with water until the washings are free from acid, then transfer the adsorbent to a tube, length 22 cm, diameter 1.2 cm, and provided with a stopcock. Allow to settle and tap the tube until the pH of the eluate is the same as that of the water.

Cover each column with a plug of glass wool and allow to drain until only a small amount of water remains above the adsorbents.

Place the column of diethylaminoethylcellulose above the other column so that the effluent runs into the carboxymethylcellulose.

Weigh accurately about 0.05 g of the substance to be examined, dissolve it in 20 ml of water, and acidify with sufficient hydrochloric acid ($\sim$70 g/l) TS to obtain a pH of 4.0. Introduce this solution to the diethylaminoethylcellulose column and allow it to run through both columns, rejecting the first colourless eluate. Elute with water, the pH of which has previously been adjusted to 4.0 with hydrochloric acid ($\sim$70 g/l) TS. Collect the coloured eluate into a 50-ml volumetric flask and adjust to volume with water. Measure the absorbance of this solution in a 1-cm layer at the maximum at about 361 nm and calculate the content of other cobalamins in mg/g, using the absorptivity value of 20.7 ($A_{1\ cm}^{1\%} = 207$); not more than 30 mg/g.

Acidic impurities. Elute the diethylaminoethylcellulose column from the above test for other cobalamins with sodium chloride (10 g/l) TS, collecting 50 ml of eluate. Measure the absorbance of this solution in a 1-cm layer at the maximum between 351 nm and 361 nm, and calculate the content of acidic impurities in mg/g, using the absorptivity value of 19.0 ($A_{1\ cm}^{1\%} = 190$); not more than 30 mg/g.

Assay

● The solutions must be protected from light throughout the assay.

Dissolve about 20 mg, accurately weighed, in sufficient acetate buffer, pH 4.5, TS to produce 500 ml. Measure the absorbance of this solution in a 1-cm layer at the maximum at about 351 nm and calculate the content of $C_{62}H_{89}CoN_{13}O_{15}P$, using the absorptivity value of 19.5 ($A_{1\ cm}^{1\%} = 195$).

HYDROXOCOBALAMINI CHLORIDUM
HYDROXOCOBALAMINI SULFAS

Hydroxocobalamin chloride
Hydroxocobalamin sulfate

Molecular formula. $C_{62}H_{90}ClCoN_{13}O_{15}P$; $C_{124}H_{180}Co_2N_{26}O_{34}P_2S$.

Relative molecular mass.   1383 (hydroxocobalamin chloride); 2791 (hydroxocobalamin sulfate).

Graphic formula for the base.

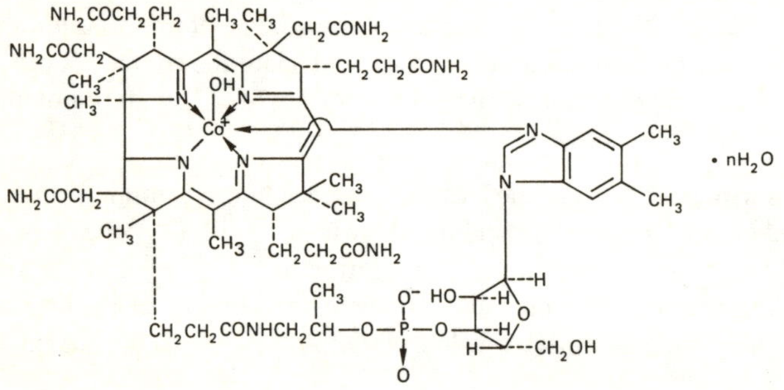

$$n = 0 \text{ (anhydrous)}$$
$$n = 1 \text{ (monohydrate)}$$

Chemical name. Cobinamide dihydroxide dihydrogen phosphate (ester), mono(inner salt), 3′-ester with 5,6-dimethyl-1-α-D-ribofuranosylbenzimidazole monohydrochloride; cobinamide dihydroxide dihydrogen phosphate (ester), mono(inner salt), 3′-ester with 5,6-dimethyl-1-α-D-ribofuranosyl-1H-benzimidazole monohydrochloride; Coα-[α-(5,6-dimethylbenzimidazolyl)]-Coβ-hydroxocobamide chloride; CAS Reg. No. 59461-30-2.
Cobinamide dihydroxide dihydrogen phosphate (ester), mono(inner salt), 3′-ester with 5,6-dimethyl-1-α-D-ribofuranosylbenzimidazole sulfate (salt) (2:1); cobinamide dihydroxide dihydrogen phosphate (ester), mono(inner salt), 3′-ester with 5,6-dimethyl-1-α-D-ribofuranosyl-1H-benzimidazole sulfate (salt) (2:1); 2(Coα-[α-(5,6-dimethylbenzimidazolyl)]-Coβ-hydroxocobamide) sulfate (salt) (2:1).

Description.   Dark red crystals or a red, crystalline powder; odourless.

Solubility.   Soluble in water.

Category.   Antianaemia drug.

Storage.   Hydroxocobalamin chloride or sulfate should be kept in a tightly closed container, protected from light, and stored in a cool place.

Labelling.   The designation on the container should state whether the substance is the chloride or the sulfate salt.

Additional information.   Even in the absence of light, Hydroxocobalamin chloride and Hydroxocobalamin sulfate are gradually degraded on exposure to a humid atmosphere, the decomposition being faster at higher temperatures.

REQUIREMENTS

General requirement.   Hydroxocobalamin chloride contains not less than 96.0% and not more than 102.0% of $C_{62}H_{90}ClCoN_{13}O_{15}P$, calculated with reference to the dried substance; Hydroxocobalamin sulfate contains not less than 96.0% and not more than 102.0% of $C_{124}H_{180}Co_2N_{26}O_{34}P_2S$, calculated with reference to the dried substance.

Identity tests

A.   The absorption spectrum of a 40 µg/ml solution in pH 4.5 acetate buffer TS, when observed between 230 nm and 550 nm, exhibits 3 maxima at about 274 nm, 351 nm, and 525 nm; the ratio of the absorbance of a 1-cm layer at 525 nm to that at 351 nm is about 0.34, and the ratio of the absorbance at 274 nm to that at .351 nm is about 0.80.

B.   Heat cautiously about 2 mg in a porcelain crucible with a few drops of sulfuric acid (~1760 g/l) TS until a faintly bluish residue is produced. Cool, add 0.05 ml of water and then a few drops of a saturated solution of ammonium thiocyanate R; a blue-green colour is produced.

C.   Place about 2 mg in a 100-ml glass-stoppered flask, dissolve in 2 ml of water and add 5 ml of phosphoric acid (~1440 g/l) TS. Insert in the flask a flat-bottomed glass tube 1 cm in diameter and 2 cm long, containing 1 ml of lithium carbonate/trinitrophenol TS. Close the flask and expose it for 4 hours to a bright light; the colour of the reagent in the glass tube remains unchanged (distinction from cyanocobalamin).

D.   For the chloride salt prepare a 20 mg/ml solution. It yields reaction B described under "General identification tests" as characteristic of chlorides (vol. 1, p. 113). For the sulfate salt prepare a 20 mg/ml solution. It yields reaction A described under "General identification tests" as characteristic of sulfates (vol. 1, p. 115).

Loss on drying.   Dry at 100 °C under reduced pressure (not exceeding 0.6 kPa or about 5 mm of mercury) for 2 hours; the chloride salt loses between 80 mg/g and 120 mg/g and the sulfate salt between 80 mg/g and 160 mg/g.

pH value. pH of a 20 mg/ml solution in carbon-dioxide-free water R, 8.0–10.0.

Other cobalamins. Carry out the test as described under "Column chromatography" (vol. 1, p. 86) shaking 20 g of diethylaminoethylcellulose R with 200 ml of sodium hydroxide (0.5 mol/l) VS, dilute with water to obtain a homogeneous suspension, allow to settle, and discard the supernatant liquid. Using a suitable filter, wash with water until the washings are free from alkali, then transfer the adsorbent to a tube, length 22 cm, diameter 1.2 cm, and provided with a stopcock. Allow to settle and tap the tube until the height of the adsorbent is about 14 cm. Wash with water until the pH of the eluate is the same as that of the water.

Similarly prepare a second column, slurrying carboxymethylcellulose R with hydrochloric acid (0.5 mol/l) VS, dilute with water, allow to settle, and discard the supernatant liquid. Using a suitable filter, wash with water until the washings are free from acid, then transfer the adsorbent to a tube, length 22 cm, diameter 1.2 cm, and provided with a stopcock. Allow to settle and tap the tube until the height of the adsorbent is about 10 cm. Wash with water until the pH of the eluate is the same as that of the water.

Cover each column with a plug of glass wool, and allow to drain until only a small amount of water remains above the adsorbents.

Place the column of diethylaminoethylcellulose above the other column so that the effluent runs into the carboxymethylcellulose.

Weigh accurately about 0.05 g of the substance to be examined, dissolve it in 20 ml of water, and acidify with sufficient hydrochloric acid ($\sim$70 g/l) TS to obtain a pH of 4.0. Introduce this solution to the diethylaminoethylcellulose column and allow it to run through both columns, rejecting the first colourless eluate. Elute with water the pH of which has previously been adjusted to 4.0 with hydrochloric acid ($\sim$70 g/l) TS. Collect the coloured eluate into a 50-ml volumetric flask and adjust to volume with water. Measure the absorbance of this solution in a 1-cm layer at the maximum at about 361 nm, and calculate the content of other cobalamins in mg/g, using the absortivity value of 20.7 ($A_{1\,cm}^{1\,\%} = 207$); not more than 30 mg/g.

Acidic impurities. Elute the diethylaminoethylcellulose column from the above test for other cobalamins with sodium chloride (10 g/l) TS, collecting 50 ml of eluate. Measure the absorbance of this solution in a 1-cm layer at the maximum between 351 nm and 361 nm, and calculate the content of acidic impurities in mg/g, using the absorptivity value of 19.0 ($A_{1\,cm}^{1\,\%} = 190$); not more than 30 mg/g.

Assay

● The solutions must be protected from light throughout the assay.

Dissolve about 20 mg, accurately weighed, in sufficient acetate buffer, pH 4.5, TS to produce 500 ml. Measure the absorbance of this solution in a 1-cm layer at the maximum at about 351 nm and calculate the content of $C_{62}H_{90}ClCoN_{13}O_{15}P$ or $C_{124}H_{180}Co_2N_{26}O_{34}P_2S$, using the absorptivity values of 19.0 or 18.8, respectively ($A_{1\ cm}^{1\%}$ = 190 or 188, respectively).

IPECACUANHAE RADIX

Ipecacuanha root

Definition. Ipecacuanha root consists of the dried rhizome and roots of *Cephaëlis ipecacuanha* (Brotero) A. Richard (Fam. Rubiaceae) or of *Cephaëlis acuminata* Karsten, or of a mixture of both species. The principal alkaloids are emetine and cephaëline.

Description. Odour, slight; taste, bitter, nauseous and acrid.

Category. Expectorant; emetic.

Storage. Ipecacuanha root should be kept in a well-closed container, protected from light.

Additional information. Even in the absence of light, the powder of Ipecacuanha root is gradually degraded on exposure to a humid atmosphere, the decomposition being faster at higher temperatures.

REQUIREMENTS

General requirement. Ipecacuanha root contains not less than 2.0% of total alkaloids, calculated as emetine.

Macroscopic characteristics

Cephaëlis ipecacuanha. Dark brick-red to very dark brown, somewhat tortuous root, seldom more than 15 cm long or 6 mm thick; the root is closely annulated externally, having rounded ridges completely encircling it; the fracture is short in the bark and splintery in the wood; a transversely cut surface shows a wide greyish bark and a small uniformly dense wood. The rhizomes are short lengths attached to roots; they are cylindrical, up to 2 mm in diameter, finely wrinkled longitudinally, and with pith occupying approximately one-sixth of the whole diameter.

Cephaëlis acuminata. In general it resembles the root of *Cephaëlis ipecacu-anha,* but differs in the following particulars: often up to 9 mm thick; external surface greyish brown or reddish brown with transverse ridges at intervals of about 1–3 mm; the ridges are about 0.5–1 mm wide, extending about half-way round the circumference and fading at the extremities into the general surface level.

Microscopic characteristics

Cephaëlis ipecacuanha. A transverse section of the root shows a narrow, brown cork layer of thin-walled polyhedral, tubular cells and a wide parenchymatous zone of phelloderm; the latter contains abundant starch, consisting of simple granules and compound granules of 2–8 components, the individual granules being oval, rounded, or roughly hemispherical, and seldom more than 15 μm in diameter; the phloem is present as a narrow unlignified zone; the xylem is dense, consisting mainly of narrow tracheids intermixed with a smaller proportion of vessels, both with numerous bordered pits in their lateral walls, the vessel element having simple circular perforations; crystal cells, each containing a bundle of raphides, 30–80 μm long, occur in the parenchymatous regions. A transverse section through an internode of the rhizome shows several layers of thin-walled cork, a somewhat collenchymatous cortex, a pericycle containing groups of large, distinctly pitted sclereids, a narrow ring of phloem, and a wide ring of xylem surrounding a pith composed of thin-walled, pitted, parenchymatous cells.

Cephaëlis acuminata. Similar to *Cephaëlis ipecacuanha* except that the individual starch granules may be up to 22 μm in diameter.

Identity test

Carry out the test as described under "Thin-layer chromatography" (vol. 1, p. 83), using silica gel R1 as the coating substance and a mixture of 93 volumes of chloroform R, 6.5 volumes of methanol R, and 0.5 volumes of ammonia (~260 g/l) TS as the mobile phase, and allow the solvent front to ascend only 10 cm above the line of application. Apply separately to the plate as bands, 20 mm by 3 mm, 10 μl of each of the following solutions: for solution A, add to 0.1 g of finely powdered test substance in a small test-tube, 0.05 ml of ammonia (~260 g/l) TS and 5 ml of chloroform R, stir vigorously with a glass rod, allow to stand for 30 minutes and filter; for solution B, dilute 1 ml of solution A to 25 ml with chloroform R; for solution C, dissolve 5 mg of emetine hydrochloride RS and 6 mg of cephaëline hydrochloride R in sufficient methanol R to produce 20 ml. After removing the plate from the chromatographic chamber, allow it to dry in air until the odour of solvent is no longer detectable, spray it with a mixture of 0.05 g of iodine R in 10 ml of chloroform R, and heat it at 60 °C for 10 minutes. Examine the chromatogram first in daylight; a lemon-yellow zone appears at about midpoint, corresponding to emetine, and below it a light brown zone, corresponding to cephaëline. Then examine the chromatogram in ultraviolet light (365 nm); the zone corresponding to emetine shows an intense yellow fluorescence, and that corresponding to cephaëline, a light blue fluorescence. The chromatogram obtained with solution A shows, in addition, several very small zones due to secondary alkaloids. The chromatogram obtained with solution B shows only 2 zones, which correspond to those obtained with solution C.

With *Cephaëlis ipecacuanha,* the zone corresponding to cephaëline obtained with solution A is much smaller than the corresponding zone obtained with solution C.

With *Cephaëlis acuminata,* the principal zones obtained with solution A correspond in position, appearance, and intensity with those obtained with solution C.

Ash.   Carry out the procedure as described under "Determination of ash" (vol. 1, p. 161); not more than 60 mg/g.

Acid-insoluble ash.   Carry out the procedure as described under "Determination of acid-insoluble ash" (vol. 1, p. 161); not more than 30 mg/g.

Foreign matter.   Weigh about 200 g and spread it in a thin layer on a glass plate. Detect the foreign matter by eye or with the use of a 6× lens, separate it from the root, and weigh it; not more than 10 mg/g.

Assay.   Weigh accurately about 7.5 g of finely powdered test substance, transfer it to a dry flask, add 100 ml of ether R, and shake for 5 minutes. Add 5 ml of ammonia (~100 g/l) TS, shake frequently during 1 hour, add 5 ml of water, and shake vigorously; decant the ether layer into a dry flask, filtering through a plug of adsorbent cotton. Wash the residue with two quantities, each of 25 ml of ether R, decanting each portion and filtering through the same plug of adsorbent cotton. Remove most of the solvent from the combined ether extracts by distillation and the remainder by gentle warming with a current of air blown into the flask. Dissolve the residue in 5 ml of previously neutralized ethanol (~710 g/l) TS by warming on a water-bath, add 15 ml of hydrochloric acid (0.1 mol/l) VS and titrate the excess of acid with sodium hydroxide (0.1 mol/l) VS, using 0.5 ml of methyl red/methylthioninium chloride TS as indicator. Each ml of hydrochloric acid (0.1 mol/l) VS is equivalent to 24.03 mg of total alkaloids, calculated as emetine.

KALII CITRAS

Potassium citrate

Molecular formula. $C_6H_5K_3O_7,H_2O$

Relative molecular mass.   324.4

Graphic formula.

$$\begin{array}{c} CH_2COOK \\ | \\ HO-C-COOK \qquad \cdot\ H_2O \\ | \\ CH_2COOK \end{array}$$

Chemical name.   Tripotassium citrate monohydrate; tripotassium 2-hydroxy-1,2,3-propanetricarboxylate monohydrate; CAS Reg. No. 6100-05-6 (monohydrate).

Description.   Transparent crystals or a white, granular powder; odourless.

Solubility.   Freely soluble in water; practically insoluble in ethanol ($\sim$750 g/l) TS.

Category.   Systemic alkalinizing substance; component of oral rehydration salt mixtures.

Storage.   Potassium citrate should be kept in a tightly closed container.

Additional information.   Potassium citrate is deliquescent when exposed to moist air.

REQUIREMENTS

General requirement.   Potassium citrate contains not less than 99.0% and not more than 101.0% of $C_6H_5K_3O_7$, calculated with reference to the anhydrous substance.

Identity tests

A.   To a 0.1 g/ml solution add 2 ml of sodium hydroxide ($\sim$80 g/l) TS; it yields the reaction described under "General identification tests" as characteristic of potassium (vol. 1, p. 114).

B.   A 0.1 g/ml solution yields reaction A described under "General identification tests" as characteristic of citrates (vol. 1, p. 113).

Heavy metals. Use 1.0 g for the preparation of the test solution as described under "Limit test for heavy metals", Procedure 1 (vol. 1, p. 118); determine the heavy metals content according to Method A (vol. 1, p. 119); not more than 10 µg/g.

Sodium. Dissolve 1 g in 10 ml of water, add 6 ml of potassium antimonate TS, and allow to stand for 15 minutes; the solution is clear or any opalescence produced is not more pronounced than that of opalescence standard TS2.

Oxalates and tartrates. Dissolve 1 g in 4 ml of hydrochloric acid ($\sim$70 g/l) TS, add 4 ml of ethanol ($\sim$750 g/l) TS and 1.0 ml of calcium chloride (55 g/l) TS; the solution remains unchanged within 1 hour.

Clarity and colour of solution. A solution of 1.0 g in 10 ml of carbon-dioxide-free water R is clear and colourless.

Readily carbonizable substances. Dissolve 0.20 g in 10 ml of sulfuric acid ($\sim$1760 g/l) TS and heat on a water-bath at 80–90 °C for 1 hour; the solution is not more intensely coloured than standard colour solutions Yw5 or Gn6 when compared as described under "Colour of liquids" (vol. 1, p. 50).

Water. Determine as described under "Determination of water by the Karl Fischer method", Method A (vol. 1, p. 135), using about 0.5 g of the substance; stir and allow it to remain in contact with the dehydrated methanol R for 15 minutes, stir again for 1 minute, and then titrate; the water content is not less than 40 mg/g and not more than 70 mg/g.

Acidity or alkalinity. Dissolve 1 g in 10 ml of carbon-dioxide-free water R and add 0.1 ml of phenolphthalein/ethanol TS; not more than 0.2 ml of hydrochloric acid (0.1 mol/l) VS or 0.2 ml of sodium hydroxide (0.1 mol/l) VS is required to change the colour of the solution.

Assay. Dissolve about 0.15 g, accurately weighed, in 20 ml of glacial acetic acid R1, heat to about 50 °C, allow to cool to room temperature, add 0.25 ml of 1-naphtholbenzein/acetic acid TS, and titrate with perchloric acid (0.1 mol/l) VS until a green colour is obtained as described under "Non-aqueous titration", Method A (vol. 1, p. 131). Each ml of perchloric acid (0.1 mol/l) VS is equivalent to 10.21 mg of $C_6H_5K_3O_7$.

LEVONORGESTRELUM

Levonorgestrel

Molecular formula. $C_{21}H_{28}O_2$

Relative molecular mass.   312.5

Graphic formula.

Chemical name. $(-)$-13-Ethyl-17-hydroxy-18,19-dinor-17α-pregn-4-en-20-yn-3-one; CAS Reg. No. 797-63-7.

Description.   A white or almost white, crystalline powder; odourless.

Solubility.   Practically insoluble in water; soluble in chloroform R; slightly soluble in ethanol ($\sim$750 g/l) TS and ether R.

Category.   Contraceptive.

Storage.   Levonorgestrel should be kept in a well-closed container, protected from light.

REQUIREMENTS

General requirement.   Levonorgestrel contains not less than 98.0% and not more than 102.0% of $C_{21}H_{28}O_2$, calculated with reference to the dried substance.

Identity tests

● Either test A or tests B and C may be applied.

A.   Carry out the examination as described under "Spectrophotometry in the infrared region" (vol. 1, p. 40). The infrared absorption spectrum is concordant with the spectrum obtained from levonorgestrel RS or with the *reference spectrum* of levonorgestrel.

B.   See the test described below under "Related substances". The principal spot obtained with solution B corresponds in position, appearance, and intensity with that obtained with solution C.

C.   Melting temperature, about 236 °C.

Specific optical rotation.   Use a 10 mg/ml solution in chloroform R; $[\alpha]_D^{20\,°C} =$ -30.0 to $-35.0°$.

Sulfated ash.   Not more than 1.0 mg/g.

Loss on drying.   Dry to constant weight at 105 °C; it loses not more than 5.0 mg/g.

Acidity or alkalinity.   Dissolve 0.10 g in 30 ml of dehydrated ethanol R and add 0.5 ml of methyl red/ethanol TS; not more than 0.15 ml of sodium hydroxide (0.01 mol/l) VS is required to obtain a yellow colour and not more than 0.30 ml of hydrochloric acid (0.01 mol/l) VS is required to obtain a red colour.

Related substances.   Carry out the test as described under "Thin-layer chromatography" (vol. 1, p. 83), using silica gel R1 as the coating substance and a mixture of 8 volumes of chloroform R and 2 volumes of acetone R as the mobile phase. Apply separately to the plate 10 µl of each of 3 solutions in chloroform R containing (A) 10 mg of the test substance per ml, (B) 0.10 mg of the test substance per ml, and (C) 0.10 mg of levonorgestrel RS per ml. After removing the plate from the chromatographic chamber, allow it to dry in air until the solvents have evaporated, spray it with a mixture of 50 ml of methanol R and 10 ml of sulfuric acid ($\sim$1760 g/l) TS, and examine the chromatogram in ultraviolet light (365 nm). Any spot obtained with solution A, other than the principal spot, is not more intense than that obtained with solution B.

Ethynyl group.   Dissolve about 0.2 g, accurately weighed, in about 40 ml of tetrahydrofuran R. Add 10 ml of silver nitrate (100 g/l) TS and titrate with sodium hydroxide (0.1 mol/l) VS, determining the endpoint potentiometrically, using a glass and a calomel electrode that contains potassium nitrate solution as the electrolyte. Repeat the operation without the substance being examined and make any necessary corrections. Each ml of sodium hydroxide (0.1 mol/l) VS is equivalent to 2.503 mg of $-C \equiv CH$; the content of ethynyl group is not less than 78.1 mg per g and not more than 81.8 mg per g.

Assay.   Dissolve about 0.05 g, accurately weighed, in sufficient methanol R to produce 100 ml; dilute 2.0 ml of this solution to 100 ml with the same solvent. Measure the absorbance of a 1-cm layer of the diluted solution at the maximum at about 241 nm. Calculate the amount of $C_{21}H_{28}O_2$ in the substance being tested by comparison with levonorgestrel RS, similarly and concurrently examined. In an adequately calibrated spectrophotometer the absorbance of the reference solution should be 0.54 ± 0.03.

LEVOTHYROXINUM NATRICUM

Levothyroxine sodium

Molecular formula. $C_{15}H_{10}I_4NNaO_4$ (anhydrous); $C_{15}H_{10}I_4NNaO_4,H_2O$ (mono-hydrate).

Relative molecular mass.   798.9 (anhydrous); 816.9 (monohydrate).

Graphic formula.

Chemical name.   Monosodium L-thyroxine; monosodium O-(4-hydroxy-3,5-diiodophenyl)-3,5-diiodo-L-tyrosine; 3-[4-(4-hydroxy-3,5-diiodophenoxy)-3,5-diiodophenyl]-L-alanine monosodium salt; CAS Reg. No. 55-03-8 (anhydrous); Monosodium L-thyroxine monohydrate; monosodium O-(4-hydroxy-3,5-diiodophenyl)-3,5-diiodo-L-tyrosine monohydrate; 3-[4-(4-hydroxy-3,5-diiodophenoxy)-3,5-diiodophenyl]-L-alanine monosodium salt monohydrate; CAS Reg. No. 31178-59-3 (monohydrate).

Other name.   Thyroxine sodium.

Description.   An almost white or slightly coloured powder, or a fine, slightly coloured, crystalline powder; odourless.

Solubility.   Very slightly soluble in water; slightly soluble in ethanol ($\sim$750 g/l) TS; practically insoluble in acetone R, chloroform R, and ether R.   It dissolves in solutions of alkali hydroxides.

Category.   Thyroid hormone.

Storage.   Levothyroxine sodium should be kept in a tightly closed container, protected from light.

Additional information.   Levothyroxine sodium may contain a variable quantity of water of crystallization; anhydrous levothyroxine sodium is hygroscopic.

REQUIREMENTS

General requirement.   Levothyroxine sodium contains not less than 97.0% and not more than 101.0% of $C_{15}H_{10}I_4NNaO_4$, calculated with reference to the dried substance.

Identity tests

A.   Dissolve 5 mg in 2.0 ml of nitric acid ($\sim$130 g/l) TS and warm the solution; a brown to violet colour is produced. Cool, add 1.0 ml of chloroform R and shake; the colour of the chloroform layer turns violet.

B.   Dissolve 5 mg in a mixture of 2.0 ml of ethanol ($\sim$750 g/l) TS and about 0.2 ml of hydrochloric acid ($\sim$70 g/l) TS, add about 0.25 ml of sodium nitrite (10 g/l) TS and allow to stand for 15 minutes or heat for 2–3 minutes in a water-bath; a yellow solution is produced. Cool and add ammonia ($\sim$100 g/l) TS to make the solution alkaline; the colour changes to red.

C.   Examine the chromatograms obtained in the test for liothyronine (see below). The principal spot in the chromatogram obtained with solution A is similar in position, colour, and size to the principal spot in the chromatogram obtained with reference solution B.

D.   When tested for sodium as described under "General identification tests" (vol. 1, p. 155), yields the characteristic reactions. If reaction B is to be used, ignite 20 mg and dissolve the residue in acetic acid ($\sim$60 g/l) TS.

Specific optical rotation.   Dissolve 0.5 g in 22 ml of a gently boiling mixture of 1 volume of hydrochloric acid (1 mol/l) VS and 4 volumes of ethanol ($\sim$750 g/l) TS. Cool and dilute to 25 ml with the same mixture of solvents. Calculate with reference to the dried substance; $[\alpha]_D^{20\,^{\circ}C} = +\,16.0$ to $+\,20.0^{\circ}$.

Loss on drying.   Dry to constant weight at 105 °C; it loses not less than 60 mg/g and not more than 120 mg/g.

Liothyronine.   Carry out the test as described under "Thin-layer chromatography" (vol. 1, p. 83), using a plate coated with a mixture of 30 g of silica gel R3 and 60 ml of a solution containing 0.75 g of soluble starch R in 100 ml of water. Use the plate directly without heating. As the mobile phase use a mixture of 20 volumes of ammonia ($\sim$260 g/l) TS, 35 volumes of 2-propanol R, and 55 volumes of ethyl acetate R. For the preparation of the test and reference solutions, make up the following solvent mixture: to 5 volumes of ammonia ($\sim$260 g/l) TS add 70 volumes of methanol R and mix. For solution A, dissolve 0.10 g of the test substance in the solvent mixture to produce 5 ml of concentrated solution, then dilute 1.0 ml of this solution with the same solvent mixture to produce 2.0 ml of diluted solution. For solution B, dissolve 50 mg of levothyroxine sodium RS in the ammonia/methanol solvent mixture to produce 5 ml. For solution C, dissolve 5 mg of liothyronine RS in the ammonia/methanol solvent mixture to produce 25 ml of concentrated solution, then dilute 1.0 ml of this solution with the same solvent mixture to produce 2.0 ml of diluted solution. For solution D, mix 1.0 ml of the concentrated solution A with 1.0 ml of the concentrated solution C. Apply separately to the plate 5 µl of each of diluted solution A, solution B, diluted solution C, and solution D. After removing the plate from the chromatographic chamber, allow it to dry in air, spray it with ferric chloride/ferricyanide/arsenite TS, and examine the chromatogram in daylight. Any spot corresponding to liothyronine in the chromatogram obtained with solution A is not more intense than the spot in the chromatogram obtained with solution C. The test is not valid unless the chromatogram obtained with solution D shows two clearly separated spots.

Soluble halides. Shake 10 mg with 10 ml of water containing about 0.05 ml of nitric acid ($\sim$130 g/l) TS for 5 minutes and filter. Dilute the filtrate to 10 ml with water and add 0.15 ml of silver nitrate (40 g/l) TS; any opalescence produced is not more intense than that of a solution simultaneously prepared by adding 0.15 ml of silver nitrate (40 g/l) TS and 0.10 ml of hydrochloric acid (0.02 mol/l) VS to 10 ml of water (7 mg/g as chlorides).

Assay. Carry out the combustion as described under "Oxygen flask method" (vol. 1, p. 124), using about 25 mg of the test substance, accurately weighed, and 10 ml of sodium hydroxide (10 g/l) TS as the absorbing liquid. When the process is complete, proceed as described under the "Determination of iodine" (vol. 1, p. 125). Each ml of sodium thiosulfate (0.05 mol/l) VS is equivalent to 1.665 mg of $C_{15}H_{10}I_4NNaO_4$.

LOPERAMIDI HYDROCHLORIDUM

Loperamide hydrochloride

Molecular formula. $C_{29}H_{33}ClN_2O_2,HCl$

Relative molecular mass. 513.5

Graphic formula.

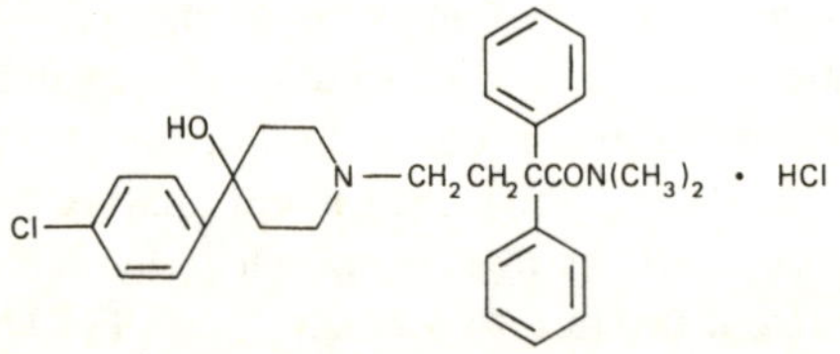

Chemical name. 4-(p-Chlorophenyl)-4-hydroxy-N,N-dimethyl-α,α-diphenyl-1-piperidinebutyramide monohydrochloride; 4-(4-chlorophenyl)-4-hydroxy-N,N-dimethyl-α,α-diphenyl-1-piperidinebutanamide monohydrochloride; CAS Reg. No. 34552-83-5.

Description. A white to slightly yellowish powder.

Solubility. Slightly soluble in water and in dilute acids; freely soluble in methanol R and chloroform R.

Category. Antidiarrhoeal drug.

Storage. Loperamide hydrochloride should be kept in a well-closed container.

REQUIREMENTS

General requirement. Loperamide hydrochloride contains not less than 98.0% and not more than 102.0% of $C_{29}H_{33}ClN_2O_2,HCl$, calculated with reference to the dried substance.

Identity tests

● Either tests A and D or tests B, C and D may be applied.

A. Carry out the examination as described under "Spectrophotometry in the infrared region" (vol. 1, p. 40). The infrared absorption spectrum is concordant with the spectrum obtained from loperamide hydrochloride RS or with the *reference spectrum* of loperamide hydrochloride.

B. Transfer about 0.04 g, accurately weighed, to a 100-ml volumetric flask, dissolve in about 50 ml of 2-propanol R, add 10 ml of hydrochloric acid (0.1 mol/l) VS and dilute to volume with 2-propanol R. The absorption spectrum of this solution against a solvent cell containing the same solvent mixture, when observed between 230 nm and 350 nm, is qualitatively similar to that of a solution of loperamide hydrochloride RS concurrently examined (maxima occur at about 253 nm, 259 nm, 265 nm, and 273 nm). The absorbances of the solutions at the respective maxima do not differ from each other by more than 3%.

C. Melting temperature, about 224 °C with decomposition.

D. A 10 mg/ml solution yields reaction A described under "General identification tests" as characteristic of chlorides (vol. 1, p. 112).

Sulfated ash. Not more than 2.0 mg/g.

Loss on drying. Dry at 80 °C under reduced pressure (not exceeding 0.6 kPa or about 5 mm of mercury) for 4 hours; it loses not more than 5.0 mg/g.

Related substances. Carry out the test as described under "Thin-layer chromatography" (vol. 1, p. 83), using silica gel R1 as the coating substance and a mixture of 85 volumes of chloroform R, 10 volumes of methanol R, and 5 volumes of formic acid (~1080 g/l) TS as the mobile phase. Apply separately to the plate 10 µl of each of 2 solutions in chloroform R containing (A) 10 mg of the test substance per ml and (B) 0.10 mg of the test substance per ml. After removing the plate from the chromatographic chamber, allow it to dry in air and expose it to iodine vapours. Examine the chromatogram in daylight. Any spot obtained with solution A, other than the principal spot, is not more intense than that obtained with solution B.

Assay. Dissolve about 0.38 g, accurately weighed, in 30 ml of glacial acetic acid R1, add 10 ml of mercuric acetate/acetic acid TS and 0.15 ml of 1-naphtholbenzein/acetic acid TS as indicator, and titrate with perchloric acid (0.1 mol/l) VS, as described under "Non-aqueous titration", Method A (vol. 1, p. 131). Each ml of perchloric acid (0.1 mol/l) VS is equivalent to 51.35 mg of $C_{29}H_{33}ClN_2O_2,HCl$.

MAGNESII HYDROXIDUM

Magnesium hydroxide

Molecular formula.　$Mg(OH)_2$

Relative molecular mass.　58.32

Chemical name.　Magnesium hydroxide; CAS Reg. No. 1309-42-8.

Description.　A white, fine, amorphous powder; odourless.

Solubility.　Practically insoluble in water and ethanol ($\sim$750 g/l) TS; soluble in dilute acids.

Category.　Antacid.

Storage.　Magnesium hydroxide should be kept in a tightly closed container.

REQUIREMENTS

General requirement.　Magnesium hydroxide contains not less than 95.0% and not more than 100.5% of $Mg(OH)_2$, calculated with reference to the dried substance.

Identity tests

A.　Dissolve 10 mg in 1.0 ml of hydrochloric acid ($\sim$70 g/l) TS, add 1.0 ml of ammonium chloride (100 g/l) TS, 0.5 ml of disodium hydrogen phosphate (100 g/l) TS, and 1.0 ml of ammonia ($\sim$100 g/l) TS; a white, crystalline precipitate is formed, which is soluble in acetic acid ($\sim$300 g/l) TS.

B.   Dissolve 10 mg in 1.0 ml of hydrochloric acid ($\sim$70 g/l) TS, and add 2.0 ml of sodium hydroxide ($\sim$80 g/l) TS; a white, gelatinous precipitate is produced, which is insoluble in an excess of sodium hydroxide ($\sim$80 g/l) TS.   Add a few drops of iodine TS; the precipitate turns dark brown.

Heavy metals.   Dissolve 1.0 g in 15 ml of hydrochloric acid ($\sim$250 g/l) TS and shake with 25 ml of methylisobutylketone R for 2 minutes.   Allow to stand, separate the layers, and evaporate the aqueous layer to dryness.   Dissolve the residue in 15 ml of water and proceed as described under "Limit test for heavy metals", Procedure 1 (vol. 1, p. 118); determine the heavy metals content according to Method A (vol. 1, p. 119); not more than 30 µg/g.

Arsenic.   Use a solution of 3.3 g in 20 ml of sulfuric acid ($\sim$100 g/l) TS and 35 ml of water and proceed as described under "Limit test for arsenic" (vol. 1, p. 122); the arsenic content is not more than 3 µg/g.

Calcium.   Dissolve 5.0 g in a mixture of 50 ml of acetic acid ($\sim$300 g/l) TS and 50 ml of water, boil for 2 minutes, cool, and dilute to 100 ml with acetic acid ($\sim$120 g/l) TS.   Filter, if necessary, through a previously ignited and tared porcelain or silica filter crucible of suitable porosity to give a clear filtrate.   Dilute 1.3 ml of the filtrate to 150 ml with water (retain the filter for the test of substances insoluble in acetic acid).   To 0.20 ml of ethanolic calcium standard (100 µg/ml Ca) TS add 0.8 ml of ammonium oxalate (50 g/l) TS.   After 1 minute add 1 ml of acetic acid ($\sim$120 g/l) TS and 15 ml of the diluted filtrate prepared above.

Prepare similarly a standard solution using a mixture of 10 ml of calcium standard (10 µg/ml Ca) TS and 5 ml of water.

After 15 minutes any opalescence produced in the test solution is not more intense than that in the standard (15 mg/g).

Iron.   Dissolve 0.15 g in 5 ml of hydrochloric acid ($\sim$70 g/l) TS and dilute to 10 ml with water.   Proceed with 4.0 ml of the resulting solution as described under "Limit test for iron" (vol. 1, p. 121); not more than 700 µg/g.

Water-soluble substances.   Mix 2.0 g with 100 ml of water and boil for 5 minutes. Filter while still hot, allow to cool, and dilute to 100 ml with water.   Evaporate 50 ml of the filtrate to dryness and dry at 105 °C to constant weight; the residue weighs not more than 20 mg.

Substances insoluble in acetic acid.   Any residue remaining on the filter used in the preparation of the solution to be examined in the limit test for calcium, when washed with water, dried and ignited at 600 °C, weighs not more than 5 mg.

Loss on ignition.   Heat 0.5 g gradually to 900 °C and ignite to constant mass; it loses not less than 0.300 g/g and not more than 0.325 g/g.

Loss on drying.   Dry to constant weight at 105 °C; it loses not more than 0.33 g/g.

Assay.   Dissolve about 0.05 g, accurately weighed, in 2 ml of hydrochloric acid ($\sim$70 g/l) TS and proceed with the titration as described under "Complexometric titrations" for magnesium (vol. 1, p. 129).   Each ml of disodium edetate (0.05 mol/l) VS is equivalent to 2.916 mg of $Mg(OH)_2$.

MAGNESII OXIDUM

Magnesium oxide

Light Magnesium oxide
Heavy Magnesium oxide

Molecular formula.   MgO

Relative molecular mass.   40.30

Chemical name.   Magnesium oxide; CAS Reg. No. 1309-48-4.

Description.   A white powder; odourless.   Light Magnesium oxide is very bulky, whereas heavy Magnesium oxide is a dense powder.

Solubility.   Practically insoluble in water and ethanol ($\sim$750 g/l) TS; soluble in dilute acids.

Category.   Antacid.

Storage.   Magnesium oxide should be kept in a tightly closed container.

Labelling.   The designation on the container should state whether it is light Magnesium oxide or heavy Magnesium oxide.

REQUIREMENTS

General requirement.   Magnesium oxide contains not less than 98.0% and not more than 100.5% of MgO, calculated with reference to the ignited substance.

Identity tests

A.   Dissolve 10 mg in 1.0 ml of hydrochloric acid ($\sim$70 g/l) TS, add 1.0 ml of ammonium chloride (100 g/l) TS, 0.5 ml of disodium hydrogen phosphate (100 g/l) TS, and 1.0 ml of ammonia ($\sim$100 g/l) TS; a white, crystalline precipitate is formed, which is soluble in acetic acid ($\sim$300 g/l) TS.

B.   Dissolve 10 mg in 1.0 ml of hydrochloric acid ($\sim$70 g/l) TS, and add 2.0 ml of sodium hydroxide ($\sim$80 g/l) TS; a white, gelatinous precipitate is produced, which is insoluble in an excess of sodium hydroxide ($\sim$80 g/l) TS. Add a few drops of iodine TS; the precipitate turns dark brown.

Heavy metals.   Dissolve 5.0 g in a mixture of 70 ml of acetic acid ($\sim$300 g/l) TS and 30 ml of water, boil for 2 minutes, cool, and dilute to 100 ml with acetic acid ($\sim$120 g/l) TS. Filter, if necessary, through a previously ignited and tared porcelain or silica filter crucible of suitable porosity to give a clear filtrate. To 20 ml of the filtrate (retain the filter for the test of substances insoluble in acetic acid and the remaining filtrate for the limit test for calcium) add 15 ml of hydrochloric acid ($\sim$250 g/l) TS and shake with 25 ml of methylisobutylketone R for 2 minutes. Allow to stand, separate the layers, and evaporate the aqueous layer to dryness. Dissolve the residue in 1 ml of acetic acid ($\sim$300 g/l) TS and dilute to 40 ml with water and mix. Determine the heavy metals content as described under "Limit test for heavy metals", according to Method A (vol. 1, p. 119); not more than 40 µg/g.

Arsenic.   Use a solution of 3.3 g in 20 ml of sulfuric acid ($\sim$100 g/l) TS and 35 ml of water and proceed as described under "Limit test for arsenic" (vol. 1, p. 122); the arsenic content is not more than 3 µg/g.

Barium.   To 0.10 g add a few drops of hydrochloric acid ($\sim$250 g/l) TS and dissolve in 20 ml of water. Add 0.10 ml of sulfuric acid ($\sim$100 g/l) TS and shake; no precipitate is produced within 10 minutes.

Calcium.   Dilute 1.3 ml of the filtrate obtained in the test for heavy metals to 150 ml with water.
    To 0.20 ml of ethanolic calcium standard (100 µg/ml Ca) TS add 0.8 ml of ammonium oxalate (50 g/l) TS. After 1 minute add 1 ml of acetic acid ($\sim$120 g/l) TS and 15 ml of the diluted filtrate prepared above.
    Prepare similarly a standard solution using a mixture of 10 ml of calcium standard (10 µg/ml Ca) TS and 5 ml of water. After 15 minutes, any opalescence produced in the test solution is not more intense than that in the standard (15 mg/g).

Iron.   Dissolve 0.15 g in 5 ml of hydrochloric acid ($\sim$70 g/l) TS and dilute to 10 ml with water. Proceed with 4.0 ml of the resulting solution as described under "Limit test for iron" (vol. 1, p. 122); not more than 500 µg/g.

Water-soluble substances.   Mix 2.0 g with 100 ml of water and boil for 5 minutes. While still hot filter through a coarse sintered-glass filter, allow to cool, and dilute to 100 ml with water. Evaporate 50 ml of the filtrate to dryness and dry at 105 °C to constant weight; the residue weighs not more than 20 mg.

Substances insoluble in acetic acid.   Any residue remaining on the filter used in the preparation of the solution to be examined in the test for heavy metals, when washed with water, dried, and ignited at 600 °C, weighs not more than 5 mg.

Loss on ignition.   Ignite 1.0 g at 900 °C to constant weight; it loses not more than 100 mg/g.

Assay.   Dissolve about 0.35 g, accurately weighed, in 20 ml of hydrochloric acid (~70 g/l) TS and proceed with the titration as described under "Complexometric titrations" for magnesium (vol. 1, p. 129).   Each ml of disodium edetate (0.05 mol/l) VS is equivalent to 2.015 mg of MgO.

MEBENDAZOLUM

Mebendazole

Molecular formula. $C_{16}H_{13}N_3O_3$

Relative molecular mass.   295.3

Graphic formula.

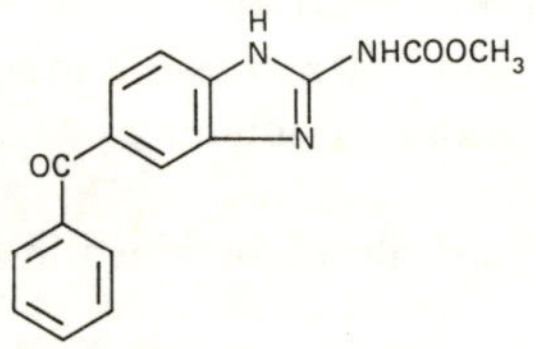

Chemical name.   Methyl 5-benzoyl-2-benzimidazolecarbamate; methyl (5-benzoyl-1*H*-benzimidazol-2-yl)carbamate; CAS Reg. No. 31431-39-7.

Description.   A white to slightly yellow powder.

Solubility.   Practically insoluble in water, dilute mineral acids, ethanol (~750 g/l) TS, ether R, and chloroform R; freely soluble in formic acid (~1080 g/l) TS.

Category.   Anthelmintic drug.

Storage.   Mebendazole should be kept in a well-closed container, protected from light.

REQUIREMENTS

General requirement.   Mebendazole contains not less than 98.0% and not more than 102.0% of $C_{16}H_{13}N_3O_3$, calculated with reference to the dried substance.

Identity tests

● Either test A alone or tests B and C may be applied.

A.   Carry out the examination as described under "Spectrophotometry in the infrared region" (vol. 1, p. 40). The infrared absorption spectrum is concordant with the spectrum obtained from mebendazole RS or with the *reference spectrum* of mebendazole.

B.   Shake 20 mg with 2.0 ml of sodium hydroxide (~80 g/l) TS, and heat the yellowish coloured suspension until it dissolves; the solution is yellow. Add a few drops of copper(II) sulfate (160 g/l) TS; a greenish precipitate is produced. Add a few drops of ammonia (~100 g/l) TS; the colour turns to greenish blue.

C.   Dissolve 20 mg in 2 ml of sulfuric acid (~1760 g/l) TS; a yellow solution is produced. Carefully dilute with 3 ml of water; the yellow colour disappears. Then add 1.0 ml of silver nitrate (40 g/l) TS; a white precipitate is formed, which does not dissolve in an excess of ammonia (~100 g/l) TS.

Heavy metals.   Use 1.0 g for the preparation of the test solution as described under "Limit test for heavy metals", Procedure 3 (vol. 1, p. 118); determine the heavy metals content according to Method A (vol. 1, p. 119); not more than 20 µg/g.

Sulfated ash.   Not more than 1.0 mg/g.

Loss on drying.   Dry at 105 °C under reduced pressure (not exceeding 0.6 kPa or about 5 mm of mercury) for 4 hours; it loses not more than 5.0 mg/g.

Related substances.   Carry out the test as described under "Thin-layer chromatography" (vol. 1, p. 83), using silica gel R6 (a precoated plate from a commercial source is suitable) as the coating substance and a mixture of 90 volumes of chloroform R, 5 volumes of methanol R, and 5 volumes of formic acid (~1080 g/l) TS as the mobile phase. Apply separately to the plate 10 µl of each of 2 solutions prepared as follows: (A) Dissolve 50 mg of the test substance in 1.0 ml of formic acid (~1080 g/l) TS in a 10-ml volumetric flask, dilute to volume with chloroform R, and mix; (B) Dilute 1.0 ml of solution A to 200 ml with a mixture of 9 volumes of chloroform R and 1 volume of formic acid (~1080 g/l) TS. After removing the plate from the chromatographic chamber, allow it to dry in air and examine the chromatogram in ultraviolet light (254 nm). Any spot obtained with solution A, other than the principal spot, is no larger or more intense than the main spot obtained with solution B.

Assay.   Dissolve about 0.22 g, accurately weighed, in 30 ml of glacial acetic acid R1, and titrate with perchloric acid (0.1 mol/l) VS, determining the endpoint potentiometrically as described under "Non-aqueous titration", Method A (vol. 1, p. 131). Each ml of perchloric acid (0.1 mol/l) VS is equivalent to 29.53 mg of $C_{16}H_{13}N_3O_3$.

METHOTREXATUM

Methotrexate

Molecular formula. $C_{20}H_{22}N_8O_5$

Relative molecular mass.   454.4

Graphic formula.

Chemical name.   (+)-N-[p-[[(2,4-Diamino-6-pteridinyl)methyl]methylamino]benzoyl]-L-glutamic acid; N-[4-[[(2,4-diamino-6-pteridinyl)methyl]methylamino]benzoyl]-L-glutamic acid; CAS Reg. No. 59-05-2.

Description.   A yellow to orange, crystalline powder.

Solubility.   Practically insoluble in water, ethanol ($\sim$750 g/l) TS, dichloroethane R, and ether R; very soluble in diluted solutions of alkali hydroxides and carbonates.

Category.   Cytotoxic drug.

Storage.   Methotrexate should be kept in a tightly closed container, protected from light.

Additional information.   Methotrexate is gradually affected by light.
CAUTION: Methotrexate must be handled with care, avoiding contact with the skin and inhalation of airborne particles.

REQUIREMENTS

General requirement.   Methotrexate contains not less than 96.0% and not more than 102.0% of $C_{20}H_{22}N_8O_5$, calculated with reference to the anhydrous substance.

Identity tests

A.   Carry out the examination as described under "Spectrophotometry in the infrared region" (vol. 1, p. 40). The infrared absorption spectrum is concordant with the spectrum obtained from methotrexate RS or with the *reference spectrum* of methotrexate.

B.   The absorption spectrum of a 10.0 µg/ml solution in sodium hydroxide (0.1 mol/l) VS, when observed between 230 nm and 380 nm, exhibits 3 maxima at about 258 nm, 303 nm, and 371 nm. The ratio of the absorbance at 303 nm to that at 371 nm is between 2.8 and 3.3.

Specific optical rotation.   Dissolve 0.25 g in 12 ml of sodium carbonate (10 g/l) TS, dilute with water to 25 ml, and calculate the result with reference to the anhydrous substance; $[a]_D^{20\,°C} = + 19$ to $+ 24°$.

Sulfated ash.   Not more than 1.0 mg/g.

Water.   Determine as described under "Determination of water by the Karl Fischer method", Method A (vol. 1, p. 135), using about 0.5 g of the substance; the water content is not more than 120 mg/g.

Assay.   Carry out the test as described on pp. 373–377 of the Amendments to vol. 1 under "High performance liquid chromatography", using a column 10 cm long and 6 mm in internal diameter packed with silica gel, 5 µm in diameter, the surface of which has been modified with chemically bonded octadecyl silyl groups.

As the mobile phase, use a mixture of 8 volumes of acetonitrile R with 92 volumes of phosphate/citrate buffer pH 6.0, TS.

Prepare the following solutions in the above-mentioned mobile phase containing (A) 0.10 mg of the test substance per ml, (B) 0.10 mg of methotrexate RS per ml, and (C) 0.10 mg of methotrexate RS and 0.10 mg of folic acid RS per ml for the system suitability test.

Operate at room temperature with a flow rate of about 1.4 ml per minute. As a detector use an ultraviolet spectrophotometer at a wavelength of about 303 nm, fitted with a low-volume flow cell (10 µl is suitable), and a suitable recorder.

Make 6 replicate injections of solution C, each of 20 µl. The resolution factor between methotrexate and folic acid should be not less than 5.0, with a relative standard deviation for the methotrexate peak of not more than 2.5% (adjust the flow rate and the ratio of the mobile phase if it does not conform).

Inject 20 µl of each of solutions A and B. Measure the peak responses and calculate the content in % of $C_{20}H_{22}N_8O_5$ using the following formula: $100(A_1M_2T)/(A_2M_1)$, in which A_1 and A_2 are the peak responses of the test substance and the reference substance, respectively, and M_1 and M_2 are the concentrations of the test solution and the reference solution, respectively, and T corresponds to the degree of purity of methotrexate RS.

METHYLTHIONINII CHLORIDUM

Methylthioninium chloride

Molecular formula. $C_{16}H_{18}ClN_3S$ (anhydrous); $C_{16}H_{18}ClN_3S,3H_2O$ (trihydrate).

Relative molecular mass.   319.9 (anhydrous); 373.9 (trihydrate).

Graphic formula.

$$\left[(CH_3)_2N-\!\!\!\underset{S}{\overset{N}{\bigcirc\!\!\!\bigcirc}}\!\!\!-N(CH_3)_2 \right] Cl^- \cdot\ nH_2O$$

n = 0 (anhydrous)
n = 3 (trihydrate)

Chemical name.   C.I. Basic Blue 9; 3,7-bis(dimethylamino)phenothiazin-5-ium chloride; CAS Reg. No. 61-73-4 (anhydrous).
C.I. Basic Blue 9 trihydrate; 3,7-bis(dimethylamino)phenothiazin-5-ium chloride trihydrate; CAS Reg. No. 7220-79-3 (trihydrate).

Other name.   Methylene blue.

Description.   Dark green crystals with a metallic lustre or a dark green, crystalline powder; odourless or almost odourless.

Solubility.   Sparingly soluble in water; slightly soluble in ethanol ($\sim$750 g/l) TS and chloroform R; practically insoluble in ether R.

Category.   Antidote.

Storage.   Methylthioninium chloride should be kept in a tightly closed container, protected from light.

Additional information.   Methylthioninium chloride is hygroscopic.

REQUIREMENTS

General requirement.   Methylthioninium chloride contains not less than 97.0% and not more than 101.0% of $C_{16}H_{18}ClN_3S$, calculated with reference to the dried substance.

Identity tests

A.   The absorption spectrum of a 5 μg/ml solution in hydrochloric acid ($\sim$70 g/l) TS, when observed between 230 nm and 800 nm, exhibits 4 maxima at about 258 nm, 288 nm, 680 nm, and 745 nm.

B.   Dissolve 1 mg in 10 ml of water; a deep blue colour is produced. Add 2.0 ml of hydrochloric acid ($\sim$70 g/l) TS and 0.25 g of zinc R powder; the colour of the solution is discharged; filter and expose the filtrate to the air; the blue colour of the solution reappears.

C.   Mix 0.05 g with 0.5 g of anhydrous sodium carbonate R in a porcelain crucible. Carefully heat the mixture to a red glow for 10 minutes. Cool, dissolve the residue in 10 ml of nitric acid ($\sim$130 g/l) TS and filter. The filtrate yields reaction A described under "General identification tests" as characteristic of chlorides (vol. 1, p. 112).

Copper or zinc.   Ignite 1.0 g in a porcelain crucible using as low a temperature as practicable, until all of the carbon is oxidized. Cool the residue, add 15 ml of nitric acid ($\sim$130 g/l) TS and boil for 5 minutes. Separately prepare a reference solution by boiling a quantity of copper(II) sulfate R, equivalent to 200 µg of Cu, with 15 ml of nitric acid ($\sim$130 g/l) TS for 5 minutes. Filter separately the cooled test and reference solutions, and wash any residue with 10 ml of water. Combine the filtrate and washings of the test solution and similarly combine the filtrate and washings of the reference solution; add to each an excess of ammonia ($\sim$100 g/l) TS and filter the solutions into 50-ml volumetric flasks. Wash the precipitates with small portions of water, adding the washings to the filtrates; dilute the contents of each flask with water to volume, mixing thoroughly. To 25 ml of each of the solutions add 10 ml of hydrogen sulfide TS; no turbidity is produced within 5 minutes (absence of zinc) and any dark colour produced in the test solution is not more intense than that of the reference solution (the copper content is not more than 0.20 mg/g).

Iron.   Mix 4 g with 200 ml of water in a long-necked, round-bottomed flask, add 15 ml of nitric acid ($\sim$1000 g/l) TS, bring gently to the boil and continue boiling until the volume of liquid is reduced to about 20 ml. Allow to cool, add 10 ml of sulfuric acid ($\sim$1760 g/l) TS and mix. Heat to boiling and add small successive quantities of nitric acid ($\sim$1000 g/l) TS, cooling before each addition, until a colourless liquid is obtained. Heat until white fumes are evolved; if darkening occurs at this stage continue the treatment with nitric acid ($\sim$1000 g/l) TS, finally heating until white fumes are again evolved. Allow the colourless liquid to cool, add 25 ml of a saturated solution of ammonium oxalate R in water, and boil until the slight froth completely subsides. Cool, dilute to 50 ml with water; 5 ml of the diluted solution complies with the "Limit test for iron" (vol. 1, p. 121); not more than 0.10 mg/g.

Sulfated ash.   Not more than 10 mg/g.

Loss on drying.   Dry to constant weight at 105 °C; it loses not less than 80 mg/g and not more than 220 mg/g.

Foreign dyes.   Carry out the test as described under "Thin-layer chromatography" (vol. 1, p. 83), using as the coating substance a slurry prepared from silica gel

R1 and a mixture of equal volumes of potassium dihydrogen phosphate (27.2 g/l) TS and disodium hydrogen phosphate (28.4 g/l) TS. As the mobile phase, use a mixture of 20 volumes of 1-propanol R, 4 volumes of anhydrous formic acid R, and 1 volume of water. Apply to the plate 2 µl of a solution prepared by dissolving 25 mg of the test substance in sufficient methanol R to produce 10 ml. After removing the plate from the chromatographic chamber, allow it to dry in an oven at 105 °C. At an R_f value of about 0.5, 3–4 spots appear, placed very close to each other, the lowest spot being violet in colour and the others red, the intensity of the colour increasing in ascending order of the spots. No other spot is detected.

Assay. Transfer about 0.3 g, accurately weighed, to a 100-ml volumetric flask, dissolve in 30 ml of water by warming on a water-bath, and allow the solution to cool. While shaking, add 50.0 ml of potassium dichromate (0.0167 mol/1) VS, dilute to volume with water, and mix. Repeat the shaking intermittently for 10 minutes, and filter; discard the first 20 ml of the filtrate. Transfer 50.0 ml of the filtrate to a glass-stoppered flask, add 40 ml of sulfuric acid (~190 g/l) TS and 1 g of potassium iodide R, mix, and allow the closed flask to stand in the dark for 5 minutes. Add 100 ml of water and titrate with sodium thiosulfate (0.1 mol/l) VS, using starch TS as indicator, until a blue-green colour is obtained. Repeat the operation without the substance being examined and make any necessary corrections. Each ml of potassium dichromate (0.0167 mol/l) VS is equivalent to 10.66 mg of $C_{16}H_{18}ClN_3S$.

METOCLOPRAMIDI HYDROCHLORIDUM

Metoclopramide hydrochloride

Molecular formula. $C_{14}H_{22}ClN_3O_2,HCl,H_2O$

Relative molecular mass. 354.3

Graphic formula.

Chemical name. 4-Amino-5-chloro-*N*-[2-(diethylamino)ethyl]-*o*-anisamide monohydrochloride monohydrate; 4-amino-5-chloro-*N*-[2-(diethylamino)-ethyl]-2-methoxybenzamide monohydrochloride monohydrate; CAS Reg. No. 54143-57-6 (monohydrate).

Description.　A white or almost white, crystalline powder; odourless or almost odourless.

Solubility.　Very soluble in water; freely soluble in ethanol ($\sim$750 g/l) TS; sparingly soluble in chloroform R; practically insoluble in ether R.

Category.　Antiemetic drug.

Storage.　Metoclopramide hydrochloride should be kept in a well-closed container, protected from light.

REQUIREMENTS

General requirement.　Metoclopramide hydrochloride contains not less than 98.0% and not more than 101.0% of $C_{14}H_{22}ClN_3O_2,HCl$, calculated with reference to the anhydrous substance.

Identity tests

● Either tests A and D or tests B, C and D may be applied.

A.　Carry out the examination as described under "Spectrophotometry in the infrared region" (vol. 1, p. 40). The infrared absorption spectrum is concordant with the spectrum obtained from metoclopramide hydrochloride RS or with the *reference spectrum* of metoclopramide hydrochloride.

B.　The absorption spectrum of a 20 µg/ml solution in hydrochloric acid (0.01 mol/l) VS, when observed between 230 nm and 350 nm, exhibits maxima at about 273 nm and 309 nm; the absorbances of a 1-cm layer at these wavelengths are about 0.79 and 0.69, respectively.

C.　Dissolve 0.05 g in 5 ml of water and add 5 ml of 4-dimethylaminobenzaldehyde TS5; a yellow-orange colour is produced.

D.　A 20 mg/ml solution yields reaction A described under "General identification tests" as characteristic of chlorides (vol. 1, p. 112).

Clarity and colour of solution.　A solution of 1.0 g in 10 ml of carbon-dioxide-free water R is clear and not more intensely coloured than standard colour solution Yw3 when compared as described under "Colour of liquids" (vol. 1, p. 50).

Sulfated ash.　Not more than 1.0 mg/g.

Water.　Determine as described under "Determination of water by the Karl Fischer Method", Method A (vol. 1, p. 135), using about 0.5 g of the substance; the water content is not less than 45 mg/g and not more than 55 mg/g.

pH value.　pH of a 0.10 g/ml solution in carbon-dioxide-free water R, 4.5–6.5.

Related substances.   Carry out the test as described under "Thin-layer chromatography" (vol. 1, p. 83), using silica gel R4 as the coating substance and a mixture of 95 volumes of 1-butanol R and 5 volumes of ammonia (~260 g/l) TS as the mobile phase.   Apply separately to the plate 5 µl of each of 2 solutions in methanol R containing (A) 50 mg of the test substance per ml and (B) 0.50 mg of the test substance per ml.   After removing the plate from the chromatographic chamber, allow it to dry in air, and examine the chromatogram in ultraviolet light (254 nm). Any spot obtained with solution A, other than the principal spot, is not more intense than that obtained with solution B.

Assay.   Dissolve about 0.3 g, accurately weighed, in 80 ml of acetic anhydride R, add 10 ml of mercuric acetate/acetic acid TS and titrate with perchloric acid (0.1 mol/l) VS, determining the endpoint potentiometrically as described under "Non-aqueous titration", Method A (vol. 1, p. 131).   Each ml of perchloric acid (0.1 mol/l) VS is equivalent to 33.63 mg of $C_{14}H_{22}ClN_3O_2,HCl$.

METRIFONATUM

Metrifonate

Molecular formula. $C_4H_8Cl_3O_4P$

Relative molecular mass.   257.4

Graphic formula.

$$\text{Cl}-\underset{\underset{\text{Cl}}{|}}{\overset{\overset{\text{Cl}}{|}}{\text{C}}}-\underset{\underset{\text{OH}}{|}}{\overset{\overset{\text{H}}{|}}{\text{C}}}-\text{PO}\begin{smallmatrix}\nearrow\text{OCH}_3\\[2pt]\searrow\text{OCH}_3\end{smallmatrix}$$

Chemical name.   Dimethyl (2,2,2-trichloro-1-hydroxyethyl)phosphonate; CAS Reg. No. 52-68-6.

Description.   A white or yellowish white, crystalline powder.

Solubility.   Sparingly soluble in water; very soluble in ethanol (~750 g/l) TS and acetone R.

Category.   Antischistosomal drug.

Storage.   Metrifonate should be kept in a tightly closed container, protected from light.

Additional information.   Even in the absence of light, Metrifonate is gradually degraded on exposure to a humid atmosphere, the decomposition being faster at higher temperatures. CAUTION: Metrifonate must be handled with care, avoiding contact with the skin and inhalation of airborne particles.

REQUIREMENTS

General requirement.   Metrifonate contains not less than 95.0% and not more than 101.0% of $C_4H_8Cl_3O_4P$, calculated with reference to the anhydrous substance.

Identity tests

A.   In a porcelain crucible mix 0.1 g with 0.2 g of a mixture composed of equal parts of potassium nitrate R and anhydrous sodium carbonate R, heat it carefully to a red glow for 3 minutes, cool the residue, and dissolve it in a mixture of 7 ml of water and 3 ml of nitric acid ($\sim$1000 g/l) TS. Keep 2 ml of this solution for test B. To 5 ml add 2 ml of ammonium molybdate (95 g/l) TS and heat to boiling; a yellow, crystalline precipitate is produced.

B.   To 2 ml of the solution kept in test A add 1 ml of silver nitrate (0.1 mol/l) VS; a white precipitate is produced, which is soluble in 3 ml of ammonia ($\sim$100 g/l) TS.

Congealing temperature.   Melt 6.2 g in a water-bath at 85 °C, add 2 g of calcium sulfate R, heat again to 80 °C, and proceed as described under "Determination of congealing point" (vol. 1, p. 24); not below 73.5 °C.

Acetone-insoluble matter.   Shake 1.0 g with 20 ml of acetone R for 15 minutes, filter, wash the filter with 10 ml of acetone R and dry it at 105 °C for 1 hour; the content of insoluble matter is not more than 5.0 mg/g.

Sulfated ash.   Not more than 3.0 mg/g.

Water.   Determine as described under "Determination of water by the Karl Fischer method", Method A (vol. 1, p. 135), using about 1 g of the substance; the water content is not more than 7.5 mg/g.

pH value.   pH of a 5.0 mg/ml solution, 2.0–3.5.

Assay.   Dissolve about 1.0 g, accurately weighed, in 90 ml of methanol R. Add 10 ml of monoethanolamine R and allow the solution to stand at 20 °C ± 0.5 °C for 1 hour. Then cool it in an ice-bath for 10 minutes, add 20 ml of nitric acid ($\sim$1000 g/l) TS, and titrate at 20 °C with silver nitrate (0.1 mol/l) VS, determining the endpoint potentiometrically using a platinum electrode and a calomel reference electrode. Each ml of silver nitrate (0.1 mol/l) VS is equivalent to 25.74 mg of $C_4H_8Cl_3O_4P$.

MICONAZOLI NITRAS

Miconazole nitrate

Molecular formula. $C_{18}H_{14}Cl_4N_2O,HNO_3$

Relative molecular mass. 479.2

Graphic formula.

$$CH_2 - CH - O - CH_2$$

· HNO_3

Chemical name. 1-[2,4-Dichloro-β-[(2,4-dichlorobenzyl)oxy]-phenethyl]imidazole mononitrate; 1-[2-(2,4-dichlorophenyl)-2-[(2,4-dichlorophenyl)methoxy]-ethyl]-1*H*-imidazole mononitrate; CAS Reg. No. 22832-87-7.

Description. A white or almost white, crystalline powder; odourless or almost odourless.

Solubility. Very slightly soluble in water and ether R; soluble in 140 parts of ethanol ($\sim$750 g/l) TS; slightly soluble in chloroform R.

Category. Antifungal drug.

Storage. Miconazole nitrate should be kept in a well-closed container, protected from light.

Additional information. Miconazole nitrate melts at about 182 °C with decomposition.

REQUIREMENTS

General requirement. Miconazole nitrate contains not less than 98.5% and not more than 101.5% of $C_{18}H_{14}Cl_4N_2O,HNO_3$, calculated with reference to the dried substance.

Identity tests

● Either test A alone or tests B and C may be applied.

A. Carry out the examination as described under "Spectrophotometry in the infrared region" (vol. 1, p. 40). The infrared absorption spectrum is concordant with the spectrum obtained from miconazole nitrate RS or with the *reference spectrum* of miconazole nitrate.

B.   The absorption spectrum of a 0.40 mg/ml solution in a mixture of 9 volumes of methanol R and 1 volume of hydrochloric acid (0.1 mol/l) VS, when observed between 230 nm and 350 nm, exhibits maxima at about 264 nm, 272 nm, and 280 nm; the absorbances of a 1-cm layer at these wavelengths are about 0.40, 0.58, and 0.48, respectively.

C.   Shake 10 mg with 5 ml of water and cool in an ice-bath. Keeping the suspension cool throughout, add 0.4 ml of potassium chloride (100 g/l) TS, 0.1 ml of diphenylamine/sulfuric acid TS, and, drop by drop with shaking, 5 ml of sulfuric acid ($\sim$1760 g/l) TS; an intense blue colour is produced.

Sulfated ash.   Not more than 2.0 mg/g.

Loss on drying.   Dry to constant weight at 100 °C under reduced pressure (not exceeding 0.6 kPa or about 5 mm of mercury); it loses not more than 5.0 mg/g.

Related substances.   Carry out the test as described under "Thin-layer chromatography" (vol. 1, p. 83), using silica gel R1 as the coating substance and a mixture of 60 volumes of hexane R, 30 volumes of chloroform R, 10 volumes of methanol R, and 1 volume of ammonia ($\sim$260 g/l) TS as the mobile phase. Apply separately to the plate 50 µl of each of 2 solutions in a mixture of equal volumes of chloroform R and methanol R containing (A) 10 mg of the test substance per ml and (B) 25 µg of the test substance per ml. After removing the plate from the chromatographic chamber, allow it to dry in air, spray it with iodine/chloroform TS, and examine the chromatogram in daylight. Any spot obtained with solution A, other than the principal spot, is not more intense than that obtained with solution B.

Assay.   Dissolve about 0.35 g, accurately weighed, in 50 ml of glacial acetic acid R1 and titrate with perchloric acid (0.1 mol/l) VS, determining the endpoint potentiometrically as described under "Non-aqueous titration", Method A (vol. 1, p. 131). Each ml of perchloric acid (0.1 mol/l) VS is equivalent to 47.92 mg of $C_{18}H_{14}Cl_4N_2O,HNO_3$.

NALOXONI HYDROCHLORIDUM

Naloxone hydrochloride

Naloxone hydrochloride, anhydrous
Naloxone hydrochloride, dihydrate

Molecular formula. $C_{19}H_{21}NO_4$,HCl (anhydrous); $C_{19}H_{21}NO_4$,HCl,$2H_2O$ (dihydrate).

Relative molecular mass. 363.8 (anhydrous); 399.9 (dihydrate).

Graphic formula.

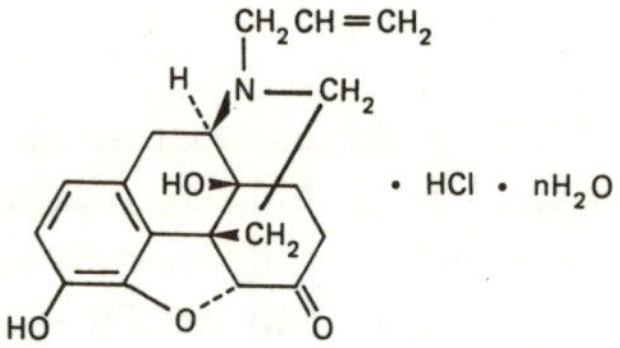

$$n = 0 \text{ (anhydrous)}$$
$$n = 2 \text{ (dihydrate)}$$

Chemical name. (–)-17-Allyl-4,5a-epoxy-3,14-dihydroxymorphinan-6-one hydrochloride; 4,5a-epoxy-3,14-dihydroxy-17-(2-propenyl)morphinan-6-one hydrochloride; (–)-12-allyl-7,7a,8,9-tetrahydro-3,7a-dihydroxy-4aH-8,9c-imino-ethanophenanthro[4,5-bcd]furan-5(6H)-one hydrochloride; CAS Reg. No. 357-08-4 (anhydrous).
(–)-17-Allyl-4,5a-epoxy-3,14-dihydroxymorphinan-6-one hydrochloride dihydrate; 4,5a-epoxy-3,14-dihydroxy-17-(2-propenyl)morphinan-6-one hydrochloride dihydrate; (–)-12-allyl-7,7a,8,9-tetrahydro-3,7a-dihydroxy-4aH-8,9c-imino-ethanophenanthro[4,5-bcd]furan-5(6H)-one hydrochloride dihydrate; CAS Reg. No. 51481-60-8 (dihydrate).

Description. A white or almost white powder.

Solubility. Soluble in water; slightly soluble in ethanol ($\sim$750 g/l) TS; practically insoluble in ether R and chloroform R.

Category. Narcotic antagonist.

Storage. Naloxone hydrochloride should be kept in a tightly closed container, protected from light.

Labelling. The designation on the container of Naloxone hydrochloride should state whether the substance is in the anhydrous form or is the dihydrate.

Additional information.   Even in the absence of light, Naloxone hydrochloride is gradually degraded on exposure to a humid atmosphere, the decomposition being faster at higher temperatures.   It melts at about 177 °C.

REQUIREMENTS

General requirement.   Naloxone hydrochloride contains not less than 98.0% and not more than 102.0% of $C_{19}H_{21}NO_4,HCl$, calculated with reference to the dried substance.

Identity tests

● Either test A or tests B and C may be applied.

A.   Carry out the examination as described under "Spectrophotometry in the infrared region" (vol. 1, p. 40).   The infrared absorption spectrum is concordant with the spectrum obtained from naloxone hydrochloride RS or with the *reference spectrum* of naloxone hydrochloride.

B.   Dissolve 0.05 g in 5 ml of hydrochloric acid (0.1 mol/l) VS and add 0.3 ml of ferric chloride (25 g/l) TS; a purplish blue colour is produced.

C.   A 0.05 g/ml solution yields reaction A described under "General identification tests" as characteristic of chlorides (vol. 1, p. 112).

Specific optical rotation.   Use a 25 mg/ml solution and calculate with reference to the dried substance; $[a]_D^{20\,°C} = -170$ to $-181°$.

Loss on drying.   Dry to constant weight at 105 °C; anhydrous Naloxone hydrochloride loses not more than 5.0 mg/g.   Naloxone hydrochloride dihydrate loses not more than 110 mg/g.

Related substances.   Carry out the test as described under "Thin-layer chromatography" (vol. 1, p. 83), using silica gel R1 as the coating substance, and as the mobile phase prepare the following solution: Shake 100 ml of 1-butanol R with 60 ml of ammonia (~17 g/l) TS, discard the lower layer, and mix 20 volumes of this saturated butanol with 1 volume of methanol R.   Apply separately to the plate 5 µl of each of 2 solutions in a mixture of 3 volumes of methanol R and 2 volumes of water containing (A) 8.0 mg of the test substance per ml and (B) 0.084 mg of noroxymorphone hydrochloride RS per ml.   After removing the plate from the chromatographic chamber, allow it to dry in air, spray it with ferric chloride/potassium ferricyanide TS and examine the chromatogram in daylight.   Any spot obtained with solution A, other than the principal spot and the spot at the origin corresponding to ammonium chloride, is not more intense than that obtained with solution B.

Chlorides content. Dissolve about 0.3 g, accurately weighed, in 50 ml of methanol R. Add 5 ml of glacial acetic acid R and 0.1 ml of eosin Y (5 g/l) TS, and titrate with silver nitrate (0.1 mol/l) VS until a pink colour is produced. Each ml of silver nitrate (0.1 mol/l) VS is equivalent to 3.545 mg of Cl; the content of chlorides is not less than 95.4 mg/g and not more than 99.4 mg/g, calculated with reference to the dried substance.

Assay. Dissolve about 0.3 g, accurately weighed, in 40 ml of glacial acetic acid R1, add 10 ml of acetic anhydride R, 10 ml of mercuric acetate/acetic acid TS, and titrate with perchloric acid (0.1 mol/l) VS as described under "Non-aqueous titration", Method A (vol. 1, p. 131). Each ml of perchloric acid (0.1 mol/l) VS is equivalent to 36.38 mg of $C_{19}H_{21}NO_4,HCl$.

NATRII CALCII EDETAS

Sodium calcium edetate

Molecular formula. $C_{10}H_{12}CaN_2Na_2O_8,2H_2O$

Relative molecular mass. 410.3

Graphic formula.

Chemical name. Disodium [(ethylenedinitrilo)tetraacetato]calciate(2–) dihydrate; (*OC*-6-21)-disodium [[*N*,*N'*-1,2-ethanediylbis[*N*-(carboxymethyl)glycinato]](4–)-*N*,*N'*,*O*,*O'*,*O^N*,*O^N'*]calciate(2–) dihydrate; calcium chelate of the disodium salt of ethylenediamine-*N*,*N*,*N'*,*N'*-tetraacetic acid dihydrate; CAS Reg. No. 6766-87-6 (dihydrate).

Description. A white or creamy white powder; almost odourless.

Solubility. Soluble in 2 parts of water; very slightly soluble in ethanol ($\sim$750 g/l) TS; practically insoluble in chloroform R and in ether R.

Category. Antidote, chelating agent for metals, mainly lead.

Storage. Sodium calcium edetate should be kept in a tightly closed container.

Additional information. Even in the absence of light, Sodium calcium edetate is gradually degraded on exposure to a humid atmosphere, the decomposition being faster at higher temperatures.

REQUIREMENTS

General requirement.   Sodium calcium edetate contains not less than 97.0% and not more than 102.0% of $C_{10}H_{12}CaN_2Na_2O_8$, calculated with reference to the anhydrous substance.

Identity tests

A.   Dissolve 2.0 g in 25 ml of water, add 2.0 ml of lead nitrate (100 g/l) TS, shake and add 6 ml of potassium iodide (80 g/l) TS; no yellow precipitate can be observed (keep the solution for test C).

B.   To 0.15 ml of ferric chloride (25 g/l) TS add 0.15 ml of ammonium thiocyanate (75 g/l) TS; to this deep red-coloured solution add about 0.05 g of the test substance; the deep red colour changes to yellow.

C.   To the solution prepared in test A, add ammonia ($\sim$100 g/l) TS, drop by drop, until an alkaline reaction is obtained with pH-indicator paper R.   Add 5 ml of ammonium oxalate (25 g/l) TS; a white precipitate is produced (distinction from disodium edetate).

D.   When tested for sodium as described under "General identification tests" (vol. 1, p. 115), yields the characteristic reactions. If reaction B is to be used, ignite a small quantity and dissolve the residue in acetic acid ($\sim$60 g/l) TS.

Heavy metals.   Use 1.0 g for the preparation of the test solution as described under "Limit test for heavy metals", Procedure 3 (vol. 1, p. 118); determine the heavy metals content according to Method A (vol. 1, p. 119); not more than 20 µg/g.

Cyanide.   Dissolve 1.0 g in 50 ml of water, add 0.1 g of potassium iodide R, 4 ml of ammonia ($\sim$100 g/l) TS, and 0.10 ml of silver nitrate (0.01 mol/l) VS, and allow to stand for 1 minute; the opalescence produced is not less than that of a standard solution containing 1 ml of nitric acid ($\sim$130 g/l) TS, 1.0 ml of hydrochloric acid (0.0001 mol/l) VS, 9 ml of water, and 0.10 ml of silver nitrate (0.1 mol/l) VS, this solution having also been allowed to stand for 1 minute.

Disodium edetate.   Dissolve 5.0 g in 20 ml of water, add 10 ml of ammonia buffer TS2 and 0.2 g of mordant black 11 indicator mixture R, and titrate with magnesium chloride (0.1 mol/l) VS.   Not more than 1.5 ml of magnesium chloride (0.1 mol/l) VS is required.

Iron.   Ignite 0.5 g and dissolve the residue in 40 ml of water.   Treat the solution as described under "Limit test for iron" (vol. 1, p. 121); not more than 80 µg/g.

Water.   Determine as described under "Determination of water by the Karl Fischer method", Method A (vol. 1, p. 135), using about 0.2 g of the substance; the water content is not more than 130 mg/g.

pH value. pH of a 0.20 g/ml solution in carbon-dioxide-free water R, 6.5–8.0.

Assay. Dissolve about 0.5 g, accurately weighed, in 90 ml of water, add 7 g of methenamine R and 5 ml of hydrochloric acid ($\sim$70 g/l) TS. Titrate with lead nitrate (0.05 mol/l) VS, using xylenol orange indicator mixture R. Each ml of lead nitrate (0.05 mol/l) VS is equivalent to 18.71 mg of $C_{10}H_{12}CaN_2Na_2O_8$.

NATRII CITRAS

Sodium citrate

Sodium citrate, anhydrous
Sodium citrate, dihydrate

Molecular formula. $C_6H_5Na_3O_7$ (anhydrous); $C_6H_5Na_3O_7,2H_2O$ (dihydrate).

Relative molecular mass. 258.1 (anhydrous); 294.1 (dihydrate).

Graphic formula.

$$\begin{array}{l} CH_2-COONa \\ \mid \\ HO-C-COONa \qquad \cdot nH_2O \\ \mid \\ CH_2-COONa \end{array}$$

$$n = 0 \text{ (anhydrous)}$$
$$n = 2 \text{ (dihydrate)}$$

Chemical name. Trisodium citrate; trisodium 2-hydroxy-1,2,3-propanetricarboxylate; CAS Reg. No. 68-04-2 (anhydrous).
Trisodium citrate dihydrate; trisodium 2-hydroxy-1,2,3-propanetricarboxylate dihydrate; CAS Reg. No. 6132-04-3 (dihydrate).

Description. Colourless crystals or a white, crystalline powder; odourless.

Solubility. Freely soluble in water and very soluble in boiling water; practically insoluble in ethanol ($\sim$750 g/l) TS and ether R.

Category. Systemic alkalinizing agent; component of oral rehydration salt mixtures.

Storage. Sodium citrate should be kept in a tightly closed container.

Labelling. The designation on the container of Sodium citrate should state whether the substance is the dihydrate or is in the anhydrous form.

Additional information. Sodium citrate is slightly deliquescent in moist air.

REQUIREMENTS

General requirement.   Sodium citrate contains not less than 99.0% and not more than 101.0% of $C_6H_5Na_3O_7$, calculated with reference to the anhydrous substance.

Identity tests

A.   When tested for sodium as described under "General identification tests" (vol. 1, p. 115), yields the characteristic reactions.   If reaction B is to be used, prepare a 20 mg/ml solution.

B.   A 20 mg/ml solution yields reaction B described under "General identification tests" as characteristic of citrates (vol. 1, p. 113).

Heavy metals.   Use 1.0 g for the preparation of the test solution as described under "Limit test for heavy metals", Procedure 1 (vol. 1, p. 118); determine the heavy metals content according to Method A (vol. 1, p. 119); not more than 10 µg/g.

Oxalates.   Dissolve 0.5 g in 4 ml of water, add 3 ml of hydrochloric acid (~420 g/l) TS and 1 g of granulated zinc R, and heat on a water-bath for 1 minute. Allow to stand for 2 minutes, decant the liquid into a test-tube containing 0.25 ml of phenylhydrazine hydrochloride (10 g/l) TS, and heat to boiling.   Cool rapidly, transfer to a graduated cylinder, and add an equal volume of hydrochloric acid (~420 g/l) TS, followed by 0.25 ml of potassium ferricyanide (50 g/l) TS.   Shake and allow to stand for 30 minutes; any pink colour produced is not more intense than that of a similarly treated solution containing 4 ml of oxalic acid (0.05 g/l) TS.

Clarity and colour of solution.   A solution of 1.0 g in 10 ml of carbon-dioxide-free water R is clear and colourless.

Water.   Determine as described under "Determination of water by the Karl Fischer method", Method A (vol. 1, p. 135).   For the anhydrous form use about 1 g of the substance; the water content is not more than 10 mg/g.   For the dihydrate use about 0.3 g of the substance; the water content is not less than 0.10 g/g and not more than 0.13 g/g.

Acidity or alkalinity.   Dissolve 1 g in 10 ml of carbon-dioxide-free water R and add 0.1 ml of phenolphthalein/ethanol TS; not more than 0.2 ml of hydrochloric acid (0.1 mol/l) VS or 0.2 ml of sodium hydroxide (0.1 mol/l) VS is required to change the colour of the solution.

Assay.   Dissolve about 0.15 g, accurately weighed, in 20 ml of glacial acetic acid R1, heat to about 50 °C, allow to cool to room temperature, add 0.25 ml of

1-naphtholbenzein/acetic acid TS, and titrate with perchloric acid (0.1 mol/l) VS until a green colour is obtained as described under "Non-aqueous titration", Method A (vol. 1, p. 131). Each ml of perchloric acid (0.1 mol/l) VS is equivalent to 8.603 mg of $C_6H_5Na_3O_7$.

NATRII CROMOGLICAS

Sodium cromoglicate

Molecular formula. $C_{23}H_{14}Na_2O_{11}$

Relative molecular mass.   512.3

Graphic formula.

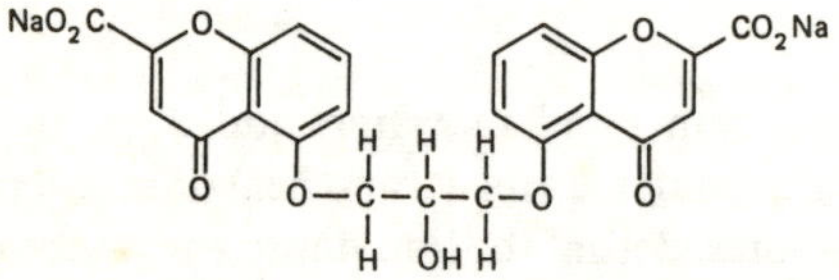

Chemical name.   Disodium 5,5'-[(2-hydroxytrimethylene)dioxy]bis[4-oxo-4H-1-benzopyran-2-carboxylate]; disodium 5,5'-[(2-hydroxy-1,3-propanediyl)bis(oxy)]-bis[4-oxo-4H-1-benzopyran-2-carboxylate]; CAS Reg. No. 15826-37-6.

Description.   A white, crystalline powder; odourless.

Solubility.   Freely soluble in water; slightly soluble in methanol R; very slightly soluble in ethanol (~750 g/l) TS; practically insoluble in chloroform R and ether R.

Category.   Antiasthmatic drug.

Storage.   Sodium cromoglicate should be kept in a tightly closed container, protected from light.

Additional information.   Sodium cromoglicate is hygroscopic.

REQUIREMENTS

General requirement.   Sodium cromoglicate contains not less than 98.0% and not more than 101.0% of $C_{23}H_{14}Na_2O_{11}$, calculated with reference to the dried substance.

Identity tests

● Either tests A and D or tests B, C and D may be applied.

A.   Carry out the examination as described under "Spectrophotometry in the infrared region" (vol. 1, p. 40). The infrared absorption spectrum is concordant with the spectrum obtained from sodium cromoglicate RS or with the reference spectrum of sodium cromoglicate.

B.   See the test described below under "Related substances". The spot obtained with solution B corresponds in position, appearance, and intensity with that obtained with solution C.

C.   Dissolve 5 mg in 0.5 ml of methanol R and add 3 ml of 4-aminoantipyrine TS1, and allow to stand for 5 minutes; an intense yellow colour is produced.

D.   When tested for sodium as described under "General identification tests" (vol. 1, p. 115), yields the characteristic reactions. If reaction B is to be used, prepare a 20 mg/ml solution.

Heavy metals.   Use 1.0 g for the preparation of the test solution as described under "Limit test for heavy metals", Procedure 3 (vol. 1, p. 118); determine the heavy metals content according to Method A (vol. 1, p. 119); not more than 20 µg/g.

Oxalates.   Dissolve 0.10 g in 20 ml of water, add 5.0 ml of iron salicylate TS and sufficient water to produce 50 ml; the absorbance at about 480 nm is not less than that of a solution containing 0.35 mg of oxalic acid R prepared in a similar manner.

Loss on drying.   Dry to constant weight at 100 °C under reduced pressure (not exceeding 0.6 kPa or about 5 mm of mercury); it loses not more than 100 mg/g.

Acidity or alkalinity.   Dissolve 1.0 g in 25 ml of carbon-dioxide-free water R and add 0.1 ml of bromothymol blue/ethanol TS; not more than 0.25 ml of sodium hydroxide (0.1 mol/l) VS or 0.25 ml of hydrochloric acid (0.1 mol/l) VS is required to obtain the midpoint of the indicator (green).

Related substances.   Carry out the test as described under "Thin-layer chromatography" (vol. 1, p. 83), using silica gel R4 as the coating substance, omitting the heating, and allowing the plate to stand overnight at room temperature. As the mobile phase use a mixture of 9 volumes of chloroform R, 9 volumes of methanol R, and 2 volumes of glacial acetic acid R. Apply separately to the plate 10 µl of each of 3 solutions in a mixture of 1 volume of acetone R, 4 volumes of tetrahydrofuran R (which has been freed from stabilizer by passage through a column of suitable alumina), and 6 volumes of water, containing (A) 20 mg of the test substance per ml, (B) 0.10 mg of the test substance per ml, and (C) 0.10 mg of sodium cromoglicate RS per ml. After removing the plate from the chromato-graphic chamber, allow it to dry in air, and examine the chromatogram in ultra-violet light (254 nm). Any spot obtained with solution A, moving ahead of the principal spot, is not more intense than that obtained with solution B.

Assay. Dissolve about 0.18 g, accurately weighed, in a mixture of 25 ml of propylene glycol R and 5 ml of 2-propanol R, warming slightly, cool and add 30 ml of dioxan R. Titrate with perchloric acid/dioxan (0.1 mol/l) VS, determining the endpoint potentiometrically as described under "Non-aqueous titration", Method A (vol. 1, p. 113). Each ml of perchloric acid/dioxan (0.1 mol/l) VS is equivalent to 25.62 mg of $C_{23}H_{14}Na_2O_{11}$.

NATRII FLUORIDUM

Sodium fluoride

Molecular formula.   NaF

Relative molecular mass.   41.99

Chemical name.   Sodium fluoride; CAS Reg. No. 7681-49-4.

Description.   A white powder; odourless.

Solubility.   Soluble in water; practically insoluble in ethanol ($\sim$750 g/l) TS.

Category.   Mineral salt.

Storage.   Sodium fluoride should be kept in a well-closed container.

REQUIREMENTS

General requirement.   Sodium fluoride contains not less than 98.0% and not more than 101.0% of NaF, calculated with reference to the dried substance.

Identity tests

A.   When tested for sodium as described under "General identification tests" (vol. 1, p. 115), yields the characteristic reactions. If reaction B is to be used, prepare a 20 mg/ml solution.

B.   Place 0.10 g in a lead or platinum crucible, add about 1 ml of sulfuric acid ($\sim$1760 g/l) TS, cover the crucible with a piece of clear polished glass, and heat on a water-bath for 15 minutes. Remove the glass cover, rinse with water and wipe dry; the surface of the glass is etched.

C.   Add a few mg of the test substance to a mixture of 0.10 ml of freshly prepared sodium alizarinsulfonate (10 g/l) TS and 0.10 ml of zirconyl nitrate TS; a red colour develops, which changes to yellow.

Heavy metals.   Use 0.5 g for the preparation of the test solution as described under "Limit test for heavy metals", Procedure 3 (vol. 1, p. 118); determine the heavy metals content according to Method A (vol. 1, p. 119); not more than 40 µg/g.

Loss on drying.   Dry to constant weight at 130 °C; it loses not more than 10 mg/g.

Acidity or alkalinity.   Dissolve 1.0 g in 20 ml of water in a platinum dish, add and dissolve into this solution 3 g of potassium nitrate R, and cool to 0 °C. Add 0.15 ml of phenolphthalein/ethanol TS; not more than 2.0 ml of sodium hydroxide (0.05 mol/l) VS or 1.0 ml of sulfuric acid (0.05 mol/l) VS is required to obtain the midpoint of the indicator (pink). (Keep the solution for the test of fluorosilicates.)

Fluorosilicates.   Heat to boiling the solution obtained in the test for acidity or alkalinity and titrate while hot with sodium hydroxide (0.05 mol/l) VS until a permanent pink colour is produced; not more than 1.5 ml of sodium hydroxide (0.05 mol/l) VS are required.

Assay.   Dissolve about 30 mg, accurately weighed, in 1.0 ml of water. Add cautiously 15 ml of acetic anhydride R and boil gently for 2 minutes, placing a small funnel on the flask to serve as a reflux condenser. Cool and titrate with perchloric acid (0.1 mol/l) VS as described under "Non-aqueous titration", Method A (vol. 1, p. 131). Each ml of perchloric acid (0.1 mol/l) VS is equivalent to 4.199 mg of NaF.

NATRII NITRIS

Sodium nitrite

Molecular formula. $NaNO_2$

Relative molecular mass.   69.00

Chemical name.   Nitrous acid, sodium salt; CAS Reg. No. 7632-00-0.

Description.   A white to slightly yellow, granular powder, or white or almost white, opaque, fused masses or sticks; odourless.

Solubility.   Freely soluble in water; sparingly soluble in ethanol ($\sim$750 g/l) TS.

Category.   Vasodilator.

Storage.   Sodium nitrite should be kept in a well-closed container, protected from light.

Additional information.   Sodium nitrite is deliquescent in air.   Even in the absence of light, it is gradually degraded on exposure to a humid atmosphere, the decomposition being faster at higher temperatures.

REQUIREMENTS

General requirement.   Sodium nitrite contains not less than 98.0% and not more than 100.5% of $NaNO_2$, calculated with reference to the dried substance.

Identity tests

A.   When tested for sodium as described under "General identification tests" (vol. 1, p. 115) yields the characteristic reactions.   If reaction B is to be used, prepare a 0.10 g/ml solution acidified with acetic acid ($\sim$300 g/l) TS.

B.   Dissolve 0.10 g in 1.0 ml of water and add 1.0 ml of ferrous sulfate ($\sim$15 g/l) TS; after a few minutes a deep brown colour is produced.

C.   Dissolve 0.20 g in 1.0 ml of water and add 1.0 ml of sulfuric acid ($\sim$100 g/l) TS; brownish red fumes are evolved.   Add a few drops of starch/iodide TS; a blue colour is produced.

Heavy metals.   Dissolve 1.0 g in 10 ml of hydrochloric acid ($\sim$70 g/l) TS, evaporate to dryness on a water-bath and until the odour of hydrochloric acid is no longer perceptible.   Proceed with the residue as described under "Limit test for heavy metals", Procedure 1 (vol. 1, p. 118); determine the heavy metals content according to Method A (vol. 1, p. 119); not more than 20 µg/g.

Chlorides.   For the preparation of the test solution, boil 2.5 g in a mixture of 3 ml of water and 2 ml of nitric acid ($\sim$1000 g/l) TS, cool, and proceed as described under "Limit test for chlorides" (vol. 1, p. 116); the chloride content is not more than 0.1 mg/g.

Loss on drying.   Dry at ambient temperature over silica gel, desiccant, R for 4 hours; it loses not more than 5.0 mg/g.

Acidity or alkalinity.   To a solution of 0.5 g in 10 ml of water add 0.1 ml of sodium hydroxide (0.01 mol/l) VS and 0.25 ml of phenol red/ethanol TS; a red colour is produced. Add 0.3 ml of hydrochloric acid (0.01 mol/l) VS; the colour changes to yellow.

Assay.   Dissolve about 0.4 g, accurately weighed, in sufficient water to produce 100 ml. To 10.0 ml of this solution add 20.0 ml of potassium permanganate (0.02 mol/l) VS and 10 ml of sulfuric acid ($\sim$1760 g/l) TS. Allow to stand for 10 minutes, add 0.5 g of potassium iodide R, swirl the flask, and titrate the liberated iodine with sodium thiosulfate (0.1 mol/l) VS, using starch TS as indicator. Each ml of sodium thiosulfate (0.1 mol/l) VS is equivalent to 3.450 mg of $NaNO_2$.

NATRII NITROPRUSSIDUM

Sodium nitroprusside

Molecular formula. $Na_2[Fe(CN)_5NO],2H_2O$

Relative molecular mass.   298.0

Graphic formula.

$$\left[\begin{array}{c} \mathrm{CN} \\ \mathrm{NC}\diagdown\diagup\mathrm{NO} \\ \mathrm{Fe} \\ \mathrm{NC}\diagup\diagdown\mathrm{CN} \\ \mathrm{CN} \end{array}\right]^{2-} \cdot\ 2Na^+ \cdot 2H_2O$$

Chemical name.   Disodium pentacyanonitrosylferrate(2–) dihydrate; disodium (*OC*-6-22)-pentakis(cyano-*C*)nitrosylferrate(2–) dihydrate; CAS Reg. No. 13755-38-9 (dihydrate).

Other names.   Sodium nitroferricyanide; sodium nitroprussiate.

Description.   Reddish brown crystals or powder; odourless or almost odourless.

Solubility.   Freely soluble in water; slightly soluble in ethanol ($\sim$750 g/l) TS; very slightly soluble in chloroform R.

Category.   Antihypertensive drug.

Storage.   Sodium nitroprusside should be kept in a tightly closed container, protected from light.

REQUIREMENTS

General requirement.   Sodium nitroprusside contains not less than 99.0% and not more than 100.5% of $Na_2[Fe(CN)_5NO]$, calculated with reference to the anhydrous substance.

Identity tests

A.   The absorption spectrum of a 4.0 mg/ml solution, when observed between 350 nm and 600 nm, exhibits a maximum at about 395 nm; the absorbance of a 1-cm layer at this wavelength is about 1.10.

B.   When tested for sodium as described under "General identification tests" (vol. 1, p. 115) yields the characteristic reactions. If reaction B is to be used, prepare a 0.10 g/ml solution acidified with acetic acid ($\sim$300 g/l) TS.

C.   Dissolve 5 mg in 2.0 ml of water, add 0.1 ml of acetone R and 0.5 ml of sodium hydroxide ($\sim$80 g/l) TS; an orange colour is produced. Add about 2 ml of acetic acid ($\sim$300 g/l) TS; the colour changes to purple.

Chlorides.   Dissolve 1.20 g in a mixture of 2 ml of nitric acid ($\sim$130 g/l) TS and 30 ml of water, and proceed as described under "Limit test for chlorides" (vol. 1, p. 116); the chloride content is not more than 0.2 mg/g.

Sulfates.   Dissolve 5.0 g in 40 ml of water and proceed as described under "Limit test for sulfates" (vol. 1, p. 116); the sulfate content is not more than 0.1 mg/g.

Ferricyanide.   Dissolve 0.50 g in 20 ml of ammonium acetate buffer, pH 4.62, TS, and divide the solution into two equal portions, A and B. To portion B add 1 ml of ferricyanide standard (50 µg/ml) TS, then add to both portions 5 ml of ferrous ammonium sulfate (1 g/l) TS and dilute to 50 ml with water. Prepare a blank solution by dissolving 0.25 g of the substance to be examined in 10 ml of ammonium acetate buffer, pH 4.62, TS, and diluting to 50 ml with water. Allow to stand for 1 hour and measure the absorbance of the solutions at the maximum at about 720 nm. The absorbance of portion A when measured against the blank is not greater than the absorbance of portion B when measured against portion A (0.2 mg/g).

Ferrocyanide.   Dissolve 2.0 g in 40 ml of water and divide the solution into two equal portions, A and B.   To portion B add 2 ml of ferrocyanide standard (100 µg/ml) TS, then add to both portions 0.2 ml of ferric chloride (50 g/l) TS and dilute to 50 ml with water. Allow to stand for 5 minutes. Prepare a blank solution by dissolving 1.0 g of the substance to be examined in sufficient water to produce 50 ml. Measure the absorbance of the solutions at the maximum at about 695 nm. The absorbance of portion A when measured against the blank is not greater than the absorbance of portion B when measured against portion A (0.2 mg/g).

Insoluble matter.   Dissolve 10.0 g in 50 ml of water, heat the solution on a water-bath for 30 minutes, filter, wash the insoluble matter with water, and dry to constant weight at 105 °C; the content of insoluble matter is not more than 0.1 mg/g.

Water.   Determine as described under "Determination of water by the Karl Fischer method", Method A (vol. 1, p. 135), using about 1 g of the substance; the water content is not less than 90 mg/g and not more than 150 mg/g.

Assay.   Dissolve about 0.35 g, accurately weighed, in 100 ml of water. Add 0.1 ml of sulfuric acid ($\sim$100 g/l) TS and 20 ml of ethanol ($\sim$750 g/l) TS.   Titrate with silver nitrate (0.1 mol/l) VS, determining the endpoint potentiometrically using a silver/silver chloride electrode system.   Each ml of silver nitrate (0.1 mol/l) VS is equivalent to 13.10 mg of $Na_2[Fe(CN)_5NO]$.

NATRII STIBOGLUCONAS

Sodium stibogluconate

Composition.   Sodium stibogluconate is a pentavalent antimony compound of indefinite composition. It has been represented by the formula $C_6H_9Na_2O_9Sb$, but it usually contains less than 2 atoms of sodium for each atom of antimony.

Chemical name.   D-Gluconic acid cyclic ester with antimonic acid ($H_8Sb_2O_9$) (2:1), trisodium salt, nonahydrate; 2,4:2',4'-*O*-(oxydistibylidyne)bis-D-gluconic acid, *Sb,Sb'*-dioxide, trisodium salt, nonahydrate; CAS Reg. No. 16037-91-5.

Description.   A colourless, mostly amorphous powder; odourless.

Solubility.   Very soluble in water; practically insoluble in ethanol ($\sim$750 g/l) TS and ether R.

Category. Antileishmaniasis drug.

Storage. Sodium stibogluconate should be kept in a well-closed container.

REQUIREMENTS

General requirement. Sodium stibogluconate contains not less than 30.0% and not more than 34.0% of total antimony, calculated with reference to the dried substance.

Identity tests

A. Heat a small quantity of the test substance; it chars without melting. Dissolve the residue in acetic acid ($\sim$60 g/l) TS; it yields reaction B, characteristic of sodium as described under "General identification tests" (vol. 1, p. 115).

B. Dissolve 0.5 g in 10 ml of water and add a few drops of hydrogen sulfide TS; an orange precipitate is produced, which dissolves in sodium hydroxide ($\sim$80 g/l) TS.

C. A 10 mg/ml solution is dextrorotatory.

Chlorides. Dissolve 2.5 g in a mixture of 50 ml of water, 2 ml of nitric acid ($\sim$130 g/l) TS, and 75 ml of acetate buffer, pH 5.0, TS. Titrate with silver nitrate (0.1 ml/l) VS, determining the endpoint potentiometrically; not more than 3.0 ml of silver nitrate (0.1 mol/l) VS are required.

Loss on drying. Dry to constant weight at 130 °C under reduced pressure (not exceeding 0.6 kPa or about 5 mm of mercury); it loses not more than 150 mg/g.

Colour and pH value. Dissolve 0.3 g in 10 ml of water and heat the solution in an autoclave under reduced pressure (about 70 kPa) for 30 minutes; the solution is colourless or almost colourless and has a pH between 5.0 and 5.6.

Trivalent antimony. Dissolve 2.0 g in 30 ml of water, add 15 ml of hydrochloric acid ($\sim$250 g/l) TS, and titrate with potassium bromate (0.00833 mol/l) VS using methyl/orange TS as indicator; not more than 1.3 ml of potassium bromate (0.00833 mol/l) VS are required.

Undue toxicity. Carry out the test as described under "Test for undue toxicity" (vol. 1, p. 154), using 10 mice that have been deprived of food for not less than 17 hours, and injecting each intravenously with 0.3 ml of a solution containing an amount equivalent to 28 mg of total antimony per ml of sterile water R. After injection, allow the mice access to food and water. Keep the mice under observation for 24 hours. The product meets the requirements for freedom from undue toxicity if no animal dies within that time. If one of the mice dies, repeat the test.

The requirements are met if none of the second group of mice dies within 24 hours.

Assay.   Place about 0.25 g, accurately weighed, in a 300-ml long-necked flask, add 10 ml of nitric acid ($\sim$1000 g/l) TS and 5 ml of sulfuric acid ($\sim$1760 g/l) TS, and heat cautiously over a small flame, keeping the liquid in motion by rotating the flask; remove the flask from the flame at the onset of the first vigorous reaction until this subsides. Continue to heat until white fumes are evolved and allow the liquid to cool. Add 1 ml of nitric acid ($\sim$1000 g/l) TS and again heat until white fumes are evolved. Add 1 g of ammonium sulfate R, again heat to the point of fuming, cool thoroughly, and add 1 g of tartaric acid R and 60 ml of water. To the clear, almost colourless solution add 1 g of potassium iodide R and boil the solution gently for about 5 minutes or until free iodine is expelled, the liquid becoming pure yellow in colour. Cool, add sodium hydroxide ($\sim$400 g/l) TS until just alkaline (about 15 ml), cool again, acidify with sulfuric acid ($\sim$100 g/l) TS until just acid, add an excess of sodium hydrogen carbonate R, and titrate with iodine (0.02 mol/l) VS, using starch TS as indicator if necessary. Each ml of iodine (0.02 mol/l) VS is equivalent to 2.435 mg of total antimony.

NATRII SULFAS

Sodium sulfate

Molecular formula. $Na_2SO_4,10H_2O$

Relative molecular mass.   322.2

Chemical name.   Disodium sulfate decahydrate; sulfuric acid disodium salt, decahydrate; CAS Reg. No. 7727-73-3 (decahydrate).

Other name.   Glauber's salt.

Description.   Colourless crystals or a white powder; odourless.

Solubility.   Freely soluble in water; practically insoluble in ethanol ($\sim$750 g/l) TS.

Category.   Laxative.

Storage.   Sodium sulfate should be kept in a well-closed container and preferably stored at a temperature not exceeding 30 °C.

Additional information.　Sodium sulfate partially dissolves in its own water of crystallization at about 33 °C.

REQUIREMENTS

General requirement.　Sodium sulfate contains not less than 99.0 % and not more than 100.5 % of Na_2SO_4, calculated with reference to the dried substance.

Identity tests

A.　When tested for sodium as described under "General identification tests" (vol. 1, p. 115), yields the characteristic reactions.　If reaction B is to be used, prepare a 0.05 g/ml solution.

B.　A 0.05 g/ml solution yields reaction A described under "General identification tests" as characteristic of sulfates (vol. 1, p. 115).

Heavy metals.　Use 1.0 g for the preparation of the test solution as described under "Limit test for heavy metals", Procedure 1 (vol. 1, p. 118); determine the heavy metals content according to Method A (vol. 1, p. 119); not more than 20 µg/g.

Ammonium salts.　Transfer 1 g to a test-tube, add about 0.3 g of potassium hydroxide R and heat the mixture; a moistened red litmus paper R placed in the evolved vapours does not turn blue.

Arsenic.　Use a solution of 5 g in 35 ml of water and proceed as described under "Limit test for arsenic" (vol. 1, p. 122); the arsenic content is not more than 2 µg/g.

Calcium.　To two separate comparison tubes transfer 0.2 ml of ethanolic calcium standard (100 µg/ml Ca) TS, add 1.5 ml of ammonium oxalate (25 g/l) TS, allow to stand for 1 minute, and then add 1 ml of acetic acid (~120 g/l) TS.　To one tube add a solution of the substance to be examined containing 0.5 g in 15 ml of water, and to the second tube add 10 ml of calcium standard (10 µg/ml Ca) TS and 5 ml of water.　Observe any opalescence produced after 15 minutes; the opalescence in the first tube is not more intense than that in the second tube (200 µg/g).

Chlorides.　Dissolve 1.25 g in a mixture of 2 ml of nitric acid (~130 g/l) TS and 30 ml of water and proceed as described under "Limit test for chlorides" (vol. 1, p. 116); the chloride content is not more than 0.2 mg/g.

Iron.　Using 1.0 g prepare a solution in 40 ml of water and proceed as described under "Limit test for iron" (vol. 1, p. 121); not more than 40 µg/g.

Magnesium.　Dissolve 0.5 g in 10 ml of water, add 1 ml of glycerol R, 0.15 ml of titan yellow TS, 0.2 ml of ammonium oxalate (50 g/l) TS, and 5 ml of sodium hydroxide (~80 g/l) TS, and shake; any pink colour produced is not more intense than that of a similarly treated mixture of 5 ml of magnesium standard (10 µg/ml Mg) TS and 5 ml of water.

Clarity and colour of solution.   A solution of 0.50 g in 10 ml of carbon-dioxide-free water R is clear and colourless.

Reducing substances.   Dissolve 0.5 g in 5 ml of water, add 1 ml of sulfuric acid ($\sim$100 g/l) TS and 0.20 ml of potassium permanganate (0.002 mol/l) VS. Allow to stand for 15 minutes; no discoloration is observed.

Loss on drying.   Dry at 30 °C for 1 hour and then to constant weight at 130 °C; it loses not less than 0.52 g/g and not more than 0.57 g/g.

Acidity or alkalinity.   Dissolve 0.5 g in 10 ml of carbon-dioxide-free water R and add 0.1 ml of bromothymol blue/ethanol TS; not more than 0.5 ml of carbonate-free sodium hydroxide (0.01 mol/l) VS or 0.5 ml of hydrochloric acid (0.01 mol/l) VS is required to obtain the midpoint of the indicator (green).

Assay.   Dissolve about 0.25 g, accurately weighed, in 250 ml of water, add 10 ml of hydrochloric acid ($\sim$70 g/l) TS, heat to boiling and add a sufficient quantity of barium chloride (50 g/l) TS. Heat on a water-bath for 30 minutes, stirring occasionally. Collect the precipitate, wash, dry and ignite at 600 °C. Each g of residue is equivalent to 0.608 g of Na_2SO_4.

NATRII SULFAS ANHYDRICUS

Sodium sulfate, anhydrous

Molecular formula. Na_2SO_4

Relative molecular mass.   142.0

Chemical name.   Disodium sulfate; sulfuric acid disodium salt, anhydrous; CAS Reg. No. 7757-82-6 (anhydrous).

Description.   A white powder; odourless.

Solubility.   Freely soluble in water; practically insoluble in ethanol ($\sim$750 g/l) TS.

Category.   Laxative.

Storage.   Anhydrous sodium sulfate should be kept in a well-closed container.

Additional information.   Anhydrous sodium sulfate is hygroscopic.

REQUIREMENTS

General requirement. Anhydrous sodium sulfate contains not less than 99.0% and not more than 100.5% of Na_2SO_4, calculated with reference to the dried substance.

Identity tests

A. When tested for sodium as described under "General identification tests" (vol. 1, p. 115), yields the characteristic reactions. If reaction B is to be used, prepare a 20 mg/ml solution.

B. A 20 mg/ml solution yields reaction A described under "General identification tests" as characteristic of sulfates (vol. 1, p. 115).

Heavy metals. Use 0.5 g for the preparation of the test solution as described under "Limit test for heavy metals", Procedure 1 (vol. 1, p. 118); determine the heavy metals content according to Method A (vol. 1, p. 119); not more than 45 µg/g.

Ammonium salts. Transfer 0.5 g to a test-tube, add about 0.3 g of potassium hydroxide R and heat the mixture; a moistened red litmus paper R placed in the evolved vapours does not turn blue.

Arsenic. Use a solution of 2.0 g in 35 ml of water and proceed as described under "Limit test for arsenic" (vol. 1, p. 122); the arsenic content is not more than 5 µg/g.

Calcium. To two separate comparison tubes transfer 0.2 ml of ethanolic calcium standard (100 µg/ml Ca) TS, add 1.5 ml of ammonium oxalate (25 g/l) TS, allow to stand for 1 minute, and then add 1 ml of acetic acid (~120 g/l) TS. To one tube add a solution of the substance to be examined containing 0.22 g in 15 ml of water, and to the second tube add 10 ml of calcium standard (10 µg/ml Ca) TS and 5 ml of water. Observe any opalescence produced after 15 minutes; the opalescence in the first tube is not more intense than that in the second tube (450 µg/g).

Chlorides. Dissolve 0.55 g in a mixture of 2 ml of nitric acid (~130 g/l) TS and 30 ml of water and proceed as described under "Limit test for chlorides" (vol. 1, p. 116); the chloride content is not more than 0.45 mg/g.

Iron. Using 0.44 g prepare a solution in 40 ml of water and proceed as described under "Limit test for iron" (vol. 1, p. 121); not more than 90 µg/g.

Magnesium. Dissolve 0.22 g in 10 ml of water, add 1 ml of glycerol R, 0.15 ml of titan yellow TS, 0.25 ml of ammonium oxalate (50 g/l) TS, and 5 ml of sodium hydroxide (~80 g/l) TS, and shake; any pink colour produced is not more intense than that of a similarly treated mixture of 5 ml of magnesium standard (10 µg/ml Mg) TS and 5 ml of water.

Clarity and colour of solution. A solution of 0.22 g in 10 ml of carbon-dioxide-free water R is clear and colourless.

Reducing substances. Dissolve 0.25 g in 5 ml of water, add 1 ml of sulfuric acid ($\sim$100 g/l) TS and 0.20 ml of potassium permanganate (0.002 mol/l) VS. Allow to stand for 15 minutes; no discoloration is observed.

Loss on drying. Dry to constant weight at 130 °C; it loses not more than 50 mg/g.

Acidity or alkalinity. Dissolve 0.22 g in 10 ml of carbon-dioxide-free water R and add 0.1 ml of bromothymol blue/ethanol TS; not more than 0.5 ml of carbonate-free sodium hydroxide (0.01 mol/l) VS or 0.5 ml of hydrochloric acid (0.01 mol/l) VS is required to obtain the midpoint of the indicator (green).

Assay. Dissolve about 0.1 g, accurately weighed, in 250 ml of water, add 10 ml of hydrochloric acid ($\sim$70 g/l) TS, heat to boiling, and add a sufficient quantity of barium chloride (50 g/l) TS. Heat on a water-bath for 30 minutes, stirring occasionally. Collect the precipitate, wash, dry and ignite at 600 °C. Each g of residue is equivalent to 0.608 g of Na_2SO_4.

NATRII THIOSULFAS

Sodium thiosulfate

Molecular formula. $Na_2S_2O_3,5H_2O$

Relative molecular mass. 248.2

Chemical name. Disodium thiosulfate pentahydrate; disodium thiosulfate ($Na_2S_2O_3$) pentahydrate; thiosulfuric acid ($H_2S_2O_3$), disodium salt, pentahydrate; CAS Reg. No. 10102-17-7 (pentahydrate).

Description. Transparent, colourless crystals; odourless.

Solubility. Very soluble in water; practically insoluble in ethanol ($\sim$750 g/l) TS.

Category. Antidote.

Storage. Sodium thiosulfate should be kept in a tightly closed container.

Additional information. Sodium thiosulfate effloresces in dry air at temperatures exceeding 33 °C and dissolves in its water of crystallization at about 49 °C.

REQUIREMENTS

General requirement. Sodium thiosulfate contains not less than 99.0% and not more than 101.0% of $Na_2S_2O_3,5H_2O$.

Identity tests

A. Dissolve 1.0 g in 10 ml of water (use this solution also for tests B and C). To 2 ml add 1.0 ml of iodine TS; the colour of the solution is discharged. Add 0.25 ml of barium chloride (50 g/l) TS; the solution remains clear.

B. To 2 ml of the solution prepared in test A add 1.0 ml of hydrochloric acid ($\sim$70 g/l) TS; an odour of sulfur dioxide is perceptible and a precipitate of sulfur is produced (proceed with caution).

C. To 2 ml of the solution prepared in test A add 2 ml of silver nitrate (0.1 mol/l) VS; a white precipitate is formed, but quickly becomes yellowish, then black.

D. When tested for sodium as described under "General identification tests" (vol. 1, p. 115) yields the characteristic reactions. If reaction B is to be used, prepare a 0.10 g/ml solution.

Heavy metals. Dissolve 1.0 g in 10 ml of water, add slowly 5 ml of hydrochloric acid ($\sim$70 g/l) TS, and evaporate to dryness on a water-bath. Add 15 ml of water to the residue, boil gently for 2 minutes and filter. Heat the filtrate to boiling, add sufficient bromine TS1 to the hot filtrate to produce a clear solution and provide a slight excess of bromine. Boil the solution to expel the excess bromine. Cool, add 0.05 ml of phenolphthalein/ethanol TS and neutralize with sodium hydroxide (1 mol/l) VS. Adjust the pH to 3–4 with acetic acid ($\sim$60 g/l) TS, dilute to 40 ml with water, and determine the heavy metals content as described under "Limit test for heavy metals", according to Method A (vol. 1, p. 119); not more than 20 µg/g.

Chlorides. Dissolve 1.20 g in a mixture of 20 ml of water and 2 ml of nitric acid ($\sim$130 g/l) TS, boil gently for 3–4 minutes, cool, filter, and proceed with the filtrate as described under "Limit test for chlorides" (vol. 1, p. 116); the chloride content is not more than 0.2 mg/g.

Sulfates and sulfites. Dissolve 0.25 g in 10 ml of water, add 5 ml of iodine TS, and gradually more iodine TS, drop by drop, until a very faint persistent yellow colour is produced. Proceed as described under "Limit test for sulfates" (vol. 1, p. 116); the sulfate content is not more than 2 mg/g.

Sulfides. Dissolve 1 g in 10 ml of water and add 0.05 ml of sodium nitroprusside (45 g/l) TS; the solution does not become violet.

Clarity and colour. A solution of 1.0 g in 10 ml of carbon-dioxide-free water R is clear and colourless.

pH value. pH of a 0.10 g/ml solution in carbon-dioxide-free water R, 6.0–8.4.

Assay. Dissolve about 0.5 g, accurately weighed, in 25 ml of water and titrate with iodine (0.05 mol/l) VS using starch TS as indicator, added towards the end of the titration. Each ml of iodine (0.05 mol/l) VS is equivalent to 24.82 mg of $Na_2S_2O_3,5H_2O$.

NATRII VALPROAS

Sodium valproate

Molecular formula. $C_8H_{15}NaO_2$

Relative molecular mass. 166.2

Graphic formula.

$$CH_3CH_2CH_2CHCO_2Na$$
$$|$$
$$CH_3CH_2CH_2$$

Chemical name. Sodium 2-propylvalerate; sodium 2-propylpentanoate; CAS Reg. No. 1069-66-5.

Description. A white or almost white, crystalline powder; odourless or almost odourless.

Solubility. Freely soluble in water and ethanol (~750 g/l) TS.

Category. Antiepileptic drug.

Storage. Sodium valproate should be kept in a well-closed container.

Additional information. Sodium valproate is deliquescent.

REQUIREMENTS

General requirement. Sodium valproate contains not less than 98.0% and not more than 101.0% of $C_8H_{15}NaO_2$, calculated with reference to the dried substance.

Identity tests

A.   Dissolve 0.5 g in 5 ml of water, add 5 ml of chloroform R and 1 ml of hydrochloric acid (~70 g/l) TS, shake vigorously for 1 minute, allow to separate, dry the lower layer with anhydrous sodium sulfate R, filter, and evaporate to dryness. Carry out the examination of a thin film of the residue as described under "Spectrophotometry in the infrared region" (vol. 1, p. 40). The infrared absorption spectrum is concordant with the spectrum obtained from valproic acid RS or with the *reference spectrum* of valproic acid.

B.   Dissolve 0.5 g in 5 ml of water and add 1 ml of cobalt(II) nitrate (100 g/l) TS; a purple precipitate is produced, which is soluble in carbon tetrachloride R.

C.   A 20 mg/ml solution yields reaction B, described under "General identification tests" as characteristic of sodium (vol. 1, p. 115).

Heavy metals.   Use 1.0 g for the preparation of the test solution as described under "Limit test for heavy metals", Procedure 3 (vol. 1, p. 118); determine the heavy metals content according to Method A (vol. 1, p. 119); not more than 20 μg/g.

Arsenic.   Use a solution of 5.0 g in 35 ml of water and proceed as described under "Limit test for arsenic" (vol. 1, p. 122); the arsenic content is not more than 2 μg/g.

Chlorides.   Dissolve 1.20 g in a mixture of 2 ml of nitric acid (~130 g/l) TS and 20 ml of water, and proceed as described under "Limit test for chlorides" (vol. 1, p. 116); the chloride content is not more than 0.2 mg/g.

Iron.   Using 0.2 g prepare a solution in 40 ml of water and proceed as described under "Limit test for iron" (vol. 1, p. 121); not more than 50 μg/g.

Sulfates.   Dissolve 2.5 g in 20 ml of water and proceed as described under "Limit test for sulfates" (vol. 1, p. 116); the sulfate content is not more than 0.2 mg/g.

Clarity and colour of solution.   The opalescence of a solution of 2.0 g in 10 ml of carbon-dioxide-free water R is not more intense than that of opalescence standard TS2 and the solution is colourless.

Loss on drying.   Dry to constant weight at 105 °C; it loses not more than 20 mg/g.

Acidity or alkalinity.   Dissolve 2.0 g in 20 ml of carbon-dioxide-free water R and add 0.1 ml of phenolphthalein/ethanol TS; not more than 1.5 ml of sodium hydroxide (0.1 mol/l) VS or 1.5 ml of hydrochloric acid (0.1 mol/l) VS is required to obtain the midpoint of the indicator (pink).

Related substances.   Carry out the test as described under "Gas chromatography" (vol. 1, p. 94) using 3 solutions:

Solution 1.   0.20 mg of octanoic acid R (internal standard) per ml of dichloromethane R.

Solution 2.   Dissolve 0.50 g of the substance being examined in 10 ml of water, acidify with sulfuric acid ($\sim$190 g/l) TS, and shake with 3 quantities, each of 20 ml, of dichloromethane R. Wash the combined dichloromethane extracts with 10 ml of water, shake with anhydrous sodium sulfate R, filter and evaporate the filtrate at a temperature not exceeding 30 °C to a volume of about 10 ml, using a rotary evaporator.

Solution 3.   Dissolve 0.50 g of the substance being examined in 10 ml of a mixture of 2.0 mg of octanoic acid R in 10 ml of sodium hydroxide (0.1 mol/l) VS, acidify with sulfuric acid ($\sim$190 g/l) TS, and shake with 3 quantities, each of 20 ml, of dichloromethane R. Wash the combined dichloromethane extracts with 10 ml of water, shake with anhydrous sodium sulfate R, filter and evaporate the filtrate at a temperature not exceeding 30 °C to a volume of about 10 ml, using a rotary evaporator.

For the procedure use a glass column, 1.5 m long and 0.4 cm in internal diameter, packed with an adequate quantity of an adsorbent composed of 15 g of a phase consisting of an ester of macrogol 20M and terephthalic acid, together with 1 g of phosphoric acid ($\sim$1440 g/l) TS supported on 84 g of acid-washed, silanized diatomaceous support R (150–180 µm). Maintain the column at 170 °C, use nitrogen R as the carrier gas and a flame ionization detector. In the chromatogram obtained with solution 3, the total area of all the peaks, excluding the main peak and those due to the solvent and the internal standard, is not greater than the area of the peak due to the internal standard.

Assay.   Dissolve about 0.25 g, accurately weighed, in 30 ml of glacial acetic acid R1, add 0.15 ml of 1-naphtholbenzein/acetic acid TS as indicator and titrate with perchloric acid (0.1 mol/l) VS, as described under "Non-aqueous titration", Method A (vol. 1, p. 131). Each ml of perchloric acid (0.1 mol/l) VS is equivalent to 16.62 mg of $C_8H_{15}NaO_2$.

NEOMYCINI SULFAS

Neomycin sulfate

Composition.   Neomycin sulfate is a mixture of sulfate salts of substances produced by the growth of *Streptomyces fradiae,* the main components of which are neomycin B and its stereoisomer neomycin C.

Chemical name.   Neomycin sulfate; CAS Reg. No. 1405-10-3.

Description.   A white or yellowish white powder; odourless or almost odourless.

Solubility.   Freely soluble in water; very slightly soluble in ethanol ($\sim$750 g/l) TS; practically insoluble in acetone R, chloroform R, and ether R.

Category.   Antiinfective drug.

Storage.   Neomycin sulfate should be kept in a tightly closed container, protected from light, and stored at a temperature not exceeding 30 °C.

Additional information.   Neomycin sulfate is hygroscopic. Even in the absence of light, it is gradually degraded on exposure to a humid atmosphere, the decomposition being faster at higher temperatures. An aqueous solution is dextrorotatory.

REQUIREMENTS

General requirement.   Neomycin sulfate contains not less than 600 International Units of neomycin per mg, calculated with reference to the dried substance.

Identity tests

A.   Carry out the test as described under "Thin-layer chromatography" (vol. 1, p. 83), using silica gel R3 as the coating substance and freshly prepared ammonium acetate (40 g/l) TS as the mobile phase. Apply separately to the plate 1 µl of each of 2 solutions containing (A) 20 mg of the test substance per ml, and (B) 20 mg of neomycin B sulfate RS per ml. After removing the plate from the chromatographic chamber, allow it to dry in air for 10 minutes, heat at 105 °C for 1 hour, and spray with triketohydrindene/butanol TS. Heat it again at 105 °C for 5 minutes and examine the chromatogram in daylight. The principal red spot obtained with solution A corresponds in position and appearance with that obtained with solution B.

B.   Dissolve 10 mg in 5 ml of water, add 0.1 ml of pyridine R and 2 ml of triketohydrindene hydrate (1 g/l) TS, and heat on a water-bath at a temperature between 65 and 70 °C for 10 minutes; a deep violet colour is produced.

C.   A 0.05 g/ml solution yields reaction A described under "General identification tests" as characteristic of sulfates (vol. 1, p. 115).

Sulfated ash.   Not more than 10 mg/g.

Loss on drying.   Dry at 60 °C under reduced pressure (not exceeding 0.6 kPa or about 5 mm of mercury) over phosphorus pentoxide R for 3 hours; it loses not more than 80 mg/g.

pH value. pH of a 0.10 g/ml solution in carbon-dioxide-free water R, 5.0–7.5.

Neamine. Carry out the test as described under "Thin-layer chromatography" (vol. 1, p. 83), using a plate prepared as follows: Mix 0.3 g of carbomer R with 240 ml of water and allow to stand for 1 hour with occasional moderate shaking. Adjust the pH to 7 by slowly adding, with continuous shaking, sodium hydroxide (~80 g/l) TS, then add 30 g of silica gel R3. Coat the plate with a layer of 0.75 mm thickness, heat the plate at 110 °C for 1 hour, allow to cool, and use immediately. As the mobile phase, use potassium dihydrogen phosphate (100 g/l) TS. Apply separately to the plate 10 µl of each of 2 solutions containing (A) 2.5 mg of the test substance per ml and (B) 0.05 mg of neamine RS per ml. After removing the plate from the chromatographic chamber, allow it to dry in a current of warm air, spray it with triketohydrindene/stannous chloride TS, and heat it at 110 °C for 15 minutes. Examine the chromatogram in daylight. Any spot obtained with solution A corresponding to neamine is not more intense than that obtained with solution B.

Content of sulfates. Dissolve 1 g in 200 ml of water, add 3 ml of hydrochloric acid (~420 g/l) TS, heat to boiling, and add 25 ml of hot barium chloride (50 g/l) TS. Heat on a water-bath for 4 hours with stirring, collect the precipitate, wash with water, dry, ignite, and weigh. Each g of residue is equivalent to 411.6 mg of sulfates; the sulfate content is not less than 250 mg/g and not more than 310 mg/g.

Assay. Carry out the assay as described under "Microbiological assay of antibiotics" (vol. 1, p. 145), using either (*a*) *Bacillus pumilus* (NCTC 8241; ATCC 14884) as the test organism, culture medium Cm1 with a final pH of 8.0–8.1, sterile phosphate buffer pH 8.0 TS1 or TS2, an appropriate concentration of neomycin (usually between 2 and 14 IU per ml), and an incubation temperature of 35–39 °C; or (*b*) *Staphylococcus aureus* (ATCC 29737) as the test organism, culture medium Cm1 with a final pH of 7.8–8.0, sterile phosphate buffer pH 8.0 TS1 or TS2, an appropriate concentration of neomycin (usually between 2 and 20 IU per ml), and an incubation temperature of 35–39 °C; or (*c*) *Staphylococcus epidermidis* (ATCC 12228) as the test organism, culture medium Cm1 with a final pH of 8.0–8.1, sterile phosphate buffer pH 8.0 TS1 or TS2, an appropriate concentration of neomycin (usually between 0.5 and 2 IU per ml), and an incubation temperature of 35–39 °C. The precision of the assay is such that the fiducial limits of error of the estimated potency ($P = 0.95$) are not less than 95% and not more than 105% of the estimated potency. The upper fiducial limit of error of the estimated potency ($P = 0.95$) is not less than 600 IU of neomycin per mg, calculated with reference to the dried substance.

NEOSTIGMINI METILSULFAS

Neostigmine metilsulfate

Molecular formula. $C_{13}H_{22}N_2O_6S$

Relative molecular mass.   334.4

Graphic formula.

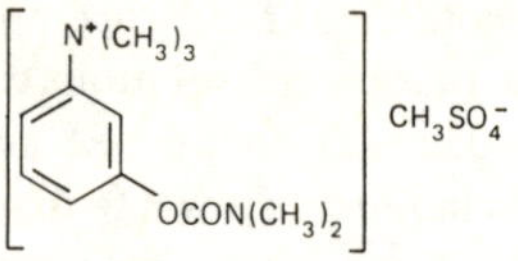

$$\left[\ \underset{\text{OCON(CH}_3)_2}{\overset{\text{N}^+(\text{CH}_3)_3}{\bigcirc}}\ \right] \text{CH}_3\text{SO}_4^-$$

Chemical name.   (*m*-Hydroxyphenyl)trimethylammonium methyl sulfate dimethylcarbamate; 3-[[(dimethylamino)carbonyl]oxy]-*N*,*N*,*N*-trimethylbenzenaminium methyl sulfate; CAS Reg. No. 51-60-5.

Description.   A white, crystalline powder; odourless.

Solubility.   Very soluble in water; freely soluble in ethanol (~750 g/l) TS.

Category.   Cholinergic.

Storage.   Neostigmine metilsulfate should be kept in a tightly closed container, protected from light.

REQUIREMENTS

General requirement.   Neostigmine metilsulfate contains not less than 98.0% and not more than 100.5% of $C_{13}H_{22}N_2O_6S$, calculated with reference to the dried substance.

Identity tests

● Either tests A and D or tests B, C and D may be applied.

A.   Carry out the examination as described under "Spectrophotometry in the infrared region" (vol. 1, p. 40). The infrared absorption spectrum is concordant with the spectrum obtained from neostigmine metilsulfate RS or with the *reference spectrum* of neostigmine metilsulfate.

B.   See the test described under "Related substances". The spot obtained with solution B corresponds in position, appearance, and intensity with that obtained with solution C.

C.   Heat 0.05 g with 0.4 g of potassium hydroxide R and 2 ml of ethanol (~750 g/l) TS on a water-bath for 3 minutes. Adjust to the original volume with ethanol (~750 g/l) TS, cool, and add 2 ml of water and 2 ml of diazobenzenedisulfonic acid TS; a red colour is produced.

D.   Mix 20 mg with 0.5 g of sodium carbonate R and heat to fusion in a small crucible; boil the fused mass with 10 ml of water until it has disintegrated, then filter.   Add 0.2 ml of bromine TS1 to the filtrate, heat to boiling, acidify with hydrochloric acid (~70 g/l) TS, and expel the excess of bromine by boiling; the resulting solution yields reaction A described under "General identification tests" as characteristic of sulfates (vol. 1, p. 115).

Melting range.   144–149 °C, after drying at 105 °C for 3 hours.

Chlorides.   Dissolve 0.20 g in 10 ml of water, add 1 ml of nitric acid (~130 g/l) TS and 1 ml of silver nitrate (40 g/l) TS; no immediate appearance of opalescence is observed.

Sulfates.   Dissolve 0.20 g in 10 ml of water, add 1.5 ml of hydrochloric acid (~70 g/l) TS and 1 ml of barium chloride (50 g/l) TS; no ready appearance of turbidity is produced.

Clarity and colour of solution.   A solution of 0.20 g in 10 ml of water is clear and not more intensely coloured than standard colour solution Bn1 when compared as described under "Colour of liquids" (vol. 1, p. 50).

Sulfated ash.   Not more than 1.0 mg/g.

Loss on drying.   Dry to constant weight at 105 °C; it loses not more than 10 mg/g.

Acidity.   Dissolve 0.20 g in 10 ml of water and add 0.1 ml of phenolphthalein/ethanol TS; the test solution is colourless.   Add 0.30 ml of sodium hydroxide (0.01 mol/l) VS; the solution turns red.

Related substances.   Carry out the test as described under "Thin-layer chromatography" (vol. 1, p. 83), using silica gel R1 as the coating substance and a mixture of 67 volumes of water, 30 volumes of methanol R, and 3 volumes of diethylamine R as the mobile phase (a certain type of precoated plate may not be suitable with this mobile phase).   Apply separately to the plate 10 μl of each of 3 solutions containing (A) 20 mg of the test substance per ml, (B) 0.10 mg of the test substance per ml, and (C) 0.10 mg of neostigmine metilsulfate RS per ml. After removing the plate from the chromatographic chamber allow it to dry in a current of warm air, spray it with 4-nitroaniline TS2 and then with sodium hydroxide (0.1 mol/l) VS. Dry the plate again in a current of warm air, spray it with potassium iodobismuthate TS2, and examine the chromatogram in daylight.   Any spot obtained with solution A, other than the principal spot, is not more intense than that obtained with solution B.

Assay. Dissolve about 0.15 g, accurately weighed, in 20 ml of water, transfer to an ammonia semi-micro distillation apparatus, and add 25 ml of sodium hydroxide ($\sim$400 g/l) TS. Pass a current of steam through the mixture and collect the distillate in 50 ml of sulfuric acid (0.01 mol/l) VS until the total volume reaches about 200 ml. Titrate the excess of acid with sodium hydroxide (0.02 mol/l) VS using methyl red/ethanol TS as indicator. Repeat the operation without the substance being tested; the difference between the titrations represents the amount of acid required to neutralize the dimethylamine formed from the neostigmine. Each ml of sulfuric acid (0.01 mol/l) VS is equivalent to 6.688 mg of $C_{13}H_{22}N_2O_6S$.

NIFURTIMOXUM

Nifurtimox

Molecular formula. $C_{10}H_{13}N_3O_5S$

Relative molecular mass. 287.3

Graphic formula.

Chemical name. 3-Methyl-4-[(5-nitrofurfurylidene)amino]thiomorpholine 1,1-dioxide; 3-methyl-*N*-[(5-nitro-2-furanyl)methylene]-4-thiomorpholinamine 1,1-dioxide; CAS Reg. No. 23256-30-6.

Description. A yellow to orange-yellow, crystalline powder; odourless.

Solubility. Practically insoluble in water and ether R; freely soluble in dimethylformamide R; sparingly soluble in dioxan R and chloroform R.

Category. Antitrypanosomal drug.

Storage. Nifurtimox should be kept in a well-closed container.

REQUIREMENTS

General requirement. Nifurtimox contains not less than 98.0% and not more than 102.0% of $C_{10}H_{13}N_3O_5S$, calculated with reference to the dried substance.

Identity tests

● Either test A alone or tests B and C may be applied.

A. Carry out the examination as described under "Spectrophotometry in the infrared region" (vol. 1, p. 40). The infrared absorption spectrum is concordant with the spectrum obtained from nifurtimox RS or with the *reference spectrum* of nifurtimox.

B. See the test described below under "Related substances". The principal spot obtained with solution B corresponds in position, appearance, and intensity with that obtained with solution C.

C. Dissolve 20 mg in a mixture of 2.0 ml of dimethylformamide R and 2.0 ml of water. Add 0.25 ml of copper(II) sulfate (160 g/l) TS and 4 drops of pyridine R; a dark green colour is produced. Add 5 ml of chloroform R and shake; the green colour remains in the aqueous layer.

Melting range. 178–182 °C.

Sulfated ash. Not more than 1.0 mg/g.

Loss on drying. Dry to constant weight at 105 °C; not more than 5.0 mg/g.

Related substances. Carry out the test as described under "Thin-layer chromatography" (vol. 1, p. 83), using silica gel R6 as the coating substance (a precoated plate from a commercial source is suitable) and a mixture of equal volumes of ethyl acetate R and hexane R as the mobile phase. Apply separately to the plate the following 3 solutions in acetone R: (A) 10 µl containing 10 mg of the test substance per ml, (B) 2 µl containing 1.0 mg of the test substance per ml, and (C) 2 µl containing 1.0 mg of nifurtimox RS per ml. Allow the spots to dry before placing the plate into an unsaturated chromatographic chamber and develop the plate for a distance of 10 cm. After removing the plate from the chromatographic chamber, allow it to dry in air, and examine the chromatogram in ultraviolet light (254 nm). Any spot obtained with solution A, other than the principal spot, is not more intense than that obtained with solution B.

Assay. Dissolve about 0.1 g, accurately weighed, in 20 ml of dimethylformamide R and 80 ml of ethanol (~750 g/l) TS. Add 5 ml of hydrochloric acid (~250 g/l) TS and start to bubble carbon dioxide R into the solution, keeping it up throughout the determination. After 3 minutes add 30.0 ml of titanium trichloride (0.1 mol/l) VS and 3 ml of potassium thiocyanate (200 g/l) TS. Allow to stand for 15 minutes and titrate the excess titanium trichloride with ferric ammonium sulfate (0.1 mol/l) VS. Each ml of titanium trichloride (0.1 mol/l) VS is equivalent to 4.788 mg of $C_{10}H_{13}N_3O_5S$.

NIRIDAZOLUM

Niridazole

Molecular formula. $C_6H_6N_4O_3S$

Relative molecular mass.   214.2

Graphic formula.

Chemical name.   1-(5-Nitro-2-thiazolyl)-2-imidazolidinone; CAS Reg. No. 61-57-4.

Description.   A yellow, crystalline powder; odourless or almost odourless.

Solubility.   Practically insoluble in water, chloroform R, and ether R; soluble in dimethylformamide R and pyridine R; slightly soluble in ethanol ($\sim$750 g/l) TS and acetone R.

Category.   Antischistosomal drug.

Storage.   Niridazole should be kept in a tightly closed container.

REQUIREMENTS

General requirement.   Niridazole contains not less than 97.0% and not more than 103.0% of $C_6H_6N_4O_3S$, calculated with reference to the dried substance.

Identity tests

● Either test A alone or tests B, C and D may be applied.

A.   Carry out the examination as described under "Spectrophotometry in the infrared region" (vol. 1, p. 40). The infrared absorption spectrum is concordant with the spectrum obtained from niridazole RS or with the *reference spectrum* of niridazole.

B.   See the test described below under "Related substances". The principal spot obtained with solution A corresponds in position, appearance, and intensity with that obtained with solution B.

C.   Dissolve 20 mg in 2.0 ml of acetone R, add 2.0 ml of sodium hydroxide (~80 g/l) TS, shake, and allow to stand for 10 minutes; a dark red colour is produced in the lower layer.

D.   Melting temperature, about 264 °C with decomposition.

Heavy metals.   Use 1.0 g for the preparation of the test solution as described under "Limit test for heavy metals", Procedure 3 (vol. 1, p. 118); determine the heavy metals content according to Method A (vol. 1, p. 119); not more than 20 µg/g.

Sulfates.   Add 0.5 g of the test substance to a mixture of 2.0 ml of hydrochloric acid (~70 g/l) TS and 8.0 ml of water, heat to boiling, cool to room temperature, filter, and dilute the filtrate to 10 ml with water; the solution is clear. Add 1.0 ml of barium chloride (0.5 mol/l) VS and again heat to boiling.

Similarly prepare a comparison solution containing 0.10 ml of sulfuric acid (0.01 mol/l) VS, 2.0 ml of hydrochloric acid (~70 g/l) TS, 8.0 ml of water, 1.0 ml of barium chloride (0.5 mol/l) VS, and heat to boiling.

Allow both solutions to stand for 1 hour; the opalescence in the solution prepared from the test substance is not more intense than that produced in the comparison solution.

Solution in dimethylformamide.   A solution of 0.10 g in 10 ml of dimethylformamide R is clear.

Sulfated ash.   Not more than 3.0 mg/g.

Loss on drying.   Dry at 100 °C under reduced pressure (not exceeding 0.6 kPa or about 5 mm of mercury) for 3 hours; it loses not more than 5.0 mg/g.

Related substances.   Carry out the test as described under "Thin-layer chromatography" (vol. 1, p. 83), using silica gel R6 as the coating substance (a precoated plate from a commercial source is suitable) and a mixture of 12 volumes of toluene R and 8 volumes of acetone R as the mobile phase. Apply separately to the plate 5 µl of each of 4 solutions in pyridine R containing (A) 10 mg of the test substance per ml (heat slightly to dissolve, if necessary), (B) 10 mg of niridazole RS per ml (heat slightly to dissolve, if necessary), (C) 20 µg of 2-amino-5-nitrothiazole RS per ml, and (D) 40 µg of niridazole-chlorethylcarboxamide RS per ml. After removing the plate from the chromatographic chamber, allow it to dry in a current of air; examine the chromatogram immediately in ultraviolet light (365 nm) and again after 15 minutes' irradiation. Any spot obtained with solution A, other than the principal spot, is not more intense than that obtained with solution C viewed immediately and not more intense than that obtained with solution D viewed after 15 minutes.

Assay.   Dissolve about 40 mg, accurately weighed, in 4 ml of dimethylformamide R and dilute with sufficient dehydrated ethanol R to produce 200 ml; dilute 5.0 ml of this solution to 100 ml with the same solvent. Measure the absorbance of a 1-cm layer of the diluted solution at the maximum at about 359 nm. Calculate the amount of $C_6H_6N_4O_3S$ in the substance being tested by comparison with niridazole RS, similarly and concurrently examined. In an adequately calibrated spectrophotometer the absorbance of a 10 µg/ml solution of niridazole RS should be 0.70 ± 0.03.

NITRAZEPAMUM

Nitrazepam

Molecular formula. $C_{15}H_{11}N_3O_3$

Relative molecular mass.   281.3

Graphic formula.

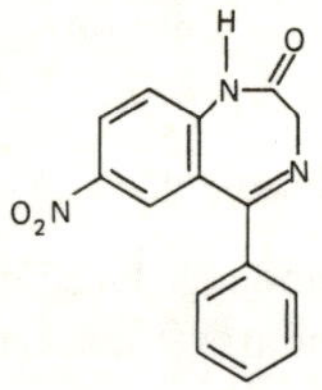

Chemical name.   1,3-Dihydro-7-nitro-5-phenyl-2H-1,4-benzodiazepin-2-one; CAS Reg. No. 146-22-5.

Description.   A yellow, crystalline powder; odourless or almost odourless.

Solubility.   Practically insoluble in water; sparingly soluble in chloroform R; slightly soluble in ethanol ($\sim$750 g/l) TS; very slightly soluble in ether R.

Category.   Sedative; hypnotic.

Storage.   Nitrazepam should be kept in a well-closed container, protected from light.

REQUIREMENTS

General requirement.   Nitrazepam contains not less than 98.5% and not more than 101.0% of $C_{15}H_{11}N_3O_3$, calculated with reference to the dried substance.

Identity tests

A. NOTE: Carry out the following operations in subdued light. Prepare a 0.005 mg/ml solution in a mixture of 1 volume of hydrochloric acid (1 mol/l) VS and 9 volumes of methanol R and examine immediately. The absorption spectrum, when observed between 230 nm and 350 nm, exhibits a maximum only at about 280 nm; the absorbance of a 1-cm layer at this wavelength is about 0.45.

B. Dissolve 10 mg in 1 ml of methanol R, warming if necessary, and add 0.05 ml of sodium hydroxide (~80 g/l) TS; an intense yellow colour is produced.

C. Dissolve 20 mg in a mixture of 5 ml of hydrochloric acid (~420 g/l) TS and 10 ml of water, boil for 5 minutes, cool, and add 2 ml of sodium nitrite (1 g/l) TS. Allow to stand for 1 minute, add 1 ml of sulfamic acid (5 g/l) TS, mix, allow to stand for 1 minute, and add 1 ml of N-(1-naphthyl)ethylenediamine hydrochloride (1 g/l) TS; a red colour is produced.

D. Melting temperature, about 227 °C with decomposition.

Heavy metals. Use 1.0 g for the preparation of the test solution as described under "Limit test for heavy metals", Procedure 3 (vol. 1, p. 118); determine the heavy metals content according to Method A (vol. 1, p. 119); not more than 20 µg/g.

Sulfated ash. Not more than 1.0 mg/g.

Loss on drying. Dry at 105 °C for 4 hours; it loses not more than 5.0 mg/g.

Related substances. Carry out the test in subdued light as described under "Thin-layer chromatography" (vol. 1, p. 83), using silica gel R4 as the coating substance and a mixture of 85 volumes of nitromethane R and 15 volumes of ethyl acetate R as the mobile phase. Apply separately to the plate 10 µl of each of 2 freshly prepared solutions in a mixture of equal volumes of chloroform R and methanol R containing (A) 25 mg of the test substance per ml and (B) 25 µg of the test substance per ml. Develop the plate for a distance of 12 cm. After removing the plate from the chromatographic chamber, allow it to dry in air and examine the chromatogram in ultraviolet light (254 nm). Any spot obtained with solution A, other than the principal spot, is not more intense than that obtained with solution B.

Assay. Dissolve about 0.25 g, accurately weighed, in 30 ml of acetic anhydride R, and titrate with perchloric acid (0.1 mol/l) VS, determining the endpoint potentiometrically as described under "Non-aqueous titration", Method A (vol. 1, p. 131). Each ml of perchloric acid (0.1 mol/l) VS is equivalent to 28.13 mg of $C_{15}H_{11}N_3O_3$.

NITROFURANTOINUM

Nitrofurantoin

Nitrofurantoin, anhydrous
Nitrofurantoin monohydrate

Molecular formula. $C_8H_6N_4O_5$ (anhydrous); $C_8H_6N_4O_5,H_2O$ (monohydrate).

Relative molecular mass.   238.2 (anhydrous); 256.2 (monohydrate).

Graphic formula.

$$O_2N\ \text{—furan—}CH=N-N\ \text{(hydantoin ring)}\quad \cdot\ nH_2O$$

n = 0 (anhydrous)
n = 1 (monohydrate)

Chemical name.   1-[(5-Nitrofurfurylidene)amino]hydantoin; 1-[[(5-nitro-2-furanyl)methylene]amino]-2,4-imidazolidinedione; CAS Reg. No. 67-20-9 (anhydrous).
1-[(5-Nitrofurfurylidene)amino]hydantoin monohydrate; 1-[[(5-nitro-2-furanyl)-methylene]amino]-2,4-imidazolidinedione monohydrate; CAS Reg. No. 17140-81-7 (monohydrate).

Other name.   Furadoninum.

Description.   Lemon-yellow crystals or a yellow, crystalline powder; odourless or almost odourless.

Solubility.   Practically insoluble in water; very slightly soluble in ethanol (~750 g/l) TS; soluble in dimethylformamide R.

Category.   Antibacterial drug.

Storage.   Nitrofurantoin should be kept in a well-closed container, protected from light, and stored at a temperature not exceeding 25 °C.

Labelling.   The designation on the container of Nitrofurantoin should state whether the substance is the monohydrate or is in the anhydrous form.

Additional information.   Nitrofurantoin melts at about 271 °C with decomposition. Nitrofurantoin and its solutions are discoloured by alkali and by exposure to light and are decomposed upon contact with metals other than stainless steel and aluminium.

REQUIREMENTS

General requirement.   Nitrofurantoin contains not less than 98.0% and not more than 102.0% of $C_8H_6N_4O_5$, calculated with reference to the dried substance.

Identity tests

● Either test A alone or tests B, C and D may be applied.

A.   Carry out the examination as described under "Spectrophotometry in the infrared region" (vol. 1, p. 40). For Nitrofurantoin monohydrate, the substance must be previously dried to constant weight at 105 °C. The infrared absorption spectrum is concordant with the spectrum obtained from nitrofurantoin RS or with the *reference spectrum* of nitrofurantoin.

B.   NOTE: Carry out the following operations in subdued light.

Prepare a blank solution by dissolving 3.6 g of sodium acetate R in 20 ml of water, adding 0.3 ml of glacial acetic acid R, and diluting with sufficient water to produce 200 ml. Dissolve 0.12 g in 50 ml of dimethylformamide R and add sufficient water to produce 1000 ml. Dilute 5 ml of this solution to 100 ml with the blank solution prepared above. Measure the absorption spectrum of the resulting solution against 10 ml of the blank solution to which 0.05 ml of dimethylformamide R has been added. When observed between 220 nm and 400 nm, the absorption spectrum exhibits maxima at about 266 nm and 367 nm. The absorbances of a 1-cm layer at these wavelengths are about 0.32 and 0.46, respectively. The ratio of the absorbance at 367 nm to that at 266 nm is between 1.36 and 1.42.

C.   Dissolve 0.2 g in a mixture of 10 ml of dimethylformamide R and 1 drop of glacial acetic acid R. To 0.5 ml of this solution add 2 ml of water, 0.15 ml of copper(II) sulfate (80 g/l) TS, and 0.2 ml of pyridine R; shake with 3 ml of chloroform R and allow the layers to separate; a green colour is produced in the chloroform layer.

D.   Dissolve 5 mg in 5 ml of sodium hydroxide (0.1 mol/l) VS; a deep yellow solution is produced, which becomes deep orange-red on standing.

Sulfated ash.   Not more than 1.0 mg/g.

Loss on drying.   Dry to constant weight at 105 °C; anhydrous Nitrofurantoin loses not more than 10 mg/g. Nitrofurantoin monohydrate loses not less than 50 mg/g and not more than 71 mg/g.

Related substances.   Carry out the test as described under "Thin-layer chromatography" (vol. 1, p. 83), using silica gel R2 as the coating substance and a mixture of 90 volumes of nitromethane R and 10 volumes of methanol R as the mobile phase. Apply separately to the plate 10 µl of each of 2 solutions: (A) dissolve 0.25 g of the test substance in a minimum volume of dimethylformamide R and dilute to

10 ml with acetone R; (B) dilute 1 ml of solution A to 100 ml with acetone R. After removing the plate from the chromatographic chamber, allow it to dry in air and heat it at 105 °C for 5 minutes. Spray the warm plate with phenylhydrazine/hydrochloric acid TS, heat it again at 105 °C for 10 minutes, and examine the chromatogram in ultraviolet light (254 nm). Any spot obtained with solution A, other than the principal spot, is not more intense than that obtained with solution B.

Assay. Dissolve about 0.4 g, accurately weighed, in a mixture of 10 ml of dimethylformamide R and 10 ml of dioxan R, add 0.10 ml of thymol blue/dimethylformamide TS and titrate with lithium methoxide (0.1 mol/l) VS to a dark green endpoint, as described under "Non-aqueous titration", Method B (vol. 1, p. 132). Each ml of lithium methoxide (0.1 mol/l) VS is equivalent to 23.82 mg of $C_8H_6N_4O_5$.

NOSCAPINUM

Noscapine

Molecular formula. $C_{22}H_{23}NO_7$

Relative molecular mass. 413.4

Graphic formula.

Chemical name. Narcotine; (5*R*)-5-[(1*S*)-6,7-dimethoxyphthalidyl]-5,6,7,8-tetrahydro-4-methoxy-6-methyl-1,3-dioxolo[4,5-*g*]isoquinoline; [*S*-(*R**,*S**)]-6,7-dimethoxy-3-(5,6,7,8-tetrahydro-4-methoxy-6-methyl-1,3-dioxolo[4,5-*g*]isoquinolin-5-yl)-1(3*H*)-isobenzofuranone; CAS Reg. No. 128-62-1.

Description. Colourless crystals or a white, crystalline powder; odourless or almost odourless.

Solubility. Practically insoluble in water; sparingly soluble in boiling water; soluble in chloroform R; slightly soluble in ethanol ($\sim$750 g/l) TS and ether R.

Category. Antitussive drug.

Storage. Noscapine should be kept in a well-closed container.

REQUIREMENTS

General requirement.   Noscapine contains not less than 98.5% and not more than 101.0% of $C_{22}H_{23}NO_7$, calculated with reference to the dried substance.

Identity tests

● Either test A alone or tests B, C and D may be applied.

A.   Carry out the examination as described under "Spectrophotometry in the infrared region" (vol. 1, p. 40). The infrared absorption spectrum is concordant with the spectrum obtained from noscapine RS or with the *reference spectrum* of noscapine.

B.   The absorption spectrum of a 0.050 mg/ml solution in methanol R, when observed between 230 nm and 350 nm, exhibits 2 maxima at about 291 nm and 310 nm and a minimum at about 263 nm. The ratio of the absorbance at 310 nm to that at 291 nm is about 1.2.

C.   To 10 mg add about 0.5 ml of sulfuric acid ($\sim$1760 g/l) TS and mix; a greenish yellow solution is formed, which becomes red and finally violet on heating.

D.   Melting temperature, about 175 °C.

Specific optical rotation.   Use a 20 mg/ml solution in hydrochloric acid (0.1 mol/l) VS; $[\alpha]_D^{20\,°C} = +42$ to $+48°$.

Sulfated ash.   Not more than 1.0 mg/g.

Loss on drying.   Dry to constant weight at 105 °C; it loses not more than 10 mg/g.

Related substances.   Carry out the test as described under "Thin-layer chromatography" (vol. 1, p. 83), using silica gel R5 as the coating substance and a mixture of 45 volumes of acetone R, 45 volumes of toluene R, 7 volumes of ethanol ($\sim$750 g/l) TS, and 3 volumes of ammonia ($\sim$260 g/l) TS as the mobile phase. Apply separately to the plate 10 μl of each of 2 solutions in ethanol ($\sim$750 g/l) TS containing (A) 20 mg of the test substance per ml and (B) 0.20 mg of the test substance per ml. After removing the plate from the chromatographic chamber, allow it to dry in air, spray it with iodine (0.1 mol/l) VS, and examine the chromatogram in daylight. Any spot obtained with solution A, other than the principal spot, is not more intense than that obtained with solution B.

Assay.   Dissolve about 0.5 g, accurately weighed, in 40 ml of glacial acetic acid R1, warming gently, and titrate with perchloric acid (0.1 mol/l) VS as described under "Non-aqueous titration", Method A (vol. 1, p. 131). Each ml of perchloric acid (0.1 mol/l) VS is equivalent to 41.34 mg of $C_{22}H_{23}NO_7$.

NOSCAPINI HYDROCHLORIDUM

Noscapine hydrochloride

Molecular formula. $C_{22}H_{23}NO_7,HCl,H_2O$

Relative molecular mass.   467.9

Graphic formula.

Chemical name.   Narcotine hydrochloride monohydrate; $(5R)$-5-[$(1S)$-6,7-di-methoxyphthalidyl]-5,6,7,8-tetrahydro-4-methoxy-6-methyl-1,3-dioxolo[4,5-g]isoquinoline hydrochloride monohydrate; [S-(R^*,S^*)]-6,7-dimethoxy-3-(5,6,7,8-tetrahydro-4-methoxy-6-methyl-1,3-dioxolo[4,5-g]isoquinolin-5-yl)-1($3H$)-isobenzofuranone hydrochloride monohydrate; CAS Reg. No. 912-60-7 (anhydrous).

Description.   Colourless crystals or a white, crystalline powder; odourless.

Solubility.   Freely soluble in water, ethanol ($\sim$750 g/l) TS, and chloroform R; practically insoluble in ether R.

Category.   Antitussive drug.

Storage.   Noscapine hydrochloride should be kept in a well-closed container, protected from light.

Additional information.   Noscapine hydrochloride is hygroscopic.

REQUIREMENTS

General requirement.   Noscapine hydrochloride contains not less than 98.5% and not more than 101.0% of $C_{22}H_{23}NO_7,HCl$, calculated with reference to the dried substance.

Identity tests

• Either tests A and D or tests B, C and D may be applied.

A.   Dissolve 0.1 g in 10 ml of water, make the solution alkaline with ammonia (~100 g/l) TS, and shake it with 10 ml of chloroform R. Separate the chloroform layer, wash it with 5 ml of water, and filter. Evaporate the filtrate almost to dryness on a water-bath, add 1 ml of dehydrated ethanol R, and evaporate to dryness. Carry out the examination using the dried residue as described under "Spectrophotometry in the infrared region" (vol. 1, p. 40). The infrared absorption spectrum is concordant with the spectrum obtained from noscapine RS or with the *reference spectrum* of noscapine.

B.   Dilute 5 ml of ammonia (~35 g/l) TS to 100 ml with methanol R; then dilute further 1 ml of this solution to 100 ml with methanol R. The absorption spectrum of a 0.050 mg/ml solution in the prepared ammonia/methanol mixture, when observed between 230 nm and 350 nm, exhibits 2 maxima at about 291 nm and 310 nm and a minimum at about 263 nm. The ratio of the absorbance at 310 nm to that at 291 nm is between 1.2 and 1.3.

C.   Place about 0.1 g on a porcelain dish, add drop by drop sulfuric acid (~1760 g/l) TS and mix; a greenish yellow colour is obtained, which turns red and finally violet on heating.

D.   A 20 mg/ml solution yields reaction A described under "General identification tests" as characteristic of chlorides (vol. 1, p. 112).

Specific optical rotation.   Use a 20 mg/ml solution in hydrochloric acid (0.01 mol/l) VS and calculate with reference to the dried substance; $[\alpha]_D^{20\,°C} = + 38.5$ to $+ 44.0°$.

Sulfated ash.   Not more than 1.0 mg/g.

Loss on drying.   Dry to constant weight at 105 °C; it loses not more than 65 mg/g.

Related substances.   Carry out the test as described under "Thin-layer chromatography" (vol. 1, p. 83), using silica gel R5 as the coating substance and a mixture of 45 volumes of acetone R, 45 volumes of toluene R, 7 volumes of ethanol (~750 g/l) TS, and 3 volumes of ammonia (~260 g/l) TS as the mobile phase. Apply separately to the plate 10 µl of each of 2 solutions in ethanol (~750 g/l) TS containing (A) 20 mg of the test substance per ml, and (B) 0.20 mg of the test substance per ml. After removing the plate from the chromatographic chamber, allow it to dry in air, spray it with iodine (0.1 mol/l) VS, and examine the chromatogram in daylight. Any spot obtained with solution A, other than the principal spot, is not more intense than that obtained with solution B.

Assay.   Dissolve about 0.5 g, accurately weighed, in 50 ml of a mixture of 7 volumes of acetic anhydride R and 3 volumes of glacial acetic acid R1, add 10 ml of mercuric acetate/acetic acid TS and titrate with perchloric acid (0.1 mol/l) VS as described under "Non-aqueous titration", Method A (vol. 1, p. 131). Each ml of perchloric acid (0.1 mol/l) VS is equivalent to 44.99 mg of $C_{22}H_{23}NO_7,HCl$.

NYSTATINUM

Nystatin

Composition. Nystatin is a mixture of substances produced by the growth of certain strains of *Streptomyces noursei,* the main component of which is nystatin A_1.

Chemical name.   Nystatin; CAS Reg. No. 1400-61-9.

Description.   A yellow to light brown powder.

Solubility.   Very slightly soluble in water; sparingly soluble in ethanol ($\sim$750 g/l) TS and methanol R; practically insoluble in chloroform R and ether R.

Category.   Antifungal drug.

Storage.   Nystatin should be kept in a tightly closed container, protected from light and stored at a temperature not exceeding 5 °C.

Additional information.   Nystatin is hygroscopic. Even in the absence of light, it is gradually degraded on exposure to a humid atmosphere, the decomposition being faster at higher temperatures. The potency of Nystatin may fall at a rate of 1% per month when it is stored under the conditions mentioned above.

REQUIREMENTS

General requirement.   Nystatin contains not less than 4400 International Units per mg, calculated with reference to the dried substance.

Identity tests

A.   Dissolve 0.10 g in a mixture of 50 ml of methanol R and 5 ml of glacial acetic acid R, add sufficient methanol R to produce 100 ml, and dilute 1 ml to 100 ml with methanol R. The absorption spectrum of the resulting solution, when observed between 240 nm and 350 nm, exhibits 3 maxima at about 291 nm, 305 nm, and 319 nm; the ratio of the absorbance of a 1-cm layer at 291 nm to that at 305 nm is between 0.61 and 0.73, and the ratio of the absorbance at 291 nm to that at 319 nm is between 0.83 and 0.96.

B.   Shake 30 mg with 5 ml of water for 2 minutes, add 2 ml of a solution prepared by dissolving 0.1 g of pyrogallol R in 100 ml of decolorized fuchsin TS, heat on a water-bath until a dark pink colour is produced, cool, and allow to stand for 1 hour; the pink colour is retained.

Loss on drying.   Dry to constant weight at 60 °C under reduced pressure (not exceeding 0.6 kPa or about 5 mm of mercury); it loses not more than 50 mg/g.

pH value.   Shake 0.3 g with 10 ml of carbon-dioxide-free water R; pH of the suspension, 6.5 – 8.0.

Undue toxicity.   Carry out the test as described under "Test for undue toxicity" (vol. 1, p. 154), injecting intraperitoneally 0.5 ml of a suspension in acacia (5 g/l) TS containing a quantity equivalent to 600 IU.

Assay.   Carry out the assay as described under "Microbiological assay of antibiotics" (vol. 1, p. 145), using Petri dishes or rectangular trays filled to a depth of 1 – 2 mm with culture medium Cm3 having a final pH of 6.0 – 6.2 and inoculated with *Saccharomyces cerevisiae* (NCYC 87; ATCC 9763) as the test organism, adding an appropriate concentration of nystatin (usually between 25 and 300 IU per ml) and incubating at a temperature of 29 – 33 °C. Prepare the solutions of the test substance by dissolving 75 mg in sufficient dimethylformamide R to produce 50 ml and dilute 10 ml to 200 ml with sterile phosphate buffer pH 6.0, TS3. Protect the solutions from light throughout the assay. The precision of the assay is such that the fiducial limits of error of the estimated potency ($P = 0.95$) are not less than 95% and not more than 105% of the estimated potency. The upper fiducial limit of error of the estimated potency ($P = 0.95$) is not less than 4400 IU of nystatin per mg, calculated with reference to the dried substance.

OXAMNIQUINUM

Oxamniquine

Molecular formula. $C_{14}H_{21}N_3O_3$

Relative molecular mass.   279.3

Graphic formula.

Chemical name.   1,2,3,4-Tetrahydro-2-[(isopropylamino)methyl]-7-nitro-6-quinolinemethanol; 1,2,3,4-tetrahydro-2-[[(1-methylethyl)amino]methyl]-7-nitro-6-quinolinemethanol; CAS Reg. No. 21738-42-1.

Description.   A yellow-orange, crystalline powder.

Solubility.   Sparingly soluble in water, soluble in methanol R, acetone R, and chloroform R.

Category.   Antischistosomal.

Storage.   Oxamniquine should be kept in a well-closed container.

REQUIREMENTS

General requirement.   Oxamniquine contains not less than 97.0% and not more than 103.0% of $C_{14}H_{21}N_3O_3$, calculated with reference to the anhydrous substance.

Identity tests

● Either test A or tests B and C may be applied.

A.   Carry out the examination as described under "Spectrophotometry in the infrared region" (vol. 1, p. 40). The infrared absorption spectrum is concordant with the spectrum obtained from oxamniquine RS or with the *reference spectrum* of oxamniquine.

B.   To 10 mg add 10 mg of zinc R powder, 1.0 ml of water, and about 0.5 ml of hydrochloric acid ($\sim$250 g/l) TS. Heat in a water-bath for 5 minutes, cool in ice, add 1 ml of sodium nitrite (100 g/l) TS, and remove the excess nitrite by adding sufficient sulfamic acid (50 g/l) TS. Add 0.5 ml of the resulting solution to a mixture of 0.5 ml of 2-naphthol TS1 and 2.0 ml of sodium hydroxide ($\sim$80 g/l) TS; an orange-red colour is produced.

C.   Melting temperature, about 151 °C.

Heavy metals.   Use 0.5 g for the preparation of the test solution as described under "Limit test for heavy metals", Procedure 3 (vol. 1, p. 118); determine the heavy metals content according to Method A (vol. 1, p. 119); not more than 50 µg/g.

Iron.   Ignite 1.0 g; cool and dissolve the residue in 5 ml of hydrochloric acid ($\sim$250 g/l) FeTS and 30 ml of water. Treat the solution as described under "Limit test for iron" (vol. 1, p. 121); the iron content is not more than 50 µg/g.

Sulfated ash.   Not more than 2.0 mg/g.

Water.   Determine as described under "Determination of water by the Karl Fischer method", Method A (vol. 1, p. 135), using about 0.5 g of the substance; the water content is not more than 20 mg/g.

pH value.   Shake 0.1 g with 10 ml of carbon-dioxide-free water R; pH of the suspension, 8.0–10.0.

Related substances.   Carry out the test as described under "Thin-layer chromatography" (vol. 1, p. 83), using silica gel R6 as the coating substance (a precoated plate from a commercial source is suitable) and 20 volumes of chloroform R, 10 volumes of hexane R, 2 volumes of 2-propanol R, and 0.5 volume of isopropylamine R as the mobile phase. Apply separately to the plate 10 µl of each of 2 solutions in a mixture of equal volumes of chloroform R and methanol R containing (A) 25 mg of the test substance per ml and (B) 0.25 mg of the test substance per ml. After removing the plate from the chromatographic chamber, allow it to dry in air for 10 minutes until the solvents have evaporated. Examine the chromatogram in ultraviolet light first at 254 nm then at 365 nm. Any spot obtained with solution A, other than the principal spot, is not more intense than that obtained with solution B.

Assay.   Dissolve about 0.3 g, accurately weighed, in 30 ml of glacial acetic acid R1, previously neutralized to oracet blue R/acetic acid TS. Titrate with perchloric acid (0.1 mol/l) VS as described under "Non-aqueous titration", Method A (vol. 1, p. 131). Each ml of perchloric acid (0.1 mol/l) VS is equivalent to 27.93 mg of $C_{14}H_{21}N_3O_3$.

OXYTETRACYCLINI DIHYDRAS

Oxytetracycline dihydrate

Oxytetracycline dihydrate (non-injectable)
Oxytetracycline dihydrate, sterile

Molecular formula. $C_{22}H_{24}N_2O_9,2H_2O$

Relative molecular mass.   496.5

Graphic formula.

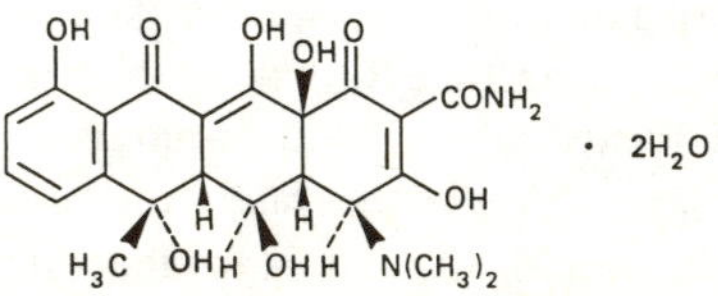

OH O OH OH O CONH$_2$ OH H$_3$C OH H OH H N(CH$_3$)$_2$ H H · 2H$_2$O

Chemical name.   (4S,4aR,5S,5aR,6S,12aS)-4-(Dimethylamino)-1,4,4a,5,5a,6, 11,12a-octahydro-3,5,6,10,12,12a-hexahydroxy-6-methyl-1,11-dioxo-2-naphthacenecarboxamide dihydrate; [4S-(4α,4aα,5α,5aα,6β,12aα)]-4-(dimethylamino)-1,4,4a,5,5a,6,11,12a-octahydro-3,5,6,10,12,12a-hexahydroxy-6-methyl-1,11-dioxo-2naphthacenecarboxamide dihydrate; CAS Reg. No. 6153-64-6 (dihydrate).

Description. A pale yellow, crystalline powder; odourless.

Solubility. Very slightly soluble in water; sparingly soluble in ethanol ($\sim$750 g/l) TS; freely soluble in dilute acids and alkalis.

Category. Antibacterial drug.

Storage. Oxytetracycline dihydrate should be kept in a tightly closed container, protected from light.

Labelling. The designation sterile Oxytetracycline dihydrate indicates that the substance complies with the additional requirements for sterile Oxytetracycline dihydrate and may be used for parenteral administration or for other sterile applications.

Additional information. Oxytetracycline dihydrate darkens on exposure to strong sunlight. It deteriorates in solutions having a pH below 2 and is rapidly destroyed by alkali hydroxide solutions.

REQUIREMENTS

General requirement. Oxytetracycline dihydrate contains not less than 920 International Units of oxytetracycline per mg, calculated with reference to the anhydrous substance.

Identity tests

A. Carry out the test as described under "Thin-layer chromatography" (vol. 1, p. 83), using a kieselguhr coating prepared as follows: To 25 g of kieselguhr R1 add 50 ml of a mixture of 2.5 ml of glycerol R and 47.5 ml of disodium edetate (0.1 mol/l) VS previously adjusted to pH 7 with ammonia ($\sim$100 g/l) TS. Coat the plates with this mixture and allow them to dry at room temperature for about 70–90 minutes, or until sufficiently dry to give a satisfactory separation. As the mobile phase, take 200 ml of a mixture of 2 volumes of ethyl acetate R, 2 volumes of chloroform R, and 1 volume of acetone R, shake with 25 ml of disodium edetate (0.1 mol/l) VS previously adjusted to pH 7 with ammonia ($\sim$100 g/l) TS, allow to settle, and use the lower layer. Apply separately to the plate 1 µl of each of 3 solutions in methanol R containing (A) 0.50 mg of the test substance per ml, (B) 0.50 mg of oxytetracycline dihydrate RS per ml, and (C) a mixture of 0.50 mg of chlortetracycline hydrochloride RS per ml, 0.50 mg of oxytetracycline dihydrate RS per ml, and 0.50 mg of tetracycline hydrochloride RS per ml. After removing the plate from the chromatographic chamber, allow it to dry in air, expose it to the vapour of ammonia ($\sim$260 g/l) TS, and examine the chromatogram in ultraviolet light (365 nm). The principal spot obtained with solution A corresponds in position, appearance, and intensity with that obtained with solution B. The test is not valid unless the chromatogram obtained with solution C shows 3 clearly separated spots.

B.   To about 1 mg add 2 ml of sulfuric acid ($\sim$1760 g/l) TS; a deep red colour is produced, which changes to yellow on the addition of 0.1 ml of water.

Specific optical rotation.   Dissolve 0.25 g in sufficient hydrochloric acid (0.1 mol/l) VS to produce 25 ml, and allow to stand for 60 minutes. Measure the rotation and calculate with reference to the anhydrous substance; $[\alpha]_D^{20\,°C} = -203$ to $-216°$.

Sulfated ash.   Not more than 5.0 mg/g.

Water.   Determine as described under "Determination of water by the Karl Fischer method", Method A (vol. 1, p. 135), using about 0.25 g of the substance; the water content is not less than 40 mg/g and not more than 75 mg/g.

pH value.   pH of a 10 mg/ml solution in carbon-dioxide-free water R, 4.5 – 7.5.

Absorption in the ultraviolet region.   The absorption spectrum of a 20 µg/ml solution in hydrochloric acid (0.1 mol/l) VS, when observed between 230 nm and 400 nm, exhibits 2 maxima at about 268 nm and 353 nm. The absorbance of a 1-cm layer at 353 nm is not less than 0.54 and not more than 0.58.

Light-absorbing impurities.   Prepare a 2.0 mg/ml solution in a mixture of 1 volume of hydrochloric acid (1 mol/l) VS and 99 volumes of methanol R and measure within 1 hour of preparation the absorbance of a 1-cm layer at 430 nm; the absorbance does not exceed 0.25. Prepare a 10 mg/ml solution in a mixture of 1 volume of hydrochloric acid (1 mol/l) VS and 99 volumes of methanol R, and measure within 1 hour of preparation the absorbance of a 1-cm layer at 490 nm; the absorbance does not exceed 0.20.

Assay.   Carry out the assay as described under "Microbiological assay of antibiotics" (vol. 1, p. 145), using either (a) *Bacillus pumilus* (NCTC 8241 or ATCC 14884) as the test organism, culture medium Cml with a final pH of 6.5 – 6.6, sterile phosphate buffer, pH 4.5 TS, an appropriate concentration of oxytetracycline (usually between 2 and 20 IU per ml), and an incubation temperature of 37 – 39 °C, or (b) *Bacillus cereus* (ATCC 11778) as the test organism, culture medium Cml with a final pH of 5.9 – 6.0, sterile phosphate buffer, pH 4.5 TS, an appropriate concentration of oxytetracycline (usually between 0.5 and 2 IU per ml), and an incubation temperature of 30 – 33 °C. The precision of the assay is such that the fiducial limits of error of the estimated potency ($P = 0.95$) are not less than 95 % and not more than 105 % of the estimated potency. The upper fiducial limit of error of the estimated potency ($P = 0.95$) is not less than 900 IU of oxytetracycline per mg, calculated with reference to the anhydrous substance.

Additional Requirements for Sterile Oxytetracycline Dihydrate

Undue toxicity.   Carry out the test as described under "Test for undue toxicity" (vol. 1, p. 154), using 0.5 ml of a solution prepared as follows: Dissolve 40 mg of the substance to be tested in 2.0 ml of hydrochloric acid (0.1 mol/l) VS and dilute with sufficient sterile water R to produce 20 ml.

Pyrogens.   Carry out the test as described under "Test for pyrogens" (vol. 1, p. 155), injecting per kg of the rabbit's mass, 1 ml of a solution prepared as follows: Dissolve 50 mg of the substance to be tested in 2.5 ml of hydrochloric acid (0.1 mol/l) VS and dilute with sufficient sterile water R to produce 10.0 ml.

Sterility.   Complies with the "Sterility testing of antibiotics" (vol. 1, p. 152), applying the membrane filtration test procedure and using a diluting fluid containing 1 ml of macrogol *p*-isooctylphenyl ether R per litre of peptone (1 g/l) TS.

OXYTETRACYCLINI HYDROCHLORIDUM

Oxytetracycline hydrochloride

Oxytetracycline hydrochloride (non-injectable)
Oxytetracycline hydrochloride, sterile

Molecular formula. $C_{22}H_{24}N_2O_9,HCl$

Relative molecular mass.   496.9

Graphic formula.

Chemical name.   (4*S*,4a*R*,5*S*,5a*R*,6*S*,12a*S*)-4-(Dimethylamino)1,4,4a,5,5a,6, 11,12a-octahydro-3,5,6,10,12,12a-hexahydroxy-6-methyl-1,11-dioxo-2-naphthacenecarboxamide monohydrochloride; [4*S*-(4α,4aα,5α,5aα,6β,12aα)]-4-(dimethylamino)-1,4,4a,5,5a,6,11,12a-octahydro-3,5,6,10,12,12a-hexahydroxy-6-methyl1,11-dioxo-2-naphthacenecarboxamide monohydrochloride; CAS Reg. No. 2058-46-0.

Description.   A yellow, crystalline powder; odourless.

Solubility.   Soluble in 2 parts of water and in 45 parts of ethanol (~750 g/l) TS; practically insoluble in chloroform R and in ether R.

Category.   Antibacterial drug.

Storage.   Oxytetracycline hydrochloride should be kept in a tightly closed container, protected from light.

Labelling.   The designation sterile Oxytetracycline hydrochloride indicates that the substance complies with the additional requirements for sterile Oxytetracycline hydrochloride and may be used for parenteral administration or for other sterile applications.

Additional information.   Oxytetracycline hydrochloride is hygroscopic. Even in the absence of light, it is gradually degraded on exposure to a humid atmosphere, the decomposition being faster at higher temperatures. Dissolved in water it becomes turbid on standing owing to the separation of the base caused through partial hydrolysis of the hydrochloride. It deteriorates in solutions of pH below 2, and is rapidly destroyed by alkali hydroxide solutions.

REQUIREMENTS

General requirement.   Oxytetracycline hydrochloride contains not less than 870 International Units of oxytetracycline per mg, calculated with reference to the anhydrous substance.

Identity tests

A.   Carry out the test as described under "Thin-layer chromatography" (vol. 1, p. 83), using a kieselguhr coating prepared as follows: To 25 g of kieselguhr R1 add 50 ml of a mixture of 2.5 ml of glycerol R and 47.5 ml of disodium edetate (0.1 mol/l) VS previously adjusted to pH 7 with ammonia (~100 g/l) TS. Coat the plates with this mixture, and allow them to dry at room temperature for about 70–90 minutes, or until sufficiently dry to give a satisfactory separation. As the mobile phase, take 200 ml of a mixture of 2 volumes of ethyl acetate R, 2 volumes of chloroform R, and 1 volume of acetone R, shake with 25 ml of disodium edetate (0.1 mol/l) VS previously adjusted to pH 7 with ammonia (~100 g/l) TS, allow to settle, and use the lower layer. Apply separately to the plate 1 µl of each of 3 solutions in methanol R containing (A) 0.50 mg of the test substance per ml, (B) 0.50 mg of oxytetracycline hydrochloride RS per ml, and (C) a mixture of 0.50 mg of chlortetracycline hydrochloride RS per ml, 0.50 mg of oxytetracycline hydrochloride RS per ml, and 0.50 mg of tetracycline hydrochloride RS per ml. After removing the plate from the chromatographic chamber, allow it to dry in air, expose it to the vapour of ammonia (~260 g/l) TS, and examine the chromatogram in ultraviolet light (365 nm). The principal spot obtained with solution A corresponds in position, appearance, and intensity with that obtained with solution B. The test is not valid unless the chromatogram obtained with solution C shows 3 clearly separated spots.

B.   To about 1 mg add 2 ml of sulfuric acid ($\sim$1760 g/l) TS; a deep red colour is produced, which changes to yellow on the addition of 0.1 ml of water.

C.   A 0.05 g/ml solution yields reaction B described under "General identification tests" as characteristic of chlorides (vol. 1, p. 113).

Specific optical rotation.   Dissolve 0.25 g in sufficient hydrochloric acid (0.1 mol/l) VS to produce 25 ml and allow to stand for 60 minutes. Measure the rotation and calculate with reference to the anhydrous substance;
$[\alpha]_D^{20\,^\circ C} = -188$ to -200°.

Sulfated ash.   Not more than 5.0 mg/g.

Water.   Determine as described under "Determination of water by the Karl Fischer method", Method A (vol. 1, p. 135), using about 0.25 g of the substance; the water content is not more than 20 mg/g.

pH value.   pH of a 10 mg/ml solution, 2.0–3.0.

Absorption in the ultraviolet region.   The absorption spectrum of a 20 µg/ml solution in hydrochloric acid (0.1 mol/l) VS, when observed between 230 nm and 400 nm, exhibits 2 maxima at about 268 nm and 353 nm. The absorbance of a 1-cm layer at 353 nm is not less than 0.54 and not more than 0.58.

Light-absorbing impurities.   Prepare a 2.0 mg/ml solution in a mixture of 1 volume of hydrochloric acid (1 mol/l) VS and 99 volumes of methanol R and measure within 1 hour of preparation the absorbance of a 1-cm layer at 430 nm; the absorbance does not exceed 0.50.

Prepare a 10 mg/ml solution in a mixture of 1 volume of hydrochloric acid (1 mol/l) VS and 99 volumes of methanol R and measure within 1 hour of preparation the absorbance of a 1-cm layer at 490 nm; the absorbance does not exceed 0.20.

Assay.   Carry out the assay as described under "Microbiological assay of antibiotics" (vol. 1, p. 145), using either (*a*) *Bacillus pumilus* (NCTC 8241 or ATCC 14884) as the test organism, culture medium Cm1 with a final pH of 6.5–6.6, sterile phosphate buffer, pH 4.5 TS, an appropriate concentration of oxytetracycline (usually between 2 and 20 IU per ml), and an incubation temperature of 37–39 °C, or (*b*) *Bacillus cereus* (ATCC 11778) as the test organism, culture medium Cm1 with a final pH of 5.9–6.0, sterile phosphate buffer, pH 4.5 TS, an appropriate concentration of oxytetracycline (usually between 0.5 and 2 IU), and an incubation temperature of 30–33 °C. The precision of the assay is such that the fiducial limits of error of the estimated potency ($P = 0.95$) are not less than 95% and not more than 105% of the estimated potency. The upper fiducial limit of error of the estimated potency ($P = 0.95$) is not less than 870 IU of oxytetracycline per mg, calculated with reference to the anhydrous substance.

Additional Requirements for Sterile Oxytetracycline Hydrochloride

Undue toxicity.   Carry out the test as described under "Test for undue toxicity" (vol. 1, p. 154), using 0.5 ml of a solution in sterile water R containing a quantity equivalent to 2 mg of oxytetracycline per ml.

Pyrogens.   Carry out the test as described under "Test for pyrogens" (vol. 1, p. 155), injecting per kg of the rabbit's mass, 5 ml of a solution in sterile water R containing 1 mg of the substance to be examined per ml.

Sterility.   Complies with the "Sterility testing of antibiotics" (vol. 1, p. 152), applying the membrane filtration test procedure.

PARACETAMOLUM

Paracetamol

Molecular formula. $C_8H_9NO_2$

Relative molecular mass.   151.2

Graphic formula.

$$HO\!-\!\langle\ \rangle\!-\!NHCOCH_3$$

Chemical name.   4′-Hydroxyacetanilide; *N*-(4-hydroxyphenyl)acetamide; CAS Reg. No. 103-90-2.

Other name.   Acetaminophen.

Description.   A white, crystalline powder; odourless.

Solubility.   Sparingly soluble in water; freely soluble in ethanol ($\sim$750 g/l) TS and acetone R; practically insoluble in ether R.

Category.   Analgesic; antipyretic.

Storage.   Paracetamol should be kept in a tightly closed container, protected from light.

REQUIREMENTS

General requirement.   Paracetamol contains not less than 98.5% and not more than 101.0% of $C_8H_9NO_2$, calculated with reference to the dried substance.

Identity tests

A. Dissolve 0.05 g in 100 ml of methanol R. To 1 ml of this solution add 0.5 ml of hydrochloric acid (0.1 mol/l) VS and dilute to 100 ml with methanol R. Protect the solution from light and immediately measure the absorbance of a 1-cm layer at the maximum wavelength of about 249 nm; about 0.88.

B. Dissolve 0.1 g in 10 ml of water and add 0.05 ml of ferric chloride (25 g/l) TS; a violet-blue colour is produced.

C. Boil 0.1 g with 1 ml of hydrochloric acid ($\sim$70 g/l) TS for 3 minutes, add 10 ml of water and cool; no precipitate is formed. Add 0.05 ml of potassium dichromate (0.0167 mol/l) VS; a violet colour, which does not turn to red (distinction from phenacetin) is slowly produced.

Melting range.   168–172 °C.

Heavy metals. Use 1.0 g and a mixture of 85 volumes of acetone R and 15 volumes of water for the preparation of the test solution as described under "Limit test for heavy metals", Procedure 2 (vol. 1, p. 118); determine the heavy metals content according to Method A (vol. 1, p. 119); not more than 10 µg/g.

Sulfated ash.   Not more than 1.0 mg/g.

Loss on drying. Dry to constant weight at 105 °C; it loses not more than 5.0 mg/g.

4-Aminophenol.   Dissolve 0.5 g in a mixture of equal volumes of methanol R and water and dilute to 10 ml with this solvent mixture. Add 0.2 ml of alkaline sodium nitroprusside TS, mix, and allow to stand for 30 minutes. Prepare similarly a reference solution containing 0.5 g of 4-aminophenol-free paracetamol R and 0.5 ml of a solution containing 0.050 mg/ml of 4-aminophenol R in the same solvent mixture. The colour of the test solution is not more intense than that of the reference solution (0.05 mg/g).

Related substances.   Carry out the test as described under "Thin-layer chromatography", using silica gel R4 as the coating substance and a mixture of 65 volumes of chloroform R, 25 volumes of acetone R, and 10 volumes of toluene R as the mobile phase. Allow the solvent front to ascend 14 cm above the line of application, using an unlined chromatographic chamber. Prepare the following 4 test solutions: For solution (A) transfer 1.0 g of finely powdered substance to be examined to a glass-stoppered tube, add 5 ml of ether R, and shake mechanically for 30 minutes. Centrifuge the tube until a clear supernatant liquid is obtained and separate this from the solid. For solution (B) dilute 1 ml of solution A to 10 ml with ethanol ($\sim$750 g/l) TS. For solution (C) dissolve 25 mg of 4-chloroacetanilide R in 50 ml of ethanol ($\sim$750 g/l) TS. For solution (D) dissolve 0.25 g of 4-chloroace-tanilide R and 0.1 g of the substance to be examined in sufficient ethanol ($\sim$750 g/l) TS to produce 100 ml. Apply separately to the plate 200 µl of solution A and 40 µl of each of the remaining 3 solutions. After removing the plate from the chromatographic chamber, allow it to dry in a current of warm air and examine the chromatogram in ultraviolet light (254 nm). Any spot due to 4-chloroacetanilide obtained with solution A is not more intense than the corresponding spot obtained with solution C. Any spot obtained with solution B, other than the principal spot and the spot corresponding to 4-chloroacetanilide, is not more intense than the spot obtained with solution C. The test is valid only if the chromatogram obtained with solution D shows two distinctly separated spots corresponding to 4-chloroacetanilide and the substance being examined, the latter having a lower R_f value.

Assay. Transfer about 0.25 g, accurately weighed, to a flask, add 10 ml of hydrochloric acid ($\sim$70 g/l) TS and boil under a reflux condenser for 1 hour. Wash the condenser with 30 ml of water, add 1 g of potassium bromide R to the combined solution, and proceed as described under "Nitrite titration" (vol. 1, p. 133), titrating with sodium nitrite (0.1 mol/l) VS. Each ml of sodium nitrite (0.1 mol/l) VS is equivalent to 15.12 mg of $C_8H_9NO_2$.

PAROMOMYCINI SULFAS

Paromomycin sulfate

Molecular formula. $C_{23}H_{45}N_5O_{14},xH_2SO_4$

Graphic formula.

Chemical name. O-2,6-Diamino-2,6-dideoxy-β-L-idopyranosyl-(1→3)-O-β-D-ribofuranosyl-(1→5)-O-[2-amino-2-deoxy-α-D-glucopyranosyl-(1→4)]-2-deoxy-streptamine sulfate (salt); O-2-amino-2-deoxy-α-D-glucopyranosyl-(1→4)-O-

[*O*-2,6-diamino-2,6-dideoxy-β-L-idopyranosyl-(1→3)-β-D-ribofuranosyl-(1→5)]-2-deoxy-D-streptamine sulfate (salt); CAS Reg. No. 1263-89-4.

Description.   A creamy white to light yellow powder; odourless or almost odourless.

Solubility.   Very soluble in water; practically insoluble in ethanol (~750 g/l) TS, chloroform R, and ether R.

Category.   Antiamoebic drug.

Storage.   Paromomycin sulfate should be kept in a tightly closed container, protected from light.

Additional information.   Paromomycin sulfate is very hygroscopic. Even in the absence of light, it is gradually degraded on exposure to a humid atmosphere, the decomposition being faster at higher temperatures.

REQUIREMENTS

General requirement.   Paromomycin sulfate contains not less than 675 International Units of paromomycin per mg, calculated with reference to the dried substance.

Identity tests

A.   Carry out the test as described under "Thin-layer chromatography" (vol. 1, p. 83), using silica gel R3 as the coating substance and a freshly prepared ammonium acetate (40 g/l) TS as the mobile phase. Apply separately to the plate 1 µl of each of 2 solutions containing (A) 20 mg of the test substance per ml and (B) 20 mg of paromomycin sulfate RS per ml. After removing the plate from the chromatographic chamber, allow it to dry in air for 10 minutes, heat it at 105 °C for 1 hour, and spray it with triketohydrindene/butanol TS. Heat it again at 105 °C for 5 minutes and examine the chromatogram in daylight. The principal red spot obtained with solution A corresponds in position and appearance with that obtained with solution B.

B.   A 0.05 g/ml solution yields reaction A described under "General identification tests" as characteristic of sulfates (vol. 1, p. 115).

Specific optical rotation.   Use a 50 mg/ml solution and calculate with reference to the dried substance; $[\alpha]_D^{20\,°C} = +50$ to $+55°$.

Sulfated ash.   Not more than 20 mg/g.

Loss on drying.   Dry to constant weight at 50 °C under reduced pressure (not exceeding 0.6 kPa or about 5 mm of mercury); it loses not more than 50 mg/g.

pH value.   pH of a 30 mg/ml solution in carbon-dioxide-free water R, 5.0–7.5.

Assay.   Carry out the assay as described under "Microbiological assay of antibiotics" (vol. 1, p. 145), using either (*a*) *Bacillus subtilis* (NCTC 10400) as the test organism, culture medium Cm1 with a final pH of 8.0, sterile phosphate buffer pH 7.8, TS, an appropriate concentration of paromomycin (usually between 1 and 4 IU per ml), and an incubation temperature of 37–39 °C; or (*b*) *Bacillus subtilis* (ATCC 6633) as the test organism, culture medium Cm11 with a final pH of 7.8, sterile phosphate buffer pH 8.0, TS1 or TS2, an appropriate concentration of paromomycin (usually between 2 and 8 IU per ml), and an incubation temperature of 36–38 °C.   The precision of the assay is such that the fiducial limits of error of the estimated potency ($P = 0.95$) are not less than 95% and not more than 105% of the estimated potency.   The upper fiducial limit of error of the estimated potency ($P = 0.95$) is not less than 675 IU of paromomycin per mg, calculated with reference to the dried substance.

PENICILLAMINUM

Penicillamine

Molecular formula. $C_5H_{11}NO_2S$

Relative molecular mass.   149.2

Graphic formula.

$$\text{HS} - \underset{\underset{\textstyle CH_3}{|}}{\overset{\overset{\textstyle CH_3}{|}}{C}} - \underset{\underset{\textstyle NH_2}{|}}{\overset{\overset{\textstyle H}{|}}{C}} - \text{COOH}$$

Chemical name.   3-Mercapto-D-valine; 3,3-dimethyl-D-cysteine; CAS Reg. No. 52-67-5.

Description.   A white or almost white, crystalline powder; odour, characteristic.

Solubility.   Soluble in 9 parts of water; slightly soluble in ethanol (~750 g/l) TS; practically insoluble in chloroform R and ether R.

Category.   Antidote.

Storage.   Penicillamine should be kept in a tightly closed container, protected from light.

Additional information.   Even in the absence of light, Penicillamine is gradually degraded on exposure to a humid atmosphere, the decomposition being faster at higher temperatures.

REQUIREMENTS

General requirement.   Penicillamine contains not less than 95.0% and not more than 100.5% of $C_5H_{11}NO_2S$, calculated with reference to the dried substance.

Identity tests

A.   Dissolve 20 mg in 4 ml of water, add 2 ml of phosphotungstic acid TS and allow to stand for a few minutes; a deep blue colour is produced.

B.   Dissolve 20 mg in 5 ml of water, add 0.05 ml of sodium hydroxide ($\sim$200 g/l) TS and 20 mg of triketohydrindene hydrate R; an intense blue or violet-blue colour is produced immediately.

Specific optical rotation.   Use a 50 mg/ml solution in sodium hydroxide (1 mol/l) VS; $[\alpha]_D^{20\,^\circ C} = -58$ to -68°.

Sulfated ash.   Not more than 1.0 mg/g.

Loss on drying.   Dry to constant weight at 60 °C under reduced pressure (not exceeding 0.6 kPa or about 5 mm of mercury); it loses not more than 5 mg/g.

pH value.   pH of a 10 mg/ml solution, 4.0–6.0.

Mercury

● NOTE. The operations described below must be carried out in subdued light.

Transfer about 0.5 g, accurately weighed, to a 650-ml long-necked flask containing a few glass beads, incline the flask at an angle of about 45°, and add 2.5 ml of nitric acid ($\sim$1000 g/l) TS through a small funnel placed in the mouth of the flask. Allow the mixture to stand at room temperature until nitrous oxide fumes are evolved and the vigorous reaction subsides (5–30 minutes). Add 2.5 ml of sulfuric acid ($\sim$1760 g/l) TS through the funnel and heat, gently at first and then to the production of fumes of sulfur trioxide. Cool, then add cautiously 2.5 ml of nitric acid ($\sim$1000 g/l) TS, heat again to the production of sulfur trioxide fumes, and cool. Repeat this treatment once more, then add 50 ml of water, rinsing the funnel, and collecting the rinsings in the flask. Remove the funnel, boil the solution down to approximately half its volume (about 25 ml), and cool to room temperature. Transfer to a 250-ml separating funnel with the aid of water and dilute with water to 50 ml. Add 1 ml of disodium edetate (20 g/l) TS and 1 ml of glacial acetic acid R and extract with small portions of chloroform R until the last chloroform extract remains colourless. Discard the chloroform extract and add 50 ml of sulfuric acid (0.125 mol/l) VS, 90 ml of water, and 10 ml of hydroxylamine hydrochloride (200 g/l) TS. Add dithizone standard TS, in portions of 0.3–0.5 ml, from a 10-ml burette. After each addition, shake the mixture well, allow the chloroform layer to separate, and discard it. Continue until an addition of dithizone standard TS remains green after shaking.

From the volume of the dithizone standard TS used, calculate the amount of mercury present in the test substance. It contains not more than 20 µg of Hg per g.

Assay. Dissolve about 0.1 g, accurately weighed, in 50 ml of water, add 5 ml of sodium hydroxide (1 mol/l) VS and 0.2 ml of dithizone TS and titrate with mercuric nitrate (0.02 mol/l) VS. Each ml of mercuric nitrate (0.02 mol/l) VS is equivalent to 5.968 mg of $C_5H_{11}NO_2S$.

PENTAMIDINI ISETIONAS

Pentamidine isetionate

Molecular formula. $C_{19}H_{24}N_4O_2,2C_2H_6O_4S$

Relative molecular mass. 592.7

Graphic formula.

HN=C(—NH₂)—C₆H₄—O—(CH₂)₅—O—C₆H₄—C(=NH)—NH₂ · 2 CH₂OH—CH₂—SO₃H

Chemical name. 4,4′-(Pentamethylenedioxy)dibenzamidine bis(2-hydroxy-ethanesulfonate); 4,4′-[1,5-pentanediylbis(oxy)]bis[benzenecarboximidamide]-bis(2-hydroxyethanesulfonate); CAS Reg. No. 140-64-7.

Description. A white, or almost white, crystalline powder; odourless.

Solubility. Soluble in 10 parts of water; slightly soluble in ethanol (~750 g/l) TS; practically insoluble in chloroform R and ether R.

Category. Antitrypanosomal drug; antileishmaniasis drug.

Storage. Pentamidine isetionate should be kept in a well-closed container.

Additional information. Pentamidine isetionate is hygroscopic.

REQUIREMENTS

General requirement.   Pentamidine isetionate contains not less than 98.5% and not more than 102.5% of $C_{19}H_{24}N_4O_2,2C_2H_6O_4S$, calculated with reference to the dried substance.

Identity tests

A.   The absorption spectrum of a 10 µg/ml solution in hydrochloric acid (0.01 mol/l) VS, when observed between 230 nm and 350 nm, exhibits a maximum at about 262 nm; the absorbance of a 1-cm layer at this wavelength is about 0.47.

B.   To 0.5 g add 5 ml of water and heat to 80 °C to dissolve. Add 10 ml of sodium hydroxide (~50 g/l) TS, cool in ice, and filter. To 2 ml of the filtrate add 0.2 ml of nitric acid (~1000 g/l) TS followed by 0.2 ml of ceric ammonium nitrate TS; a red-orange colour is produced.

C.   Melting temperature, about 190 °C.

Sulfated ash.   Not more than 1.0 mg/g.

Loss on drying.   Dry to constant weight at 105 °C; it loses not more than 40 mg/g.

pH value.   pH of a 0.05 g/ml solution, 4.5–6.5.

Related substances.   Carry out the test as described under "Thin-layer chromatography" (vol. 1, p. 83), using silica gel R6, activated at 105 °C for 1 hour, as the coating substance (a precoated plate from a commercial source is suitable), and as the mobile phase the upper layer obtained by shaking together 10 volumes of water, 8 volumes of 1-butanol R, and 2 volumes of glacial acetic acid R. Apply separately to the plate 10 µl of each of 2 solutions in methanol R containing (A) 50 mg of the test substance per ml and (B) 0.25 mg of the test substance per ml. After removing the plate from the chromatographic chamber, allow it to dry in air, and examine the chromatogram in ultraviolet light (254 nm). Any spot obtained with solution A, other than the principal spot, is not more intense than that obtained with solution B.

Assay.   Carry out Method A as described under "Determination of nitrogen" (vol. 1, p. 136), using about 0.4 g of the test substance, accurately weighed, and 9 ml of nitrogen-free sulfuric acid (~1760 g/l) TS. Each ml of sulfuric acid (0.05 mol/l) VS is equivalent to 14.82 mg of $C_{19}H_{24}N_4O_2,2C_2H_6O_4S$.

PENTAMIDINI MESILAS

Pentamidine mesilate

Molecular formula. $C_{19}H_{24}N_4O_2,2CH_4O_3S$

Relative molecular mass. 532.6

Graphic formula.

$$HN=\underset{H_2N}{\overset{}{C}}-\langle C_6H_4\rangle-O-(CH_2)_5-O-\langle C_6H_4\rangle-\underset{NH_2}{\overset{NH}{C}} \cdot 2CH_3SO_3H$$

Chemical name. 4,4'-(Pentamethylenedioxy)dibenzamidine dimethanesulfon-ate; 4,4'-[1,5-pentanediylbis(oxy)]bis[benzenecarboximidamide] dimethanesul-fonate; CAS Reg. No. 6823-79-6.

Description. A white or light pink, granular powder; almost odourless.

Solubility. Slightly soluble in water and ethanol ($\sim$750 g/l) TS; practically inso-luble in ether R, acetone R, and chloroform R.

Category. Antitrypanosomal drug; antileishmaniasis drug.

Storage. Pentamidine mesilate should be kept in a well-closed container.

REQUIREMENTS

General requirement. Pentamidine mesilate contains not less than 98.5% and not more than 102.5% of $C_{19}H_{24}N_4O_2,2CH_4O_3S$, calculated with reference to the dried substance.

Identity tests

A. To 0.5 g add 5 ml of water and heat to 80 °C to dissolve. Add 10 ml of sodium hydroxide ($\sim$50 g/l) TS, cool in ice, and filter. To 2 ml of the filtrate add 0.2 ml of nitric acid ($\sim$1000 g/l) TS followed by 0.2 ml of ceric ammonium nitrate TS; a yellow colour is produced.

B. Heat 0.5 g with 1 ml of sodium hydroxide ($\sim$400 g/l) TS in a test-tube; ammonia, perceptible by its odour, is evolved.

C. Dissolve 1 g in 10 ml of water at 80 °C, add 10 ml of sodium hydroxide ($\sim$50 g/l) TS, cool in ice, filter (keep the filtrate for test D), wash with 10 ml of water, and dry the precipitate at 105 °C; melting temperature, about 188 °C.

D.   Transfer 10 ml of the filtrate obtained in test C to a platinum crucible, add 2.5 ml of hydrogen peroxide ($\sim$60 g/l) TS, mix with the help of a glass rod and evaporate to dryness on a water-bath. Dissolve the residue in 1 ml of water, add 1 ml of glacial acetic acid R and again evaporate to dryness on a water-bath, then ignite until free from carbon. Cool, mix the residue with 5 ml of water and filter, if necessary. Neutralize with hydrochloric acid ($\sim$70 g/l) TS and add an excess of 3 ml. Boil for 30 seconds, cool and proceed with reaction A described under "General identification tests" as characteristic of sulfates (vol. 1, p. 115).

Sulfated ash.   Not more than 1.0 mg/g.

Loss on drying.   Dry to constant weight at 105 °C; it loses not more than 15 mg/g.

pH value.   pH of a 0.05 g/ml solution prepared in warm water and then cooled, 4.5–6.5.

Related substances.   Carry out the test as described under "Thin-layer chromatography" (vol. 1, p. 83), using silica gel R6, activated at 105 °C for 1 hour, as the coating substance (a precoated plate from a commercial source is suitable), and as the mobile phase the upper layer obtained by shaking together 10 volumes of water, 8 volumes of 1-butanol R, and 2 volumes of glacial acetic acid R. Apply separately to the plate 10 µl of each of 2 solutions in methanol R containing (A) 50 mg of the test substance per ml (warm, if necessary) and (B) 0.25 mg of the test substance per ml. After removing the plate from the chromatographic chamber, allow it to dry in air and examine the chromatogram in ultraviolet light (254 nm). Any spot obtained with solution A, other than the principal spot, is not more intense than that obtained with solution B.

Assay.   Carry out Method A as described under "Determination of nitrogen" (vol. 1, p. 136), using about 0.4 g, accurately weighed, and 9 ml of nitrogen-free sulfuric acid ($\sim$1760 g/l) TS. Each ml of sulfuric acid (0.05 mol/l) VS is equivalent to 13.32 mg of $C_{19}H_{24}N_4O_2,2CH_4O_3S$.

PETHIDINI HYDROCHLORIDUM

Pethidine hydrochloride

Molecular formula. $C_{15}H_{21}NO_2,HCl$

Relative molecular mass.   283.8

Graphic formula.

Chemical name.   Ethyl 1-methyl-4-phenylisonipecotate hydrochloride; ethyl 1-methyl-4-phenyl-4-piperidinecarboxylate hydrochloride; CAS Reg. No. 50-13-5.

Other name.   Meperidine hydrochloride.

Description.   A white, crystalline powder; odourless.

Solubility.   Very soluble in water; soluble in ethanol ($\sim$750 g/l) TS; practically insoluble in ether R.

Category.   Narcotic analgesic.

Storage.   Pethidine hydrochloride should be kept in a well-closed container, protected from light.

Additional information.   Even in the absence of light, Pethidine hydrochloride is gradually degraded on exposure to a humid atmosphere, the decomposition being faster at higher temperatures.

REQUIREMENTS

General requirement.   Pethidine hydrochloride contains not less than 98.0% and not more than 101.0% of $C_{15}H_{21}NO_2,HCl$, calculated with reference to the dried substance.

Identity tests

A.   Dissolve 5 mg in 0.5 ml of water, add about 0.1 ml of formaldehyde TS and 2 ml of sulfuric acid ($\sim$1760 g/l) TS; an orange-red colour is produced.

B.   Dissolve 0.1 g in 5 ml of ethanol ($\sim$750 g/l) TS and add 15 ml of trinitrophenol (7 g/l) TS; a yellow, crystalline precipitate is produced. Collect the precipitate on a filter, wash with water, and dry at 105 °C; melting temperature, about 190 °C (picrate). (Keep a portion of the picrate for test C.)

C.   Mix 5 mg of the picrate obtained in test B with 5 mg of the substance being examined; melting temperature, not less than 20 °C lower than that of the picrate alone.

D.   A 10 mg/ml solution yields reaction A described under "General identification tests" as characteristic of chlorides (vol. 1, p. 112).

Melting range.   After drying to constant weight at 105 °C, 187–190 °C.

Clarity and colour of solution.   A solution of 0.20 g in 10 ml of water is clear and colourless.

Sulfated ash.   Not more than 1.0 mg/g.

Loss on drying.   Dry to constant weight at 105 °C; it loses not more than 5.0 mg/g.

pH value.   pH of a 0.05 g/ml solution, 4.0–6.0.

Related substances.   Carry out the test as described under "Thin-layer chromatography" (vol. 1, p. 83), using kieselguhr R1 as the coating substance and a mixture of 1 volume of 2-phenoxyethanol R and 9 volumes of acetone R to impregnate the plate, dipping it about 5 mm into the liquid. After the solvent has reached a height of a least 15 cm, remove the plate from the chromatographic chamber and allow the acetone to evaporate. Use the impregnated plate immediately, carrying out the chromatography in the same direction as the impregnation. Prepare the mobile phase by shaking together 1 volume of diethylamine R, 100 volumes of light petroleum R1, and 8 volumes of 2-phenoxyethanol R, allow to settle, and use the supernatant liquid. For the preparation of the test solutions, dissolve 0.10 g in 5 ml of water, add 0.5 ml of sodium hydroxide (~400 g/l) TS, 2 ml of ether R, and shake. Allow the layers to separate and use the upper layer as solution A. Dilute 0.5 ml of solution A to 50 ml with ether R and use as solution B. Apply separately to the plate 5 µl of each of solutions A and B. After removing the plate from the chromatographic chamber, allow it to dry in air for 10 minutes, return it to the chamber, and allow the solvent mixture to ascend a second time 12 cm above the line of application. Remove the plate, allow it to dry in air for 10 minutes, and spray it with dichlorofluorescein TS. Allow it to stand for 5 minutes and examine the chromatogram in daylight; red to orange spots on a white to almost white background are obtained. Then examine the chromatogram in ultraviolet light (365 nm). Any spot obtained with solution A, other than the principal spot, is not more intense than that obtained with solution B.

Assay. Dissolve about 0.20 g, accurately weighed, in 30 ml of glacial acetic acid R1, add 10 ml of mercuric acetate/acetic acid TS, and titrate with perchloric acid (0.1 mol/l) VS as described under "Non-aqueous titration", Method A (vol. 1, p. 131). Each ml of perchloric acid (0.1 mol/l) VS is equivalent to 28.38 mg of $C_{15}H_{21}NO_2,HCl$.

PHYTOMENADIONUM

Phytomenadione

Molecular formula. $C_{31}H_{46}O_2$

Relative molecular mass. 450.7

Graphic formula.

$$\text{structural formula of phytomenadione}$$

Chemical name. Phylloquinone; [R-[R*,R*-(E)]]-2-methyl-3-(3,7,11,15-tetra-methyl-2-hexadecenyl)-1,4-naphthalenedione; 2-methyl-3-phytyl-1,4-naphtho-quinone; CAS Reg. No. 84-80-0.

Other names. Phytonadione; Vitamin K_1.

Description. A clear, yellow to amber-coloured, very viscous liquid; odourless or almost odourless.

Miscibility. Practically immiscible with water; sparingly miscible with ethanol ($\sim$750 g/l) TS; freely miscible with chloroform R and ether R.

Category. Anticoagulant.

Storage. Phytomenadione should be kept in a tightly closed container, protected from light.

REQUIREMENTS

General requirement. Phytomenadione contains not less than 97.0% and not more than 102.0% of $C_{31}H_{46}O_2$.

Identity tests

A.   The absorption spectrum of a 10 µg/ml solution in 2,2,4-trimethylpentane R, when observed between 230 nm and 350 nm, exhibits 4 maxima at about 243 nm, 249 nm, 261 nm, and 270 nm. The absorbances at those wavelengths using 1-cm cells are about 0.40, 0.42, 0.38, and 0.39, respectively. The spectrum also exhibits minima at about 246 nm, 254 nm, and 266 nm. The ratio of the absorbance at the minimum of about 254 nm to that at the maximum of about 249 nm is between 0.70 and 0.75.

B.   The absorption spectrum of a 0.10 mg/ml solution in 2,2,4-trimethylpentane R, when observed between 230 nm and 350 nm, exhibits a maximum at about 327 nm and a minimum at about 285 nm. The absorbance of a 1-cm layer at the maximum is about 0.70, and at the minimum about 0.22.

C.   Mix about 0.05 g of the test liquid with 5 ml of ethanol ($\sim$750 g/l) TS and add 1.0 ml of potassium hydroxide/ethanol TS1; a green colour is produced. Allow to stand for 15 minutes; the colour of the solution turns to red-brown.

Refractive index. $n_D^{20} = 1.525 - 1.529$.

Acidity or alkalinity.   Dissolve 1 g in 20 ml of dehydrated ethanol R; the solution is neutral to litmus paper R.

Related substances.   Carry out, in subdued light, the test described under "Thin-layer chromatography" (vol. 1, p. 83), using silica gel R4 as the coating substance and a mixture of 80 volumes of cyclohexane R, 20 volumes of ether R, and 1 volume of methanol R as the mobile phase. Apply separately to the plate 10 µl of each of 2 solutions in 2,2,4-trimethylpentane R containing (A) 5 mg of the test substance per ml and (B) 0.05 mg of menadione R per ml. After removing the plate from the chromatographic chamber, allow it to dry in air and examine the chromatogram in ultraviolet light (254 nm). Any spot obtained with solution A, other than the principal spot, is not more intense than that obtained with solution B.

Assay

NOTE. Carry out the following operations in subdued light.

Dissolve about 0.1 g, accurately weighed, in sufficient 2,2,4-trimethylpentane R to produce 100 ml. Dilute 10 ml to 100 ml with 2,2,4-trimethylpentane R and further dilute 10 ml of this solution to 100 ml with the same solvent. Measure the absorbance of this solution in a 1-cm layer at the maximum at about 249 nm and calculate the content of $C_{31}H_{46}O_2$, using the absorptivity value of 42 ($A_{1\ cm}^{1\%} = 420$).

PIX LITHANTHRACIS

Coal tar

Composition. Coal tar is a by-product usually obtained during the destructive distillation of coal. It is a complex and undefined mixture of a great number of chemical compounds. The product is available in various compositions; CAS Reg. No. 8007-45-2.

Description. Brown-black or black, viscous liquid; odour, characteristic and strong resembling naphthalene.

Solubility. Slightly soluble in water; very slightly or partially soluble in ethanol ($\sim$750 g/l) TS, ether R, chloroform R, and hexane R.

Category. Keratoplastic agent.

Storage. Coal tar should be kept in a tightly closed container.

Additional information. Coal tar burns in air with a luminous sooty flame. On exposure to air it hardens. Even in the absence of light, it is gradually degraded on exposure to a humid atmosphere, the decomposition being faster at higher temperatures.

REQUIREMENTS

Identity test

Carefully add 0.5 g to 10 ml of light petroleum R1 and allow to stand for 30 minutes; the supernatant liquid has a blue fluorescence in daylight and a more intense fluorescence when viewed in ultraviolet light (365 nm).

Sulfated ash. Not more than 20 mg/g.

PRAZIQUANTELUM

Praziquantel

NOTE. See the statement regarding the provisional nature of this Monograph in the Preface on page 9.

Molecular formula. $C_{19}H_{24}N_2O_2$

Relative molecular mass. 312.4

Graphic formula.

Chemical name. 2-(Cyclohexylcarbonyl)-1,2,3,6,7,11b-hexahydro-4*H*-pyrazino-[2,1-*a*]isoquinolin-4-one; CAS Reg. No. 55268-74-1.

Description. A white or almost white, crystalline powder; odourless or with a faint characteristic odour.

Solubility. Very slightly soluble in water; freely soluble in ethanol ($\sim$750 g/l) TS and chloroform R.

Category. Antischistosomal drug.

Storage. Praziquantel should be kept in a well-closed container, protected from light.

REQUIREMENTS

General requirement. Praziquantel contains not less than 98.5% and not more than 101.0% of $C_{19}H_{24}N_2O_2$, calculated with reference to the dried substance.

Identity tests

● Either test A or tests B and C may be applied.

A. Carry out the examination as described under "Spectrophotometry in the infrared region" (vol. 1, p. 40). The infrared absorption spectrum is concordant with the spectrum obtained from praziquantel RS or with the *reference spectrum* of praziquantel.

B. See the test below under "Related substances". The principal spot obtained with solution A corresponds in position, appearance, and intensity with that obtained with solution B.

C. Melting temperature, about 138 °C.

Heavy metals. Use 1.0 g for the preparation of the test solution as described under "Limit test for heavy metals", Procedure 3 (vol. 1, p. 118); determine the heavy metals content according to Method A (vol. 1, p. 119); not more than 20 µg/g.

Sulfated ash. Not more than 1.0 mg/g.

Loss on drying. Dry at 50 °C under reduced pressure (not exceeding 0.6 kPa or about 5 mm of mercury) for 2 hours; it loses not more than 5.0 mg/g.

Related substances. Carry out the test as described under "Thin-layer chromatography" (vol. 1, p. 83), using silica gel R5 as the coating substance and a mixture of 85 volumes of toluene R and 15 volumes of methanol R as the mobile phase. Use an unlined chamber. Apply separately to the plate, in a current of nitrogen R, 10 µl of each of 2 solutions in chloroform R containing (A) 50 mg of the test substance per ml and (B) 50 mg of praziquantel RS per ml; further apply 2 µl of each of 2 solutions in chloroform R containing (C) 0.5 mg of praziquantel RS per ml and (D) 1.0 mg of praziquantel RS per ml. Allow the mobile phase to ascend 7 cm. After removing the plate from the chromatographic chamber, allow it to dry in a current of warm air, place the plate in a chamber with iodine vapours and allow to stand for 20 minutes. Examine the chromatogram immediately in daylight. Any spot obtained with solution A, other than the principal spot, is not more intense than that obtained with solution C, except one spot above the main spot which is not more intense than that obtained with solution D.

Assay. Carry out the assay with a suitable infrared spectrophotometer as described under "Spectrophotometry in the infrared region" (vol. 1, p. 40). Prepare a solution in carbon tetrachloride R containing 8 mg, accurately weighed, of the test substance per ml. Use a pair of matched sodium chloride cells, thickness 0.01 cm, fill both cells with carbon tetrachloride R and calibrate the instrument at 1658 cm^{-1} to 100% transmission. When shutting the sample-channel the instrument should measure 0% transmission. Fill the sample cell with the solution of the test substance and scan three times the range 1800–1550 cm^{-1}. Determine the minimum absorbance at 1720 cm^{-1} and the maximum absorbance at 1658 cm^{-1}. Calculate in percentage the amount of $C_{19}H_{24}N_2O_2$ in the substance being tested by comparison with praziquantel RS, similarly and concurrently examined using the formula: $100(C_1/C_2)(A_1/A_2)$, where C_1 is the concentration of the solution of praziquantel RS, C_2 is the concentration of the solution to be assayed, A_1 is the difference between the absorbances of the solution to be assayed and A_2 is the difference between the absorbances for the reference solution.

PREDNISOLONI ACETAS

Prednisolone acetate

Molecular formula. $C_{23}H_{30}O_6$

Relative molecular mass.   402.5

Graphic formula.

Chemical name.   11β,17,21-Trihydroxypregna-1,4-diene-3,20-dione 21-acetate; 21-(acetyloxy)-11β,17-dihydroxypregna-1,4-diene-3,20-dione; CAS Reg. No. 52-21-1.

Description.   A white or almost white, crystalline powder; odourless.

Solubility.   Practically insoluble in water; slightly soluble in ethanol ($\sim$750 g/l) TS, acetone R, and chloroform R.

Category.   Adrenal hormone.

Storage.   Prednisolone acetate should be kept in a well-closed container, protected from light.

Additional information.   Prednisolone acetate has a melting temperature of about 235 °C with decomposition.

REQUIREMENTS

General requirement.   Prednisolone acetate contains not less than 96.0% and not more than 104.0% of $C_{23}H_{30}O_6$, calculated with reference to the dried substance.

Identity tests

● Either tests A and C or tests B and C may be applied.

A.   Carry out the examination as described under "Spectrophotometry in the infrared region" (vol. 1, p. 40). The infrared absorption spectrum is concordant with the spectrum obtained from prednisolone acetate RS or with the *reference spectrum* of prednisolone acetate.

B.   Carry out the test as described under "Thin-layer chromatography" (vol. 1, p. 83), using kieselguhr R1 as the coating substance and a mixture of 10 volumes of formamide R and 90 volumes of acetone R to impregnate the plate, dipping it about 5 mm into the liquid. After the solvent has reached a height of at least 16 cm, remove the plate from the chromatographic chamber and allow it to stand at room temperature until the solvents have completely evaporated. Use the impregnated plate within 2 hours, carrying out the chromatography in the same direction as the impregnation. Use 75 volumes of toluene R and 25 volumes of chloroform R as the mobile phase. Apply separately to the plate 2 µl of each of 2 solutions in a mixture of 9 volumes of chloroform R and 1 volume of methanol R containing (A) 2.5 mg of the test substance per ml and (B) 2.5 mg of prednisolone acetate RS per ml. Develop the plate for a distance of 15 cm. After removing the plate from the chromatographic chamber, allow it to dry in air until the solvents have evaporated, heat it at 120 °C for 15 minutes, spray it with a mixture of 20 ml of sulfuric acid ($\sim$190 g/l) TS and 80 ml of ethanol ($\sim$750 g/l) TS, and then heat it at 120 °C for 10 minutes. Allow it to cool and examine the chromatogram in daylight and in ultraviolet light (365 nm). The principal spot obtained with solution A corresponds in position, appearance, and intensity with that obtained with solution B.

C. To 0.05 g add 2 ml of ethanol ($\sim$750 g/l) TS and 2 ml of sulfuric acid ($\sim$700 g/l) TS and boil gently for 1 minute; ethyl acetate, perceptible by its odour (proceed with caution), is produced.

Specific optical rotation. Use a 10 mg/ml solution in dioxan R; $[\alpha]_D^{20\,°C} = +112$ to $+119°$.

Loss on drying. Dry to constant weight at 105 °C; it loses not more than 10 mg/g.

Related substances. Carry out the test as described under "Thin-layer chromatography" (vol. 1, p. 83), using silica gel R1 as the coating substance and a mixture of 95 volumes of dichloroethane R, 5 volumes of methanol R, and 0.2 volumes of water as the mobile phase. Apply separately to the plate 1 µl of each of 2 solutions in a mixture of 9 volumes of chloroform R and 1 volume of methanol R containing (A) 15 mg of the test substance per ml and (B) 0.30 mg of the test substance per ml. After removing the plate from the chromatographic chamber, allow it to dry in air until the solvents have evaporated, then heat it at 105 °C for 10 minutes. Allow it to cool, spray it with blue tetrazolium/sodium hydroxide TS, and examine the chromatogram in daylight. Any spot obtained with solution A, other than the principal spot, is not more intense than that obtained with solution B.

Assay. Dissolve about 20 mg, accurately weighed, in sufficient methanol R to produce 100 ml; dilute 5.0 ml of this solution to 100 ml with the same solvent. Measure the absorbance of a 1-cm layer of the diluted solution at the maximum at about 243 nm. Calculate the amount of $C_{23}H_{30}O_6$ in the substance being tested by comparison with prednisolone acetate RS, similarly and concurrently examined. In an adequately calibrated spectrophotometer the absorbance of the reference solution should be 0.37 ± 0.02.

PROBENECIDUM

Probenecid

Molecular formula. $C_{13}H_{19}NO_4S$

Relative molecular mass.   285.4

Graphic formula.

$$(CH_3CH_2CH_2)_2NSO_2 - C_6H_4 - COOH$$

Chemical name.   *p*-(Dipropylsulfamoyl)benzoic acid; 4-[(dipropylamino)sulfonyl]benzoic acid; CAS Reg. No. 57-66-9.

Description.   A white or almost white, crystalline powder; odourless.

Solubility.   Practically insoluble in water; soluble in 25 parts of ethanol (~750 g/l) TS and in 12 parts of acetone R; soluble in chloroform R and in dilute solutions of alkali hydroxides.

Category.   Antigout drug.

Storage.   Probenecid should be kept in a well-closed container.

REQUIREMENTS

General requirement.   Probenecid contains not less than 98.0% and not more than 101.0% of $C_{13}H_{19}NO_4S$, calculated with reference to the dried substance.

Identity tests

● Either test A alone or tests B and C may be applied.

A.   Carry out the examination as described under "Spectrophotometry in the infrared region" (vol. 1, p. 40). The infrared absorption spectrum is concordant with the spectrum obtained from probenecid RS or with the *reference spectrum* of probenecid.

B.   See the test described below under "Related substances". The principal spot obtained with solution A (first application) corresponds in position, appearance and intensity with that obtained with solution B.

C.   Melting temperature, about 199 °C.

Heavy metals.   Use 1.0 g for the preparation of the test solution as described under "Limit test for heavy metals", Procedure 3 (vol. 1, p. 118); determine the heavy metals content according to Method A (vol. 1, p. 119); not more than 20 µg/g.

Sulfated ash.   Not more than 1.0 mg/g.

Loss on drying.   Dry to constant weight at 105 °C; it loses not more than 5.0 mg/g.

Acidity.   Heat 2.0 g with 100 ml of carbon-dioxide-free water R on a water-bath for 30 minutes, cool and filter. Add 0.15 ml of phenolphthalein/ethanol TS to the filtrate and titrate with carbonate-free sodium hydroxide (0.1 mol/l) VS; not more than 0.5 ml of the titrant is required to obtain the midpoint of the indicator.

Related substances.   Carry out the test as described under "Thin-layer chromatography" (vol. 1, p. 83), using silica gel R4 as the coating substance and a mixture of 15 volumes of 1-propanol R and 3 volumes of ammonia ($\sim$17 g/l) TS as the mobile phase. Prepare the 3 following solutions in a mixture of 1 volume of ammonia ($\sim$17 g/l) TS and 9 volumes of ethanol ($\sim$750 g/l) TS containing (A) 10 mg of the test substance per ml, (B) 10 mg of probenecid RS per ml, and (C) 0.050 mg of the test substance per ml. Apply to the plate 1 µl of each of solutions A and B. Apply separately 20 µl of each of solutions A and C. After removing the plate from the chromatographic chamber, allow it to dry in air and examine the chromatogram in ultraviolet light (254 nm). Any spot obtained with solution A (second application), other than the principal spot, is not more intense than that obtained with solution C.

Assay.   Dissolve about 1.0 g, accurately weighed, in 50 ml of neutralized ethanol TS and titrate with carbonate-free sodium hydroxide (0.1 mol/l) VS, using bromothymol blue/ethanol TS as indicator. Repeat the operation without the substance being examined and make any necessary corrections. Each ml of carbonate-free sodium hydroxide (0.1 mol/l) VS is equivalent to 28.54 mg of $C_{13}H_{19}NO_4S$.

PROCAINI BENZYLPENICILLINUM

Procaine benzylpenicillin

Procaine benzylpenicillin (non-injectable)
Procaine benzylpenicillin, sterile

Molecular formula. $C_{16}H_{18}N_2O_4S,C_{13}H_{20}N_2O_2,H_2O$

Relative molecular mass. 588.7

Graphic formula.

Chemical name. 2-(Diethylamino)ethyl *p*-aminobenzoate compound with (2*S*,5*R*,6*R*)-3,3-dimethyl-7-oxo-6-(2-phenylacetamido)-4-thia-1-azabicyclo-[3.2.0]heptane-2-carboxylic acid (1:1) monohydrate; 2-(diethylamino)ethyl 4-aminobenzoate compound with [2*S*-(2α,5α,6β)]-3,3-dimethyl-7-oxo-6-[(phenyl-acetyl)amino]-4-thia-1-azabicyclo[3.2.0]heptane-2-carboxylic acid (1:1) mono-hydrate; CAS Reg. No. 6130-64-9 (monohydrate).

Other names. Penicillin G procaine, Procaine penicillin.

Description. A white or almost white, crystalline powder; odourless or almost odourless.

Solubility. Slightly soluble in water; soluble in ethanol ($\sim$750 g/l) TS and chloroform R.

Category. Antibacterial drug.

Storage. Procaine benzylpenicillin should be kept in a tightly closed container, protected from light, and stored at a temperature not exceeding 30 °C.

Labelling. The designation sterile Procaine benzylpenicillin indicates that the substance complies with the additional requirements for sterile Procaine benzyl-penicillin and may be used for parenteral administration or for other sterile applications.

Additional information. Solutions of Procaine benzylpenicillin are dextro-rotatory. It is readily decomposed by acids, alkalis, and oxidizing agents. Even in the absence of light, it is gradually degraded on exposure to a humid atmosphere, the decomposition being faster at higher temperatures.

REQUIREMENTS

General requirement.   Procaine benzylpenicillin contains not less than 96.0% and not more than 100.5% of total penicillins calculated as $C_{16}H_{18}N_2O_4S,C_{13}H_{20}N_2O_2$ and not less than 38.5% and not more than 41.5% of $C_{13}H_{20}N_2O_2$, both calculated with reference to the anhydrous substance.

Identity tests

A.   To 2 mg in a test-tube add 0.05 ml of water followed by 2 ml of sulfuric acid ($\sim$1760 g/l) TS and mix; the solution is almost colourless. Immerse the test-tube for 1 minute in a water-bath; the solution remains almost colourless. Place 2 mg in a second test-tube, add 1 drop of water and 2 ml of formaldehyde/sulfuric acid TS and mix; the solution is almost colourless, but after a few minutes the colour changes to yellow-brown. Immerse the test-tube for 1 minute in a water-bath; a reddish brown colour is produced.

B.   Dissolve 10 mg in 10 ml of water and add 0.5 ml of neutral red/ethanol TS. Add sufficient sodium hydroxide (0.01 mol/l) VS to give a permanent orange colour and then add 1.0 ml of penicillinase TS; the colour changes rapidly to red.

C.   About 0.05 g yields the reaction described for the identification of primary aromatic amines under "General identification tests" (vol. 1, p. 111), producing a bright, orange-red precipitate.

Water.   Determine as described under "Determination of water by the Karl Fischer Method", Method A (vol. 1, p. 135), using about 0.5 g of the substance; the water content is not less than 28 mg/g and not more than 42 mg/g.

pH value.   pH of a saturated solution containing about 3.0 g in 10 ml of carbon-dioxide-free water R, 5.0–7.5.

Assay

For total penicillins.   Dissolve about 0.045 g, accurately weighed, in sufficient water to produce 1000 ml. Transfer two 2.0-ml aliquots of this solution into separate stoppered tubes. To one tube add 10.0 ml of imidazole/mercuric chloride TS, mix, stopper the tube and place in a water-bath at 60 °C for exactly 25 minutes. Cool the tube rapidly to 20 °C (solution A). To the second tube add 10.0 ml of water and mix (solution B).

Without delay measure the absorbance of a 1-cm layer at the maximum at about 314 nm against a solvent cell containing a mixture of 2.0 ml of water and 10.0 ml of imidazole/mercuric chloride TS for solution A and water for solution B.

From the difference between the absorbance of solution A and that of solution B, calculate the amount of $C_{16}H_{18}N_2O_4S,C_{13}H_{20}N_2O_2$ in the substance being tested by comparison with 0.050 g of benzylpenicillin sodium RS similarly and concurrently examined, taking into account that each mg of benzylpenicillin sodium RS ($C_{16}H_{17}N_2NaO_4S$) is equivalent to 1.601 mg of $C_{16}H_{18}N_2O_4S,C_{13}H_{20}N_2O_2$. In an adequately calibrated spectrophotometer the absorbance of the reference solution should be 0.62 ± 0.03.

For procaine. Dissolve about 0.5 g, accurately weighed, in 10 ml of water, add 5 ml of sodium carbonate (75 g/l) TS and extract with four successive quantities, each of 25 ml of chloroform R, filter the chloroform extracts, and evaporate to a small volume on a water-bath. Add 20.0 ml of hydrochloric acid (0.1 mol/l) VS and distil off the remaining chloroform. Cool, add 0.25 ml of methyl red/ethanol TS and titrate with sodium hydroxide (0.1 mol/l) VS. Each ml of hydrochloric acid (0.1 mol/l) VS is equivalent to 23.63 mg of $C_{13}H_{20}N_2O_2$.

Additional Requirements for Sterile Procaine Benzylpenicillin

Pyrogens. Carry out the test as described under "Test for pyrogens" (vol. 1, p. 155) injecting, per kg of the rabbit's mass, 5 ml of a solution in sterile water R containing 0.4 mg of the substance to be examined per ml.

Sterility. Complies with the "Sterility testing of antibiotics" (vol. 1, p. 152), applying either the membrane filtration test procedure with added penicillinase TS or the direct test procedure.

PROCARBAZINI HYDROCHLORIDUM

Procarbazine hydrochloride

Molecular formula. $C_{12}H_{19}N_3O,HCl$

Relative molecular mass.   257.8

Graphic formula.

$$(CH_3)_2CHNHC(=O)-C_6H_4-CH_2NHNHCH_3 \cdot HCl$$

Chemical name.   *N*-Isopropyl-α-(2-methylhydrazino)-*p*-toluamide monohydrochloride; *N*-(1-methylethyl)-4-[(2-methylhydrazino)methyl]benzamide monohydrochloride; CAS Reg. No. 366-70-1.

Description.   A white to yellowish, crystalline powder.

Solubility.   Soluble in water and methanol R; sparingly soluble in ethanol ($\sim$750 g/l) TS; slightly soluble in chloroform R; practically insoluble in ether R.

Category.   Cytotoxic drug.

Storage.   Procarbazine hydrochloride should be kept in a tightly closed container, protected from light.

Additional information.   Procarbazine hydrochloride melts at about 223 °C with decomposition.   Even in the absence of light, Procarbazine hydrochloride is gradually degraded on exposure to a humid atmosphere, the decomposition being faster at higher temperatures.   CAUTION: Procarbazine hydrochloride must be handled with care, avoiding contact with the skin and inhalation of airborne particles.   Wear rubber gloves while handling this substance.

REQUIREMENTS

General requirement.   Procarbazine hydrochloride contains not less than 98.5% and not more than 100.5% of $C_{12}H_{19}N_3O,HCl$, calculated with reference to the dried substance.

Identity tests

A.   Carry out the examination as described under "Spectrophotometry in the infrared region" (vol. 1, p. 40).   The infrared absorption spectrum is concordant with the spectrum obtained from procarbazine hydrochloride RS or with the *reference spectrum* of procarbazine hydrochloride.

B.   A 0.10 g/ml solution yields reaction B described under "General identification tests" as characteristic of chlorides (vol. 1, p. 113).

Heavy metals.   Use 1.0 g for the preparation of the test solution as described under "Limit test for heavy metals", Procedure 1 (vol. 1, p. 118); determine the heavy metals content according to Method A (vol. 1, p. 119); not more than 20 µg/g.

Sulfated ash.   Not more than 1.0 mg/g.

Loss on drying.   Dry to constant weight at 105 °C; it loses not more than 5.0 mg/g.

pH value.   pH of a 0.05 g/ml solution, 3.0–4.5.

Assay.   Dissolve about 0.125 g, accurately weighed, in a mixture of 5 ml of formic acid ($\sim$1080 g/l) TS and 20 ml of glacial acetic acid R1, add 5 ml of mercuric acetate/acetic acid TS, and titrate with perchloric acid (0.1 mol/l) VS as described under "Non-aqueous titration", Method A (vol. 1, p. 131).   Each ml of perchloric acid (0.1 mol/l) VS is equivalent to 25.78 mg of $C_{12}H_{19}N_3O,HCl$.

PROMETHAZINI HYDROCHLORIDUM

Promethazine hydrochloride

Molecular formula. $C_{17}H_{20}N_2S,HCl$

Relative molecular mass. 320.9

Graphic formula.

$CH_2CH(CH_3)N(CH_3)_2$ · HCl

Chemical name. 10-[2-(Dimethylamino)propyl]phenothiazine monohydrochloride; *N,N*,α-trimethyl-10*H*-phenothiazine-10-ethanamine monohydrochloride; CAS Reg. No. 58-33-3.

Other name. Diprazinum.

Description. A white or faintly yellowish, crystalline powder; odourless or almost odourless.

Solubility. Very soluble in water; freely soluble in ethanol ($\sim$750 g/l) TS and chloroform R; practically insoluble in ether R.

Category. Antiemetic drug.

Storage. Promethazine hydrochloride should be kept in a tightly closed container, protected from light.

Additional information. On prolonged exposure to air, Promethazine hydrochloride slowly oxidizes and acquires a blue colour. Even in the absence of light, it is gradually degraded on exposure to a humid atmosphere, the decomposition being faster at higher temperatures.

REQUIREMENTS

General requirement. Promethazine hydrochloride contains not less than 98.5% and not more than 101.0% of $C_{17}H_{20}N_2S,HCl$, calculated with reference to the dried substance.

Identity tests

A. Dissolve 20 mg in 5 ml of water and add 0.05 g of lead(IV) oxide R; no red coloration is observed in the supernatant liquid but it slowly turns bluish.

B.   Dissolve 0.25 g in 25 ml of water and add slowly, with stirring, 25 ml of tri-nitrophenol (7 g/l) TS. Allow the mixture to stand for 10 minutes, collect the precipitate and wash with a small quantity of water; melting temperature after recrystallization from ethanol ($\sim$750 g/l) TS and drying, about 160 °C with decomposition (picrate).

C.   Dissolve 0.05 g in 5 ml of water and add 2 ml of nitric acid ($\sim$1000 g/l) TS; a dark red colour is produced, which turns yellowish on standing. The solution yields reaction A described under "General identification tests" as characteristic of chlorides (vol. 1, p. 112).

Solution in chloroform.   A solution of 1.0 g in 10 ml of chloroform R is clear and not more intensely coloured than standard colour solution Ywl when compared as described under "Colour of liquids" (vol. 1, p. 50).

Sulfated ash.   Not more than 1.0 mg/g.

Loss on drying.   Dry to constant weight at 105 °C; it loses not more than 5.0 mg/g.

pH value.   pH of a 0.10 g/ml solution in carbon-dioxide-free water, 3.5 – 5.0.

Related impurities.   Carry out, in subdued light, the test as described under "Thin-layer chromatography" (vol. 1, p. 83), using silica gel R4 as the coating substance and a mixture of 85 volumes of hexane R, 10 volumes of acetone R, and 5 volumes of diethylamine R as the mobile phase. Apply separately to the plate 10 μl of each of 2 freshly prepared solutions in a mixture of 95 volumes of methanol R and 5 volumes of diethylamine R containing (A) 20 mg of the test substance per ml and (B) 0.20 mg of the test substance per ml. After removing the plate from the chromatographic chamber, allow it to dry in air and examine the chromatogram in ultraviolet light (254 nm). Any spot obtained with solution A, other than the principal spot, is not more intense than that obtained with solution B.

Assay.   Dissolve about 0.4 g, accurately weighed, in 200 ml of acetone R, add 10 ml of mercuric acetate/acetic acid TS and 3 ml of methyl orange/acetone TS, and titrate with perchloric acid (0.1 mol/l) VS as described under "Non-aqueous titration", Method A (vol. 1, p. 131). Each ml of perchloric acid (0.1 mol/l) VS is equivalent to 32.09 mg of $C_{17}H_{20}N_2S,HCl$.

PROTIONAMIDUM

Protionamide

Molecular formula. $C_9H_{12}N_2S$

Relative molecular mass.   180.3

Graphic formula.

$$\text{(2-propyl-4-pyridinecarbothioamide structure)}$$

Chemical name.   2-Propylthioisonicotinamide; 2-propyl-4-pyridinecarbothio-amide; CAS Reg. No. 14222-60-7.

Description.   Yellow crystals or a crystalline powder; odourless or almost odour-less.

Solubility.   Practically insoluble in water; soluble in ethanol ($\sim$750 g/l) TS and methanol R; slightly soluble in chloroform R and ether R.

Category.   Antileprosy drug.

Storage.   Protionamide should be kept in a well-closed container, protected from light.

REQUIREMENTS

General requirement.   Protionamide contains not less than 98.0% and not more than 101.0% of $C_9H_{12}N_2S$, calculated with reference to the dried substance.

Identity tests

● Either tests A and D or tests B, C and D may be applied.

A.   Carry out the examination as described under "Spectrophotometry in the infrared region" (vol. 1, p. 40). The infrared absorption spectrum is concordant with the spectrum obtained from protionamide RS or with the *reference spectrum* of protionamide.

B.   The absorption spectrum of a 10 µg/ml solution in ethanol ($\sim$750 g/l) TS, when observed between 230 nm and 350 nm, exhibits a maximum at about 291 nm; the absorbance of a 1-cm layer at this wavelength is about 0.39.

C.   Heat 0.1 g with 5 ml of hydrochloric acid (1 mol/l) VS; the vapours evolved blacken lead acetate paper R.

D.   Melting temperature, about 141 °C.

Heavy metals. Use 1.0 g for the preparation of the test solution as described under "Limit test for heavy metals", Procedure 3 (vol. 1, p. 118); determine the heavy metals content according to Method A (vol. 1, p. 119); not more than 20 µg/g.

Sulfated ash. Not more than 1.0 mg/g.

Loss on drying. Dry to constant weight at 105 °C; it loses not more than 5.0 mg/g.

Acidity. Dissolve 2.0 g in 20 ml of warm methanol R, add 20 ml of water, cool, shake until crystallization occurs, and titrate with sodium hydroxide (0.1 mol/l) VS, using cresol red/ethanol TS as indicator; not more than 0.2 ml is required to obtain the midpoint of the indicator (orange).

Related substances. Carry out the test as described under "Thin-layer chromatography" (vol. 1, p. 83), using silica gel R4 as the coating substance and a mixture of 9 volumes of chloroform R and 1 volume of methanol R as the mobile phase. Apply separately to the plate 5 µl of each of 2 solutions in methanol R containing (A) 50 mg of the test substance per ml and (B) 0.25 mg of the test substance per ml. After removing the plate from the chromatographic chamber allow it to dry in air and examine the chromatogram in ultraviolet light (254 nm). Any spot obtained with solution A, other than the principal spot, is not more intense than that obtained with solution B.

Assay. Dissolve about 0.45 g, accurately weighed, in 30 ml of glacial acetic acid R1, and titrate with perchloric acid (0.1 mol/l) VS as described under "Non-aqueous titration", Method A (vol. 1, p. 131). Each ml of perchloric acid (0.1 mol/l) VS is equivalent to 18.03 mg of $C_9H_{12}N_2S$.

PYRANTELI EMBONAS

Pyrantel embonate

Molecular formula. $C_{11}H_{14}N_2S,C_{23}H_{16}O_6$

Relative molecular mass. 594.7

Graphic formula.

Chemical name. (*E*)-1,4,5,6-Tetrahydro-1-methyl-2-[2-(2-thienyl)vinyl]pyrimidine compound with 4,4′-methylenebis[3-hydroxy-2-naphthoate] (1:1); (*E*)-1,4,5,6-tetrahydro-1-methyl-2-[2-(2-thienyl)ethenyl]pyrimidine 4,4′-methylenebis[3-hydroxy-2-naphthalenecarboxylate] (1:1); CAS Reg. No. 22204-24-6.

Other name. Pyrantel pamoate.

Description. A yellow, crystalline powder.

Solubility. Practically insoluble in water and methanol R; soluble in dimethyl sulfoxide R; slightly soluble in dimethylformamide R.

Category. Anthelmintic drug.

Storage. Pyrantel embonate should be kept in a well-closed container, protected from light.

REQUIREMENTS

General requirement. Pyrantel embonate contains not less than 97.0% and not more than 103.0% of $C_{11}H_{14}N_2S,C_{23}H_{16}O_6$, calculated with reference to the dried substance.

Identity tests

● Either tests A and D or tests B, C and D may be applied.

A. Carry out the examination as described under "Spectrophotometry in the infrared region" (vol. 1, p. 40). The infrared absorption spectrum is concordant with the spectrum obtained from pyrantel embonate RS or with the *reference spectrum* of pyrantel embonate.

B. The absorption spectrum of a 13 μg/ml solution in methanol R, when observed between 230 nm and 360 nm, exhibits 2 maxima at about 288 nm and 300 nm. The ratio of the absorbance at 288 nm to that at 300 nm is about 1.0.

C. Dissolve 5 mg in 1.0 ml of hydrochloric acid (~70 g/l) TS and add 1.0 ml of formaldehyde/sulfuric acid TS; a purple colour is produced.

D. Melting temperature, above 250 °C with decomposition.

Sulfated ash. Not more than 5.0 mg/g.

Loss on drying. Dry at 60 °C under reduced pressure (not exceeding 0.6 kPa or about 5 mm of mercury) for 3 hours; it loses not more than 20 mg/g.

Related substances. Carry out the test as described under "Thin-layer chromatography" (vol. 1, p. 83), using silica gel R2 as the coating substance and a mixture

of 20 volumes of ethyl acetate R, 5 volumes of methanol R, and 1.5 volumes of diethylamine R as the mobile phase. Apply separately to the plate 100 µl of each of 2 solutions in a mixture of 5 volumes of chloroform R, 5 volumes of methanol R, and 0.5 volumes of ammonia ($\sim$260 g/l) TS containing (A) 20 mg of the test substance per ml and (B) 0.20 mg of the test substance per ml. After removing the plate from the chromatographic chamber, allow it to dry in a current of air for 10 minutes and examine the chromatogram in ultraviolet light (254 nm). Any spot obtained with solution A, other than the principal spot, is not more intense than that obtained with solution B.

Assay

● Perform the assay in subdued light and without any prolonged interruptions, preferably using low-actinic glassware.

Transfer about 0.10 g, accurately weighed, to a 200-ml volumetric flask, dissolve in a mixture of 10 ml of dioxan R and 10 ml of ammonia ($\sim$100 g/l) TS, and dilute to volume with perchloric acid ($\sim$140 g/l) TS. Filter, discard the first 10 ml of the filtrate, and transfer 5 ml of the subsequent filtrate to a 50-ml volumetric flask. Dilute to volume with perchloric acid ($\sim$140 g/l) TS and mix. Transfer 25 ml to a 250-ml separating funnel, add 100 ml of chloroform R, and shake well. Drain off the chloroform layer into a second separating funnel. Repeat the extraction of the aqueous phase with a second 100-ml portion of chloroform R, and combine the chloroform extracts into the same separating funnel. Add 40 ml of hydrochloric acid (0.05 mol/l) VS to the combined chloroform extracts and shake well. Drain off the chloroform phase into a third separating funnel and extract with a further 40-ml portion of hydrochloric acid (0.05 mol/l) VS, discarding the chloroform phase. Combine the aqueous phases in a 100-ml volumetric flask, rinse the separating funnel, draining into the volumetric flask, and dilute to volume with hydrochloric acid (0.05 mol/l) VS. Measure the absorbance of a 1-cm layer of this solution at the maximum at about 311 nm against a solvent cell containing hydrochloric acid (0.05 mol/l) VS. Calculate the amount of $C_{11}H_{14}N_2S,C_{23}H_{16}O_6$ in the substance being tested by comparison with pyrantel embonate RS, similarly and concurrently examined.

PYRAZINAMIDUM

Pyrazinamide

Molecular formula. $C_5H_5N_3O$

Relative molecular mass.   123.1

Graphic formula.

$$\text{(pyrazine ring with CONH}_2\text{ substituent)}$$

Chemical name.   Pyrazinecarboxamide; CAS Reg. No. 98-96-4.

Description.   A white or almost white, crystalline powder; odourless.

Solubility.   Sparingly soluble in water and chloroform R; slightly soluble in ethanol (~750 g/l) TS.

Category.   Antituberculosis drug.

Storage.   Pyrazinamide should be kept in a well-closed container.

REQUIREMENTS

General requirement.   Pyrazinamide contains not less than 98.5% and not more than 101.0% of $C_5H_5N_3O$, calculated with reference to the anhydrous substance.

Identity tests

● Either test A alone or tests B, C and D may be applied.

A.   Carry out the examination as described under "Spectrophotometry in the infrared region" (vol. 1, p. 40). The infrared absorption spectrum is concordant with the spectrum obtained from pyrazinamide RS or with the *reference spectrum* of pyrazinamide.

B.   The absorption spectrum of a 10 µg/ml solution, when observed between 230 nm and 350 nm, exhibits a maximum at about 268 nm and another smaller one at 310 nm; the absorbance of a 1-cm layer at 268 nm is about 0.66.

C.   Dissolve 0.1 g in 10 ml of water and add 1 ml of ferrous sulfate (15 g/l) TS; an orange-red colour develops turning to blue on the addition of 1 ml of sodium hydroxide (~80 g/l) TS.

D.   Boil 20 mg with 5 ml of sodium hydroxide ($\sim$200 g/l) TS; ammonia, perceptible by its odour, is evolved.

Melting range.   188–191 °C.

Heavy metals.   Use 1.0 g for the preparation of the test solution as described under "Limit test for heavy metals", Procedure 3 (vol. 1, p. 118); determine the heavy metals content according to Method A (vol. 1, p. 119); not more than 20 µg/g.

Sulfated ash.   Not more than 1.0 mg/g.

Water.   Determine as described under "Determination of water by the Karl Fischer Method", Method A (vol. 1, p. 135), using about 1 g of the substance; the water content is not more than 5.0 mg/g.

pH value.   pH of a 15 mg/ml solution in carbon-dioxide-free water R, 5.0–7.0.

Ammonia.   To 20 ml of carbon-dioxide-free water R add 1.0 ml of formaldehyde TS and 0.05 ml of phenolphthalein/ethanol TS, neutralize with carbonate-free sodium hydroxide (0.1 mol/l) VS, if necessary, add 0.50 g of the test substance, and dissolve cautiously while heating. Titrate with carbonate-free sodium hydroxide (0.1 mol/l) VS until a pink colour is obtained; not more than 0.50 ml of carbonate-free sodium hydroxide (0.1 mol/l) VS is required.

Assay.   Dissolve about 0.07 g, accurately weighed, in 15 ml of chloroform R and 5 ml of acetic anhydride R, add 0.15 ml of sudan red TS as indicator, and titrate with perchloric acid (0.1 mol/l) VS as described under "Non-aqueous titration", Method A (vol. 1, p. 131). Each ml of perchloric acid (0.1 mol/l) VS is equivalent to 12.31 mg of $C_5H_5N_3O$.

PYRIMETHAMINUM

Pyrimethamine

Molecular formula. $C_{12}H_{13}ClN_4$

Relative molecular mass.   248.7

Graphic formula.

Chemical name.   2,4-Diamino-5-(*p*-chlorophenyl)-6-ethylpyrimidine; 5-(4-chlorophenyl)-6-ethyl-2,4-pyrimidinediamine; CAS Reg. No. 58-14-0.

Description.   A white, crystalline powder; odourless.

Solubility.   Practically insoluble in water; slightly soluble in ethanol ($\sim$750 g/l) TS, chloroform R, and acetone R.

Category.   Antimalarial.

Storage.   Pyrimethamine should be kept in a well-closed container, protected from light.

REQUIREMENTS

General requirement.   Pyrimethamine contains not less than 99.0% and not more than 101.0% of $C_{12}H_{13}ClN_4$, calculated with reference to the dried substance.

Identity tests

● Either tests A and D or tests B, C and D may be applied.

A.   Carry out the examination as described under "Spectrophotometry in the infrared region" (vol. 1, p. 40). The infrared absorption spectrum is concordant with the spectrum obtained with pyrimethamine RS or with the *reference spectrum* of pyrimethamine.

B.   The absorption spectrum of a 15 µg/ml solution in hydrochloric acid (0.005 mol/l) VS, when observed between 230 nm and 350 nm, exhibits a maximum at about 272 nm and a minimum at about 260 nm; the absorbance of a 1-cm layer at the maximum is about 0.48 and at the minimum about 0.45.

C.   To 0.5 g add 1 ml of a mixture of equal volumes of glacial acetic acid R and acetic anhydride R and heat under a reflux condenser for 30 minutes. Pour the warm mixture into 25 ml of water; a white, crystalline precipitate is produced. Collect the precipitate on a filter, wash with water, recrystallize from 4 ml of ethanol ($\sim$750 g/l) TS mixed with 6 ml of water, and dry at 105 °C; melting temperature, about 172 °C (2,4-diacetylpyrimethamine).

D.   Ignite 0.1 g with 0.5 g of anhydrous sodium carbonate R, extract the residue with water, and filter. Neutralize with nitric acid ($\sim$130 g/l) TS; it yields reaction A described under "General identification tests" as characteristic of chlorides (vol. 1, p. 112).

Melting range.   239–242 °C.

Sulfated ash.   Not more than 1.0 mg/g.

Loss on drying.   Dry to constant weight at 105 °C; it loses not more than 5.0 mg/g.

Acidity or alkalinity.   Boil 0.3 g with 15 ml of water, cool and filter. Add 0.25 ml of methyl red/ethanol TS to the filtrate; a yellow colour is observed. Not more than 0.1 ml of hydrochloric acid (0.05 mol/l) VS is required to change the colour of the solution to red.

Assay.   Dissolve about 0.4 g, accurately weighed, in 30 ml of glacial acetic acid R1, add 0.20 ml of quinaldine red/ethanol TS as indicator, and titrate with perchloric acid (0.1 mol/l) VS as described under "Non-aqueous titration", Method A (vol. 1, p. 131). Each ml of perchloric acid (0.1 mol/l) VS is equivalent to 24.87 mg of $C_{12}H_{13}ClN_4$.

QUINIDINI SULFAS

Quinidine sulfate

Molecular formula. $(C_{20}H_{24}N_2O_2)_2,H_2SO_4,2H_2O$

Relative molecular mass.   783.0

Graphic formula.

$$\left[\text{CH}_3\text{O}\cdots\text{HO}\cdots\text{quinidine structure, CH=CH}_2\right]_2 \cdot \text{H}_2\text{SO}_4 \cdot 2\text{H}_2\text{O}$$

Chemical name.   Quinidine sulfate (2:1) (salt), dihydrate; (9S)-6′-methoxycin-chonan-9-ol sulfate (2:1) (salt), monohydrate; CAS Reg. No. 6591-63-5 (dihy-drate).

Description.   Colourless, needle-like crystals or a white, crystalline powder; odourless.

Solubility.   Sparingly soluble in water; soluble in ethanol (~750 g/l) TS and chloroform R; practically insoluble in ether R and acetone R.

Category.   Antidysrhythmic drug.

Storage.   Quinidine sulfate should be kept in a well-closed container, protected from light.

Additional information.   Quinidine sulfate has a very bitter taste. It darkens in colour on exposure to light.

REQUIREMENTS

General requirement.   Quinidine sulfate contains not less than 99.0% and not more than 101.0% of total alkaloids, calculated as $(C_{20}H_{24}N_2O_2)_2,H_2SO_4$ and with reference to the dried substance.

Identity tests

A.   Dissolve 0.10 g in 10 ml of water; the solution produces a slight blue fluorescence (keep the remaining solution for test B). To 1.0 ml add a few drops of sulfuric acid ($\sim$100 g/l) TS, and dilute with water to 5 ml; a vivid blue fluorescence is produced.

B.   To 1.0 ml of the solution prepared for test A, add 4 ml of water, 0.15 ml of bromine TS1, and 1.0 ml of ammonia ($\sim$100 g/l) TS; an emerald-green colour is produced.

C.   Dissolve 0.05 g in 5 ml of hot water, cool, add 1 ml of silver nitrate (40 g/l) TS, and stir with a glass rod; after a few minutes a white precipitate is produced, which is soluble in nitric acid ($\sim$130 g/l) TS.

D.   A 20 mg/ml solution yields reaction A described under "General identification tests" as characteristic of sulfates (vol. 1, p. 115).

Specific optical rotation.   Use a 20 mg/ml solution in hydrochloric acid (0.1 mol/l) VS and calculate with reference to the dried substance;
$[\alpha]_D^{20\,°C} = +275$ to $+290°$.

Clarity and colour of solution.   Dissolve 0.20 g in 10 ml of hydrochloric acid (0.1 mol/l) VS; the solution is clear and not more intensely coloured than standard colour solution Yw2 when compared as described under "Colour of liquids" (vol. 1, p. 50).

Sulfated ash.   Not more than 1.0 mg/g.

Loss on drying.   Dry to constant weight at 130 °C; it loses not less than 30 mg/g and not more than 50 mg/g.

pH value.   pH of a 10 mg/ml solution in carbon-dioxide-free water R, 6.0–6.8.

Related cinchona alkaloids.   Carry out the test as described under "Thin-layer chromatography" (vol. 1, p. 83), using silica gel R1 as the coating substance and a mixture of 20 volumes of toluene R, 12 volumes of ether R, and 5 volumes of diethylamine R as the mobile phase. Apply separately to the plate 4 µl of each of 4 solutions in methanol R containing (A) 10 mg of the test substance per ml, (B) 0.25 mg of quinine R per ml, (C) 0.25 mg of cinchonine R per ml, and (D) 10 mg of the test substance dissolved in 1 ml of solution C. After removing the plate from the chromatographic chamber, allow it to dry in a current of air for 15 minutes and repeat the development. Heat the plate at 105 °C for 30 minutes, allow it to cool, spray it with potassium iodoplatinate TS, and examine the chromatogram in daylight. Any spot obtained with solution A, other than the principal spot, is not more intense than that obtained with solution B or solution C. If any spot is obtained with solution A immediately below the principal spot, it should be disregarded. The test is valid only if the chromatogram obtained with solution D shows two distinctly separated spots.

Limit of dihydroquinidine. Dissolve about 0.2 g, accurately weighed, in 20 ml of water. Add 0.5 g of potassium bromide R, 15 ml of hydrochloric acid (~ 70 g/l) TS, and 0.1 ml of methyl red/ethanol TS. Titrate with potassium bromate (0.0167 mol/l) VS until a yellow colour is produced. Add 0.5 g of potassium iodide R in 200 ml of water, stopper the flask, and allow to stand in the dark for 5 minutes. Titrate the iodine liberated by excess potassium bromate in the solution with sodium thiosulfate (0.1 mol/l) VS, adding 2 ml of starch TS when the solution has reached a light yellow colour. Each ml of potassium bromate (0.0167 mol/l) VS is equivalent to 18.67 mg of $(C_{20}H_{24}N_2O_2)_2,H_2SO_4$, calculated with reference to the dried substance. Express the results of both the above determination and the assay in percentages. The difference between the two is not more than 15%.

Assay. Dissolve about 0.20 g, accurately weighed, in 10 ml of chloroform R and 20 ml of acetic anhydride R, and titrate with perchloric acid (0.1 mol/l) VS, determining the endpoint potentiometrically as described under "Non-aqueous titration", Method A (vol. 1, p. 131). Each ml of perchloric acid (0.1 mol/l) VS is equivalent to 24.90 mg of $(C_{20}H_{24}N_2O_2)_2,H_2SO_4$.

QUININI BISULFAS

Quinine bisulfate

Molecular formula. $C_{20}H_{24}N_2O_2,H_2SO_4,7H_2O$

Relative molecular mass. 548.6

Graphic formula.

Chemical name.   Quinine sulfate (1:1) (salt), heptahydrate;
(8αS,9R)-6′-methoxycinchonan-9-ol sulfate (1:1) (salt), heptahydrate;
(8S,9R)-9-hydroxy-6′-methoxycinchonan sulfate (1:1) (salt), heptahydrate; CAS
Reg. No. 6183-68-2 (heptahydrate).

Description.   Colourless crystals or a white, crystalline powder; odourless.

Solubility.   Freely soluble in water; sparingly soluble in ethanol (∼750 g/l)
TS.

Category.   Antimalarial drug.

Storage.   Quinine bisulfate should be kept in a well-closed container, protected
from light.

Additional information.   Quinine bisulfate effloresces in dry air. Even in the
absence of light, it is gradually degraded on exposure to a humid atmosphere, the
decomposition being faster at higher temperatures.

REQUIREMENTS

General requirement.   Quinine bisulfate contains not less than 98.5% and not
more than 101.5% of total alkaloids, calculated as $C_{20}H_{24}N_2O_2,H_2SO_4$ and with
reference to the dried substance.

Identity tests

A.   Dissolve 5 mg in 10 ml of water and add 0.05 ml of sulfuric acid (∼100 g/l)
TS; a strong blue fluorescence is produced (keep the solution for test B).

B.   To the solution prepared for test A add 0.15 ml of bromine TS1 and 1.0 ml of
ammonia (∼100 g/l) TS; an emerald-green colour is produced.

C.   Dissolve 0.05 g in 5 ml of water and add 1 ml of silver nitrate (40 g/l) TS; no
white precipitate is produced.

D.   A 20 mg/ml solution yields reaction A described under "General identification tests" as characteristic of sulfates (vol. 1, p. 115).

Specific optical rotation.   Use a 30 mg/ml solution in hydrochloric acid
(0.1 mol/l) VS and calculate with reference to the dried substance;
$[\alpha]_D^{20\,°C}$ = −208 to −216°.

Clarity and colour of solution.   Dissolve 0.20 g in 10 ml of hydrochloric acid
(0.1 mol/l) VS; the solution is clear and not more intensely coloured than standard
colour solution Yw2 when compared as described under "Colour of liquids"
(vol. 1, p. 50).

Sulfated ash.   Not more than 1.0 mg/g.

Loss on drying.   Dry at 60 °C under reduced pressure (not exceeding 0.6 kPa or about 5 mm of mercury) for 18 hours; it loses not less than 190 mg/g and not more than 240 mg/g.

pH value.   pH of a 10 mg/ml solution, 2.8–3.4.

Related cinchona alkaloids.   Carry out the test as described under "Thin-layer chromatography" (vol. 1, p. 83), using silica gel R1 as the coating substance and a mixture of 20 volumes of toluene R, 12 volumes of ether R, and 5 volumes of diethylamine R as the mobile phase.   Apply separately to the plate 4 μl of each of 4 solutions in methanol R containing (A) 10 mg of the test substance per ml, (B) 0.25 mg of quinine R per ml, (C) 0.25 mg of cinchonidine R per ml, and (D) 10 mg of the test substance dissolved in 1 ml of solution C.   After removing the plate from the chromatographic chamber, allow it to dry in a current of air for 15 minutes and repeat the development.   Heat the plate at 105 °C for 30 minutes, allow it to cool, spray it with potassium iodoplatinate TS, and examine the chromatogram in daylight.   Any spot obtained with solution A, other than the principal spot, is not more intense than that obtained with solution B or solution C.   If any spot is obtained with solution A immediately below the principal spot, it should be disregarded.   The test is valid only if the chromatogram obtained with solution D shows two distinctly separated spots.

Limit of dihydroquinine.   Dissolve about 0.2 g, accurately weighed, in 20 ml of water.   Add 0.5 g of potassium bromide R, 15 ml of hydrochloric acid ($\sim$70 g/l) TS, and 0.1 ml of methyl red/ethanol TS.   Titrate with potassium bromate (0.0167 mol/l) VS until a yellow colour is produced.   Add 0.5 g of potassium iodide R in 200 ml of water, stopper the flask, and allow to stand in the dark for 5 minutes.   Titrate the iodine liberated by excess potassium bromate in the solution with sodium thiosulfate (0.1 mol/l) VS, adding 2 ml of starch TS when the solution has reached a light yellow colour.   Each ml of potassium bromate (0.0167 mol/l) VS is equivalent to 21.13 mg of $C_{20}H_{24}N_2O_2,H_2SO_4$, calculated with reference to the dried substance.   Express the results of both the above determination and the assay in percentages.   The difference between the two is not more than 10%.

Assay.   Dissolve about 0.45 g, accurately weighed, in 15 ml of water.   Add 25 ml of sodium hydroxide (0.1 mol/l) VS and extract with 3 quantities, each of 25 ml of chloroform R.   Wash the combined chloroform extracts with 20 ml of water.   Dry the chloroform extracts with anhydrous sodium sulfate R, evaporate to dryness under reduced pressure, and dissolve the residue in 50 ml of glacial acetic acid R1.   Titrate with perchloric acid (0.1 mol/l) VS as described under "Non-aqueous titration", Method A (vol. 1, p. 131).   Each ml of perchloric acid (0.1 mol/l) VS is equivalent to 21.13 mg of $C_{20}H_{24}N_2O_2,H_2SO_4$.

QUININI DIHYDROCHLORIDUM

Quinine dihydrochloride

Molecular formula. $C_{20}H_{24}N_2O_2,2HCl$

Relative molecular mass.   397.3

Graphic formula.

Chemical name.   (8αS,9R)-6′-Methoxycinchonan-9-ol dihydrochloride; (8S,9R)-9-hydroxy-6′-methoxycinchonan dihydrochloride; CAS Reg. No. 60-93-5.

Description.   A white or almost white, crystalline powder; odourless.

Solubility.   Very soluble in water; freely soluble in chloroform R; soluble in ethanol (~750 g/l) TS; practically insoluble in ether R.

Category.   Antimalarial drug.

Storage.   Quinine dihydrochloride should be kept in a well-closed container, protected from light.

Additional information.   Quinine dihydrochloride turns yellow on exposure to light. Even in the absence of light, it is gradually degraded on exposure to a humid atmosphere, the decomposition being faster at higher temperatures.

REQUIREMENTS

General requirement.   Quinine dihydrochloride contains not less than 99.0% and not more than 101.0% of total alkaloids, calculated as $C_{20}H_{24}N_2O_2,2HCl$ and with reference to the dried substance.

Identity tests

A.   Dissolve 5 mg in 10 ml of water and add 0.05 ml of sulfuric acid (~100 g/l) TS; a strong blue fluorescence is produced (keep the solution for test B).

B.   To the solution prepared for test A add 0.15 ml of bromine TS1 and 1.0 ml of ammonia (~100 g/l) TS; an emerald-green colour is produced.

C.   Dissolve 0.05 g in 5 ml of water and add 1 ml of silver nitrate (40 g/l) TS; a white precipitate is produced.

D.   A 20 mg/ml solution yields reaction A described under "General identification tests" as characteristic of chlorides (vol. 1, p. 113).

Specific optical rotation.   Use a 30 mg/ml solution in hydrochloric acid (0.1 mol/l) VS and calculate with reference to the dried substance; $[\alpha]_D^{20\,°C} = -223$ to $-229°$.

Clarity and colour of solution.   Dissolve 0.20 g in 10 ml of hydrochloric acid (0.1 mol/l) VS; the solution is clear and not more intensely coloured than standard colour solution Yw2 when compared as described under "Colour of liquids" (vol. 1, p. 50).

Sulfated ash.   Not more than 1.0 mg/g.

Loss on drying.   Dry to constant weight at 105 °C; it loses not more than 30 mg/g.

pH value.   pH of a 30 mg/ml solution, 2.0–3.0.

Related cinchona alkaloids.   Carry out the test as described under "Thin-layer chromatography" (vol. 1, p. 83), using silica gel R1 as the coating substance and a mixture of 20 volumes of toluene R, 12 volumes of ether R, and 5 volumes of diethylamine R as the mobile phase. Apply separately to the plate 4 µl of each of 4 solutions in methanol R containing (A) 10 mg of the test substance per ml, (B) 0.25 mg of quinine R per ml, (C) 0.25 mg of cinchonidine R per ml, and (D) 10 mg of the test substance dissolved in 1 ml of solution C. After removing the plate from the chromatographic chamber, allow it to dry in a current of air for 15 minutes and repeat the development. Heat the plate at 105 °C for 30 minutes, allow to cool, spray with potassium iodoplatinate TS and examine the chromatogram in daylight. Any spot obtained with solution A, other than the principal spot, is not more intense than that obtained with solution B or solution C. If any spot is obtained with solution A immediately below the principal spot, it should be disregarded. The test is valid only if the chromatogram obtained with solution D shows two distinctly separated spots.

Limit of dihydroquinine.   Dissolve about 0.2 g, accurately weighed, in 20 ml of water. Add 0.5 g of potassium bromide R, 15 ml of hydrochloric acid (~70 g/l) TS, and 0.1 ml of methyl red/ethanol TS. Titrate with potassium bromate (0.0167 mol/l) TS until a yellow colour is produced. Add 0.5 g of potassium iodide R in 200 ml of water, stopper the flask, and allow to stand in the dark for 5 minutes. Titrate the iodine liberated by excess potassium bromate in the solution with sodium thiosulfate (0.1 mol/l) VS, adding 2 ml of starch TS when the solution has reached a light yellow colour. Each ml of potassium bromate (0.0167 mol/l) VS is equivalent to 19.87 mg of $C_{20}H_{24}N_2O_2,2HCl$, calculated with reference to the dried substance. Express the results of both the above determination and the assay in percentages. The difference between the two is not more than 10%.

Assay. Dissolve about 0.3 g, accurately weighed, in 50 ml of glacial acetic acid R1, add 20 ml of acetic anhydride R and 10 ml of mercuric acetate/acetic acid TS, and titrate with perchloric acid (0.1 mol/l) VS as described under "Non-aqueous titration", Method A (vol. 1, p. 131). Each ml of perchloric acid (0.1 mol/l) VS is equivalent to 19.87 mg of $C_{20}H_{24}N_2O_2,2HCl$.

RIFAMPICINUM

Rifampicin

Molecular formula. $C_{43}H_{58}N_4O_{12}$

Relative molecular mass. 823.0

Graphic formula.

Chemical name. (2*S*,12*Z*,14*E*,16*S*,17*S*,18*R*,19*R*,20*R*,21*S*,22*S*,23*S*,24*E*)-5,6,9,17,19,21-Hexahydroxy-23-methoxy-2,4,12,16,18,20,22-heptamethyl-8-[*N*-(4-methyl-1-piperazinyl)formimidoyl]-2,7-(epoxypentadeca[1,11,13]-trienimino)naphtho[2,1-*b*]-furan-1,11-(2*H*)-dione, 21-acetate; 3-[[(4-methyl-1-piperazinyl)imino]methyl]rifamycin; CAS Reg. No. 13292-46-1.

Other name. Rifampin.

Description. A brick red to red-brown, crystalline powder; odourless or almost odourless.

Solubility. Very slightly soluble in water; freely soluble in chloroform R; soluble in methanol R; slightly soluble in acetone R, ethanol (~750 g/l) TS, and ether R.

Category. Antileprosy drug; antituberculosis drug.

Storage.   Rifampicin should be kept in a tightly closed container, protected from light and stored at a temperature not exceeding 15 °C, or in an atmosphere of nitrogen at a temperature not exceeding 30 °C.

REQUIREMENTS

General requirement.   Rifampicin contains not less than 97.0% and not more than 102.0% of $C_{43}H_{58}N_4O_{12}$, calculated with reference to the dried substance.

Identity tests

A.   Carry out the examination as described under "Spectrophotometry in the infrared region" (vol. 1, p. 40). The infrared absorption spectrum is concordant with the spectrum obtained from rifampicin RS or with the *reference spectrum* of rifampicin.

B.   Dissolve 50 mg in 50 ml of methanol R and dilute 1 ml of this solution to 50 ml with phosphate buffer, pH 7.4, TS. The absorption spectrum of the resulting solution, when observed between 220 nm and 500 nm, exhibits 4 maxima at about 237 nm, 254 nm, 334 nm, and 475 nm; the ratio of the absorbance of a 1-cm layer at the maximum at about 334 nm to that at the maximum at about 475 nm is about 1.75.

C.   Suspend 25 mg in 25 ml of water, shake for 5 minutes and filter. To 5 ml of the filtrate add 1 ml of ammonium persulfate/phosphate buffer TS and shake for a few minutes; the colour turns from orange-yellow to violet-red without the formation of a precipitate.

Heavy metals.   Place 1.0 g in a silica crucible and mix it with 4 ml of magnesium sulfate/sulfuric acid TS. Heat cautiously to ignition and continue heating until a white or at most greyish residue is obtained. Ignite at a temperature not exceeding 800 °C, allow to cool, and moisten the residue with a few drops of sulfuric acid (~100 g/l) TS. Evaporate, ignite again, and allow to cool. Next, dissolve the residue in hydrochloric acid (~70 g/l) TS, add, drop by drop, a solution of ammonia (~100 g/l) PbTS, until the pH of the solution is between 8 and 8.5, then add, also drop by drop, acetic acid (~60 g/l) PbTS to adjust the pH to 3–4, filter, dilute with water to 40 ml, and mix. Determine the heavy metals content as described under "Limit test for heavy metals", according to Method A (vol. 1, p. 119); not more than 20 µg/g.

Sulfated ash.   Not more than 1.0 mg/g.

Loss on drying.   Dry at 60 °C under reduced pressure (not exceeding 0.6 kPa or about 5 mm of mercury) for 4 hours; it loses not more than 10 mg/g.

pH value. Shake 0.10 g with 10 ml of carbon-dioxide-free water R; pH of the suspension, 4.5–6.5.

Related substances. Carry out the test as described under "Thin-layer chromatography" (vol. 1, p. 83), using silica gel R1 as the coating substance and preparing the slurry with phosphate/citrate buffer pH 6.0, TS. As the mobile phase use a mixture of 85 volumes of chloroform R and 15 volumes of methanol R. Apply separately to the plate 20 µl of each of 4 solutions in chloroform R containing (A) 20 mg of the test substance per ml, (B) 0.10 mg of 3-formylrifamycin SV RS per ml, (C) 0.30 mg of rifampicin quinone RS per ml, and (D) 0.20 mg of the test substance per ml. After removing the plate from the chromatographic chamber, allow it to dry in air and examine the chromatogram in daylight. Any coloured spots obtained with solution A, other than the principal spot, are not more intense than the corresponding spots obtained with solutions B and C. Furthermore, any other spots obtained with solution A are not more intense than that obtained with solution D.

Assay. Dissolve about 0.10 g, accurately weighed, in sufficient methanol R to produce 100 ml. Dilute 2 ml of this solution to 100 ml with phosphate buffer, pH 7.4, TS. Measure the absorbance of the resulting solution in a 1-cm layer at the maximum at about 475 nm, using as the blank phosphate buffer, pH 7.4, TS. Calculate the content of $C_{43}H_{58}N_4O_{12}$, using the absorptivity value of 18.7 ($A_{1\,cm}^{1\%} = 187$).

SALBUTAMOLUM

Salbutamol

Molecular formula. $C_{13}H_{21}NO_3$

Relative molecular mass. 239.3

Graphic formula.

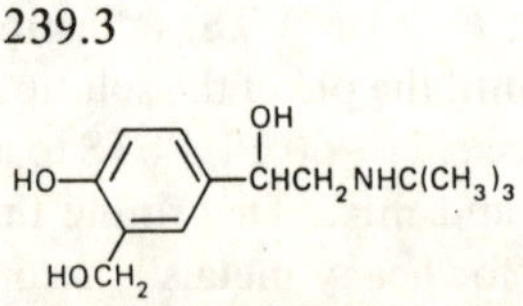

OH
HO—CHCH₂NHC(CH₃)₃
HOCH₂

Chemical name. α¹-[(*tert*-Butylamino)methyl]-4-hydroxy-*m*-xylene-α,α′-diol; α¹-[[(1,1-dimethylethyl)amino]methyl]-4-hydroxy-1,3-benzenedimethanol; CAS Reg. No. 18559-94-9.

Description. A white or almost white, crystalline powder; odourless.

Solubility.   Soluble in 70 parts of water; soluble in ethanol ($\sim$750 g/l) TS; slightly soluble in ether R.

Category.   Antiasthmatic drug.

Storage.   Salbutamol should be kept in a well-closed container, protected from light.

REQUIREMENTS

General requirement.   Salbutamol contains not less than 98.0% and not more than 101.0% of $C_{13}H_{21}NO_3$, calculated with reference to the dried substance.

Identity tests

● Either test A alone or tests B, C and D may be applied.

A.   Carry out the examination as described under "Spectrophotometry in the infrared region" (vol. 1, p. 40). The infrared absorption spectrum is concordant with the spectrum obtained from salbutamol RS or with the *reference spectrum* of salbutamol.

B.   The absorption spectrum of a 0.080 mg/ml solution in hydrochloric acid (0.1 mol/l) VS, when observed between 230 nm and 350 nm, exhibits a maximum only at about 276 nm; the absorbance of a 1-cm layer at this wavelength is about 0.56.

C.   Dissolve 0.05 g in 5 ml of water and add 0.1 ml of ferric chloride (25 g/l) TS; a reddish violet colour is produced.   Add 0.05 g of sodium hydrogen carbonate R; a fleshy precipitate is produced with an evolution of gas.   Add a few drops of sulfuric acid ($\sim$1760 g/l) TS; the solution becomes colourless.

D.   Melting temperature, about 155 °C with decomposition.

Sulfated ash.   Not more than 1.0 mg/g.

Loss on drying.   Dry to constant weight at 50 °C under reduced pressure (not exceeding 0.6 kPa or about 5 mm of mercury); it loses not more than 5.0 mg/g.

Related substances.   Carry out the test as described under "Thin-layer chromatography" (vol. 1, p. 83), using silica gel R1 as the coating substance and a mixture of 4 volumes of ammonia ($\sim$260 g/l) TS, 16 volumes of water, 30 volumes of 2-propanol R, and 50 volumes of ethyl acetate R as the mobile phase. Apply separately to the plate 5 µl of each of 2 solutions in methanol R containing (A) 20 mg of the test substance per ml and (B) 0.10 mg of the test substance per ml. After removing the plate from the chromatographic chamber, allow it to dry in air until the solvents have evaporated. Place the plate for a few minutes in an atmosphere saturated with diethylamine R, spray it with diazotized sulfanilic acid TS, and examine the chromatogram in daylight. Any spot obtained with solution A, other than the principal spot, is not more intense than that obtained with solution B.

Assay.   Dissolve about 0.4 g, accurately weighed, in 30 ml of glacial acetic acid R1 and titrate with perchloric acid (0.1 mol/l) VS as described under "Non-aqueous titration", Method A (vol. 1, p. 131). Each ml of perchloric acid (0.1 mol/l) VS is equivalent to 23.93 mg of $C_{13}H_{21}NO_3$.

SALBUTAMOLI SULFAS

Salbutamol sulfate

Molecular formula. $(C_{13}H_{21}NO_3)_2,H_2SO_4$

Relative molecular mass.   288.4

Graphic formula.

$$HO-\text{(benzene ring)}-CHCH_2NHC(CH_3)_3 \cdot \tfrac{1}{2} H_2SO_4$$

with substituents OH on the CH, and HOCH$_2$ on the ring.

Chemical name. α^1-[(*tert*-Butylamino)methyl]-4-hydroxy-*m*-xylene-α,α'-diol sulfate (2:1) (salt); α^1-[[(1,1-dimethylethyl)amino]methyl]-4-hydroxy-1,3-benzenedimethanol sulfate (2:1) (salt); CAS Reg. No. 51022-70-9.

Description.   A white or almost white powder; odourless.

Solubility.   Soluble in 4 parts of water; slightly soluble in ethanol ($\sim$750 g/l) TS, chloroform R, and ether R.

Category.   Antiasthmatic drug.

Storage.   Salbutamol sulfate should be kept in a well-closed container, protected from light.

Additional information.   Even in the absence of light, Salbutamol sulfate is gradually degraded on exposure to a humid atmosphere, the decomposition being faster at higher temperatures.

REQUIREMENTS

General requirement.   Salbutamol sulfate contains not less than 98.0% and not more than 101.0% of $C_{13}H_{21}NO_3,\frac{1}{2}H_2SO_4$, calculated with reference to the dried substance.

Identity tests

● Either tests A and D or tests B, C and D may be applied.

A.   Carry out the examination as described under "Spectrophotometry in the infrared region" (vol. 1, p. 40).   The infrared absorption spectrum is concordant with the spectrum obtained from salbutamol sulfate RS or with the *reference spectrum* of salbutamol sulfate.

B.   The absorption spectrum of a 0.080 mg/ml solution in hydrochloric acid (0.1 mol/l) VS, when observed between 230 nm and 350 nm, exhibits a maximum at about 276 nm; the absorbance of a 1-cm layer at this wavelength is about 0.46.

C.   Dissolve 0.05 g in 5 ml of water and add 0.1 ml of ferric chloride (25 g/l) TS; a reddish violet colour is produced.   Add 0.05 g of sodium hydrogen carbonate R; a fleshy precipitate is produced with an evolution of gas.   Add a few drops of sulfuric acid ($\sim$1760 g/l) TS; the solution becomes colourless.

D.   A 20 mg/ml solution yields reaction A described under "General identification tests" as characteristic of sulfates (vol. 1, p. 115).

Sulfated ash.   Not more than 1.0 mg/g.

Loss on drying.   Dry to constant weight at 100 °C under reduced pressure (not exceeding 0.6 kPa or about 5 mm of mercury); it loses not more than 5.0 mg/g.

Related substances.   Carry out the test as described under "Thin-layer chromatography" (vol. 1, p. 83), using silica gel R1 as the coating substance and a mixture of 4 volumes of ammonia ($\sim$260 g/l) TS, 16 volumes of water, 30 volumes of 2-propanol R, and 50 volumes of ethyl acetate R as the mobile phase.   Apply separately to the plate 5 µl of each of 2 solutions containing (A) 20 mg of the test substance per ml and (B) 0.10 mg of the test substance per ml.   After removing the plate from the chromatographic chamber, allow it to dry in air until the solvents have evaporated.   Place the plate for a few minutes in an atmosphere saturated with diethylamine R, spray it with diazotized sulfanilic acid TS, and examine the chromatogram in daylight.   Any spot obtained with solution A, other than the principal spot, is not more intense than that obtained with solution B.

Assay.   Dissolve about 0.9 g, accurately weighed, in 30 ml of glacial acetic acid R1 and titrate with perchloric acid (0.1 mol/l) VS as described under "Non-aqueous titration", Method A (vol. 1, p. 131). Each ml of perchloric acid (0.1 mol/l) VS is equivalent to 57.67 mg of $C_{13}H_{21}NO_3,\frac{1}{2}H_2SO_4$.

SENNAE FOLIUM

Senna leaf

Alexandrian Senna leaf
Tinnevelly Senna leaf

Composition.   Senna leaf consists of the dried leaflets of *Cassia senna* L., known as Alexandrian or Khartoum Senna (*C. acutifolia* Delile) or Tinnevelly Senna (*C. angustifolia* Vahl), or a mixture of both species.

Description.   Odour, slight; taste, first mucilaginous and sweet, then slightly bitter.

Category.   Cathartic drug.

Storage.   Senna leaf should be kept protected from light and moisture.

Additional information.   Even in the absence of light, Senna leaf is gradually degraded on exposure to a humid atmosphere, the decomposition being faster at higher temperatures.

REQUIREMENTS

General requirement.   Senna leaf contains not less than 2.5% of hydroxyanthracene derivatives, calculated as sennoside B.

Identity test

To about 0.5 g of the powdered leaf add 10 ml of sodium hydroxide/ethanol TS and boil on a water-bath, dilute with 10 ml of water, and filter. Acidify the filtrate with hydrochloric acid (~70 g/l) TS and extract with 10 ml of ether R. Separate the ether layer and shake it with 5 ml of ammonia (~100 g/l) TS; a yellowish red colour is produced in the ammonia layer.

Macroscopic examination

Alexandrian Senna leaf. Pale greyish green, thin, fragile leaflets; lanceolate, mucronate; length, 20–40 mm; width, 5–15 mm, the maximum width being at a point slightly below the centre; lamina, slightly undulant; both surfaces covered with fine, short trichomes; pinnate venation, slightly prominent midrib with lateral veins leaving the midrib at an angle of about 60° and anastomosing to form a ridge parallel to the margin.

Tinnevelly Senna leaf. Yellowish green leaflets; elongated and lanceolate; length, 25–50 mm; width at the centre, 7–20 mm; lamina, flat; both surfaces are smooth with a very small number of trichomes, and marked with impressed transverse or oblique lines.

Microscopic examination. Epidermis with polygonal cells containing mucilage; unicellular thick-walled trichomes, length, up to 260 µm, slightly curved at the base, warty; paracytic stomata on both surfaces; under the epidermal cells a single row of palisade layer; cluster crystals of calcium oxalate distributed throughout the lacunose tissue; on the adaxial surface of the leaf, sclerenchymatous fibres and a gutter-shaped group of similar fibres on the abaxial side containing prismatic crystals of calcium oxalate.

Water-soluble extractive. Shake 5 g with a mixture of 0.5 ml of chloroform R and 200 ml of water, filter, evaporate 20 ml of the filtrate and weigh; the residue is not less than 300 mg/g.

Acid-insoluble ash. Carry out the procedure as described under "Determination of acid-insoluble ash" (vol. 1, p. 161); not more than 20 mg/g.

Stems and foreign matter. Weigh about 200 g and spread it in a thin layer. Detect the stems and the foreign matter by eye or with the use of a 6× lens; separate and weigh individually the stems and the foreign matter; not more than 20 mg/g of stems and not more than 10 mg/g of foreign matter.

Assay. Place 0.15 g of the powdered leaf in a 100-ml flask. Add 30.0 ml of water, mix, weigh and place in a water-bath at 80–90 °C. Heat under a reflux condenser for 15 minutes. Allow to cool, weigh, and adjust to the original mass with water. Centrifuge and transfer 20.0 ml of the supernatant liquid to a 150-ml separating funnel. Add 0.1 ml of hydrochloric acid ($\sim$70 g/l) TS and shake with 3 quantities, each of 15 ml, of chloroform R. Allow to separate and discard the chloroform layer. Add 0.10 g of sodium hydrogen carbonate R and shake for 3 minutes. Centrifuge and transfer 10.0 ml of the supernatant liquid to a 100-ml round-bottomed flask with a ground-glass neck. Add 20 ml of ferric chloride (65 g/l) TS and mix. Heat for 20 minutes under a reflux condenser in a water-bath with the water level above that of the liquid in the flask; add 1 ml of hydrochloric acid ($\sim$420 g/l) TS and heat for a further 20 minutes, with frequent shaking, to dissolve the precipitate. Cool, transfer the mixture to a separating funnel and shake with 3 quantities, each of 25 ml, of ether R previously used to rinse the flask. Combine the ether layers and wash with 2 quantities, each of 15 ml, of water. Transfer the ether layers to a volumetric flask and dilute to 100 ml with ether R. Evaporate 10.0 ml carefully to dryness and dissolve the residue in 10.0 ml of a solution containing 5 mg of magnesium acetate R per ml of methanol R. Measure the absorbance of this solution in a 1-cm layer at the maximum at about 515 nm against a solvent cell containing methanol R. Calculate in % the amount of hydroxyanthracene derivatives as sennoside B with an absorptivity value of 24.0 $(A_{1\,cm}^{1\,\%} = 240)$ as follows: 1.25 A/W, where A is the absorbance at 515 nm and W is the mass of the material examined in g.

SENNAE FRUCTUS

Senna fruit

Alexandrian Senna fruit
Tinnevelly Senna fruit

Composition.   Alexandrian Senna fruit is the dried ripe fruit of *Cassia senna* L., (*C. acutifolia* Delile) and Tinnevelly Senna fruit is the dried ripe fruit of *Cassia angustifolia* Vahl.

Description.   Odour, slight; taste, first mucilaginous and sweet, then slightly bitter.

Category.   Cathartic drug.

Storage.   Senna fruit should be kept protected from light and moisture.

Additional information.   Even in the absence of light, Senna fruit is gradually degraded on exposure to a humid atmosphere, the decomposition being faster at higher temperatures.

REQUIREMENTS

General requirement.   Alexandrian Senna fruit contains not less than 3.4% of hydroxyanthracene derivatives and Tinnevelly Senna fruit contains not less than 2.2% of hydroxyanthracene derivatives, both calculated as sennoside B.

Identity test

Cut the fruit into small pieces or powder about 0.5 g, add 10 ml of sodium hydroxide/ethanol TS and boil on a water-bath, dilute with 10 ml of water and filter. Acidify the filtrate with hydrochloric acid (~70 g/l) TS and extract with 10 ml of ether R. Separate the ether layer and shake it with 5 ml of ammonia (~100 g/l) TS; a pink to red colour is produced in the ammonia layer.

Macroscopic examination.   Leaflike, flat and thin pods, yellowish green to yellowish brown with a dark brown central area, oblong or reniform.

Alexandrian Senna fruit.   Pale to greyish green; length, about 40–50 mm; width, 20–25 mm; stylar point at one end, containing 6–7 obovate green to pale brown seeds, with longitudinal prominent ridges on the testa.

Tinnevelly Senna fruit.   Brown to greyish black; length, about 35–60 mm; width, 14–18 mm; stylar point at one end, containing up to 10 obovate green to pale brown seeds, with indefinite transverse ridges.

Microscopic examination.   Epicarp with very thick cuticularized isodiametrical cells, occasional *anomocytic* or *paracytic* stomata, and very few unicellular and warty trichomes; hypodermis with collenchymatous cells; mesocarp with parenchymatous tissue containing a layer of calcium oxalate prisms; endocarp consisting of thick-walled fibre, mostly perpendicular to the longitudinal axis of the fruit, but the inner fibres running at an oblique angle or parallel to the longitudinal axis. Seeds, subepidermal layer of palisade cells with thick outer walls; the endosperm has polyhedral cells with mucilaginous walls.

Water-soluble extractive.   Shake 5 g with a mixture of 0.5 ml of chloroform R and 200 ml of water, filter, evaporate 20 ml of the filtrate and weigh; the residue is not less than 250 mg/g.

Acid-insoluble ash.   Carry out the procedure as described under "Determination of acid-insoluble ash" (vol .1, p. 161); not more than 20 mg/g.

Foreign matter.   Weigh about 200 g and spread it in a thin layer.   Detect the foreign matter by eye or with the use of a 6× lens, separate and weigh; not more than 10 mg/g.

Assay.   Place 0.15 g of the powdered fruit in a 100-ml flask.   Add 30.0 ml of water, mix, weigh, and place in a water-bath at 80–90 °C.   Heat under a reflux condenser for 15 minutes.   Allow to cool, weigh, and adjust to the original mass with water. Centrifuge and transfer 20.0 ml of the supernatant liquid to a 150-ml separating funnel.   Add 0.1 ml of hydrochloric acid (~70 g/l) TS and shake with 3 quantities, each of 15 ml, of chloroform R.   Allow to separate and discard the chloroform layer.   Add 0.10 g of sodium hydrogen carbonate R and shake for 3 minutes.   Centrifuge and transfer 10.0 ml of the supernatant liquid to a 100-ml round-bottomed flask with a ground-glass neck.   Add 20 ml of ferric chloride

(65 g/l) TS and mix. Heat for 20 minutes under a reflux condenser in a water-bath with the water level above that of the liquid in the flask; add 1 ml of hydrochloric acid (Λ420 g/l) TS and heat for a further 20 minutes, with frequent shaking, to dissolve the precipitate. Cool, transfer the mixture to a separating funnel and shake with 3 quantities, each of 25 ml, of ether R previously used to rinse the flask. Combine the ether layers and wash with 2 quantities, each of 15 ml, of water. Transfer the ether layers to a volumetric flask and dilute to 100 ml with ether R. Evaporate 10.0 ml carefully to dryness and dissolve the residue in 10.0 ml of a solution containing 5 mg of magnesium acetate R per ml of methanol R. Measure the absorbance of this solution in a 1-cm layer at the maximum at about 515 nm against a solvent cell containing methanol R. Calculate in % the amount of hydroxyanthracene derivatives as sennoside B with an absorptivity value of 24.0 ($A_{1\,cm}^{1\,\%} = 240$) as follows: 1.25 A/W, where A is the absorbance at 515 nm and W is the mass of the material examined in g.

SPECTINOMYCINI HYDROCHLORIDUM

Spectinomycin hydrochloride

Molecular formula. $C_{14}H_{24}N_2O_7,2HCl,5H_2O$

Relative molecular mass.   495.4

Graphic formula.

Chemical name.   (2R,4aR,5aR,6S,7S,8R,9S,9aR,10aS)-Decahydro-4a,7,9-trihydroxy-2-methyl-6,8-bis(methylamino)-4H-pyrano[2,3-b][1,4]benzodioxin-4-one dihydrochloride pentahydrate; [2R-(2α,4aβ,5aβ,6β,7β,8β,9α,9aα,10aβ)]-decahydro-4a,7,9-trihydroxy-2-methyl-6,8-bis(methylamino)-4H-pyrano[2,3-b][1,4]benzodioxin-4-one dihydrochloride pentahydrate; CAS Reg. No. 22189-32-8 (pentahydrate).

Description.   A white or almost white, crystalline powder; odourless.

Solubility.   Freely soluble in water; practically insoluble in ethanol ($\sim$750 g/l) TS, chloroform R and ether R.

Category.   Antibacterial drug.

Storage. Spectinomycin hydrochloride should be kept in a well-closed container and stored at a temperature not exceeding 30 °C.

REQUIREMENTS

General requirement. Spectinomycin hydrochloride contains not less than 600 µg of $C_{14}H_{24}N_2O_7$ per mg, calculated with reference to the anhydrous substance.

Identity tests

A. Carry out the examination as described under "Spectrophotometry in the infrared region" (vol. 1, p. 40). The infrared absorption spectrum is concordant with the spectrum obtained from spectinomycin hydrochloride RS or with the *reference spectrum* of spectinomycin hydrochloride.

B. A 20 mg/ml solution yields reaction B described under "General identification tests" as characteristic of chlorides (vol. 1, p. 113).

Specific optical rotation. Use a 0.10 g/ml solution, and calculate with reference to the anhydrous substance; $[\alpha]_D^{20\,°C} = +\,15$ to $+\,21°$.

Sulfated ash. Not more than 10 mg/g.

Water. Determine as described under "Determination of water by the Karl Fischer Method", Method A (vol. 1, p. 135), using about 0.2 g of the substance; the water content is not less than 0.16 g/g and not more than 0.20 g/g.

pH value. pH of a 0.10 g/ml solution, 3.8–5.6.

Related substances. Carry out the test as described under "Thin-layer chromatography" (vol. 1, p. 83), using silica gel R1 as the coating substance and a mixture of 10 volumes of 1-propanol R, 8 volumes of water, 1 volume of glacial acetic acid R, and 1 volume of pyridine R as the mobile phase. Apply separately to the plate 10 µl of each of 2 solutions containing (A) 20 mg of the test substance per ml and (B) 0.20 ml of the test substance per ml. After removing the plate from the chromatographic chamber, allow it to dry in air, spray it with potassium permanganate (25 g/l) TS, allow it to stand for 2–3 minutes, and examine the chromatogram in daylight. Any spot obtained with solution A, other than the principal spot, is not more intense than that obtained with solution B.

Histamine-like substances. Carry out the test as described under "Test for histamine-like substances" (vol. 1, p. 157), using 1 ml per kg of body mass of a solution in saline TS containing 25 mg of the substance to be examined per ml.

Undue toxicity.   Carry out the test as described under "Test for undue toxicity" (vol. 1, p. 154), using 0.5 ml of a solution in saline TS containing 12.5 mg of the substance to be examined.

Pyrogens.   Carry out the test as described under "Test for pyrogens" (vol. 1, p. 155) injecting, per kg of the rabbit's mass, 5 ml of a solution in saline TS containing 15 mg of the substance to be examined per ml.

Sterility.   Complies with the "Sterility testing of antibiotics" (vol. 1, p. 152), applying the membrane filtration test procedure.

Assay.   Carry out the assay described under "Gas chromatography" (vol. 1, p. 94). As an internal standard use a solution containing 2 mg of triphenylantimony R per ml of dimethylformamide R. Use the following 2 solutions: (1) to about 30 mg of spectinomycin hydrochloride RS, accurately weighed, add 10.0 ml of the internal standard and 1.0 ml of hexamethyldisilazane R, and shake intermittently for 1 hour; and (2) to 30 mg of the substance being examined add 10.0 ml of the internal standard and 1.0 ml of hexamethyldisilazane R, and shake intermittently for 1 hour. For the procedure use a flame ionization detector and a glass column 1.3 m long and 0.4 cm in internal diameter packed with an adequate quantity of an adsorbent composed of 5 g of phenyl/methylpolysiloxane R supported on 95 g of acid-washed and base-washed, silanized kieselguhr R4. Maintain the column and the detector at about 215 °C and 270 °C, respectively, and the injection part at about 265 °C. Use dry helium R as the carrier gas at a flow rate of about 90 ml per minute. Prepare chromatogram A and B injecting separately about 2.5 µl of each of solutions 1 and 2. Measure the area of the major peak in each chromatogram, and calculate the content in µg of $C_{14}H_{24}N_2O_7$ per mg in the substance being tested.

SPIRONOLACTONUM

Spironolactone

Molecular formula. $C_{24}H_{32}O_4S$

Relative molecular mass.   416.6

Graphic formula.

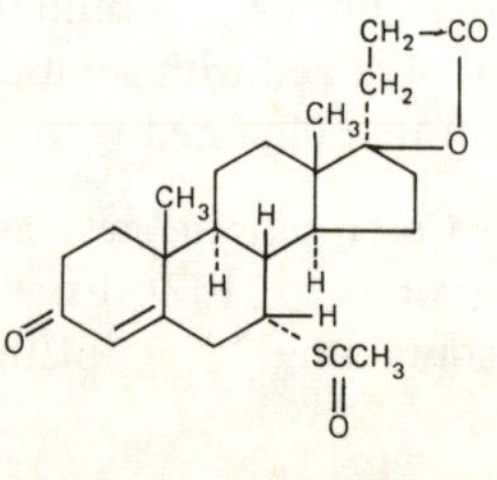

Chemical name.   17-Hydroxy-7α-mercapto-3-oxo-17α-pregn-4-ene-21-carboxylic acid γ-lactone acetate; 7α-(acetylthio)-17-hydroxy-3-oxo-17α-pregn-4-ene-21-carboxylic acid γ-lactone; CAS Reg. No. 52-01-7.

Description.   A light yellowish white to light yellowish brown powder; odourless or with a faint characteristic odour.

Solubility.   Practically insoluble in water; soluble in ethanol (~750 g/l) TS; freely soluble in chloroform R.

Category.   Diuretic.

Storage.   Spironolactone should be kept in a well-closed container, protected from light.

Additional information.   Spironolactone may show preliminary melting at about 135 °C, followed by resolidification.

REQUIREMENTS

General requirement.   Spironolactone contains not less than 97.0% and not more than 101.5% of $C_{24}H_{32}O_4S$, calculated with reference to the dried substance.

Identity tests

● Either test A alone or tests B, C and D may be applied.

A.   Carry out the examination as described under "Spectrophotometry in the infrared region" (vol. 1, p. 40). The infrared absorption spectrum is concordant with the spectrum obtained from spironolactone RS or with the *reference spectrum* of spironolactone.

B.   The absorption spectrum of a 10 μg/ml solution in methanol R, when observed between 230 nm and 350 nm, exhibits a maximum at about 238 nm; the absorbance of a 1-cm layer at this wavelength is about 0.47.

C.   Shake 10 mg with 2 ml of sulfuric acid (~700 g/l) TS; an orange solution with an intense yellowish green fluorescence is produced. Heat the solution gently; the colour changes to deep red and hydrogen sulfide, which blackens lead acetate paper R, is evolved. Pour the solution into water; a greenish yellow, opalescent solution is produced.

D.   Melting temperature, about 204 °C with decomposition.

Specific optical rotation.   Use a 10 mg/ml solution in chloroform R; $[\alpha]_D^{20\,°C} = -33.0$ to $-37.0°$.

Chromium.   Place 0.20 g with 1 g of potassium carbonate R and 0.3 g of potassium nitrate R into a platinum crucible; mix, heat gently until fused, and ignite at 600–650 °C until the carbon is removed. Cool, dissolve the residue as completely as possible in 10 ml of water using gentle heat, filter, and dilute with sufficient water to produce 20 ml. To 10 ml add 0.5 g of urea R and acidify with sulfuric acid (~190 g/l) TS, dilute to 20 ml with water, and add 0.5 ml of diphenylcarbazide TS. The colour produced is not deeper than that of a solution obtained by adding 1 ml of sulfuric acid (~190 g/l) TS to 0.50 ml of a freshly prepared solution containing 2.83 mg of potassium dichromate R in 100 ml of water, then diluting to 20 ml with water and adding 0.5 ml of diphenylcarbazide TS.

Sulfated ash.   Not more than 1.0 mg/g.

Loss on drying.   Dry to constant weight at 105 °C; it loses not more than 5.0 mg/g.

Related substances.   Carry out the test as described under "Thin-layer chromatography" (vol. 1, p. 83), using silica gel R5 as the coating substance (a precoated plate from a commercial source is suitable) and butyl acetate R as the mobile phase. Apply separately to the plate 5 µl of each of 2 solutions in chloroform R containing (A) 20 mg of the test substance per ml and (B) 0.20 mg of the test substance per ml. After removing the plate from the chromatographic chamber, allow it to dry at room temperature and develop the plate a second time allowing the solvent to ascend 15 cm above the line of application. Remove the plate, allow the solvent to evaporate at room temperature, spray it with sulfuric acid/methanol TS, and heat at 105 °C for 10 minutes. Examine the chromatogram in daylight. Any spot obtained with solution A, other than the principal spot, is not more intense than that obtained with solution B.

Mercapto compounds.   Shake 2.0 g with 20 ml of water, filter, and titrate 10 ml of the filtrate with iodine (0.005 mol/l) VS, using starch TS as indicator. Repeat the operation without the test substance and make any necessary corrections. Not more than 0.1 ml of iodine (0.005 mol/l) VS is required.

Assay.   Dissolve about 10 mg, accurately weighed, in sufficient methanol R to produce 100 ml and dilute 10 ml of this solution to 100 ml with methanol R. Measure the absorbance of this solution in a 1-cm layer at the maximum at about 238 nm, and calculate the content of $C_{24}H_{32}O_4S$, using the absorptivity value of 47 ($A_{1\ cm}^{1\ \%} = 470$).

STIBII NATRII TARTRAS

Antimony sodium tartrate

Molecular formula. $C_4H_4NaO_7Sb$

Relative molecular mass. 308.8

Graphic formula.

$$Na^+ \left[H_2O \rightarrow Sb \begin{array}{l} O-C=O \\ O-C-H \\ O-C-H \\ {}^-O-C=O \end{array} \right]$$

Chemical name. Sodium aqua[tartrato(4⁻)-O^1,O^2,O^3]antimoniate(III); CAS Reg. No. 34521-09-0.

Description. Colourless, transparent scales or an almost white powder; odourless.

Solubility. Soluble in 1.5 parts of water; practically insoluble in ethanol ($\sim$750 g/l) TS.

Category. Antischistosomal drug.

Storage. Antimony sodium tartrate should be kept in a tightly closed container, protected from light.

Additional information. Antimony sodium tartrate is hygroscopic. Even in the absence of light, it is gradually degraded on exposure to a humid atmosphere, the decomposition being faster at higher temperatures.

REQUIREMENTS

General requirement. Antimony sodium tartrate contains not less than 98.0% and not more than 101.0% of $C_4H_4NaO_7Sb$, calculated with reference to the dried substance.

Identity tests

A. When tested for sodium as described under "General identification tests" (vol. 1, p. 115), yields the characteristic reactions. If reaction B is to be used, prepare a 10 mg/ml solution.

B. Dissolve 0.05 g in 1.0 ml of hydrochloric acid ($\sim$70 g/l) TS and add 1.0 ml of hydrogen sulfide TS; an orange-red precipitate is produced, which is soluble in ammonium sulfide TS and in sodium hydroxide ($\sim$80 g/l) TS.

C. Dissolve 20 mg in 0.2 ml of water; it yields reaction B described under "General identification tests", as characteristic of tartrates (vol. 1, p. 115).

Arsenic. Dissolve 1.3 g in 10 ml of water and add 16 ml of stannated hydrochloric acid ($\sim$250 g/l) AsTS in a flask, connect to a condenser, and distil 20 ml; wash the flask and condenser, return the distillate and washings to the flask, add 0.05 ml of stannous chloride AsTS, and redistil 16 ml; proceed with the distillate as described under "Limit test for arsenic" (vol. 1, p. 122); the arsenic content is not more than 8 µg/g.

Clarity and colour of solution. A solution of 0.50 g in 10 ml of water is clear and colourless.

Loss on drying. Dry to constant weight at 105 °C; it loses not more than 60 mg/g.

Acidity or alkalinity. Dissolve 1.0 g in 50 ml of water and add a few drops of bromocresol green/ethanol TS; not more than 2 ml of either hydrochloric acid (0.01 mol/l) VS or sodium hydroxide (0.01 mol/l) VS are required to obtain the midpoint of the indicator (green) indicative of pH 4.5.

Assay. Dissolve about 0.5 g, accurately weighed, in 50 ml of water, add 5 g of potassium sodium tartrate R and 2 g of sodium tetraborate R. Titrate with iodine (0.05 mol/l) VS using starch TS as indicator, added towards the end of the titration. Each ml of iodine (0.05 mol/l) VS is equivalent to 15.44 mg of $C_4H_4NaO_7Sb$.

SULFACETAMIDUM

Sulfacetamide

Molecular formula. $C_8H_{10}N_2O_3S$

Relative molecular mass. 214.2

Graphic formula.

Chemical name. *N*-Sulfanilylacetamide; *N*-[(4-aminophenyl)sulfonyl]acetamide; CAS Reg. No. 144-80-9.

Description. A white or almost white, crystalline powder; odourless.

Solubility.   Very slightly soluble in water and chloroform R; freely soluble in acetone R and methanol R; soluble in ethanol (~750 g/l) TS.

Category.   Antiinfective agent.

Storage.   Sulfacetamide should be kept in a well-closed container, protected from light.

REQUIREMENTS

General requirement.   Sulfacetamide contains not less than 99.0% and not more than 101.0% of $C_8H_{10}N_2O_3S$, calculated with reference to the dried substance.

Identity tests

● Either test A alone or tests B and C may be applied.

A.   Carry out the examination as described under "Spectrophotometry in the infrared region" (vol. 1, p. 40). The infrared absorption spectrum is concordant with the spectrum obtained from sulfacetamide RS or with the *reference spectrum* of sulfacetamide.

B.   See the test described below under "Related substances". The principal spot obtained with solution A corresponds in position, appearance, and intensity with that obtained with solution B.

C.   Dissolve 0.10 g in 5 ml of ethanol (~750 g/l) TS, add about 0.2 ml of sulfuric acid (~1760 g/l) TS and heat; ethyl acetate, perceptible by its odour (proceed with caution), is produced.

Melting range.   181–184 °C.

Heavy metals.   For the preparation of the test solution use 1.0 g dissolved in a mixture of 10 ml of water and 1.0 ml of acetic acid (~300 g/l) TS, heat until dissolved, cool, and filter. Dilute to 40 ml with water and determine the heavy metals content as described under "Limit test for heavy metals", according to Method A (vol. 1, p. 119); not more than 20 µg/g.

Solution in alkali.   Dissolve 0.5 g in 10 ml of sodium hydroxide (1 mol/l) VS; the solution is clear or any opalescence produced is not more pronounced than that of opalescence standard TS2, and the solution is not more intensely coloured than standard colour solution Yw3 when compared as described under "Colour of liquids" (vol. 1, p. 50).

Solution in acid.   A solution of 1.0 g in 10 ml of hydrochloric acid (1 mol/1) VS is clear or any opalescence produced is not more pronounced than that of opalescence standard TS2.

Sulfated ash. Not more than 1.0 mg/g.

Loss on drying. Dry to constant weight at 105 °C; it loses not more than 5.0 mg/g.

Related substances. Carry out the test as described under "Thin-layer chromatography" (vol. 1, p. 83), using silica gel R3 as the coating substance and a mixture of 20 volumes of chloroform R, 2 volumes of methanol R, and 1 volume of dimethylformamide R as the mobile phase. Apply separately to the plate 10 μl of each of 3 solutions in a mixture of 9 volumes of ethanol (~750 g/l) TS and 1 volume of ammonia (~260 g/l) TS containing (A) 2.5 mg of the test substance per ml, (B) 2.5 mg of sulfacetamide RS per ml, and (C) 12.5 μg of sulfanilamide RS per ml. After removing the plate from the chromatographic chamber, allow it to dry in air until the solvents have evaporated. Spray the dried plate with sulfuric acid/ethanol TS, heat it at 105 °C for 30 minutes, and immediately expose it to nitrous fumes in a closed chamber for 15 minutes (the nitrous fumes may be generated by adding sulfuric acid (~700 g/l) TS drop by drop to a solution containing 10 g of sodium nitrite R and 3 g of potassium iodide R in 100 ml). Place the plate in a current of warm air for 15 minutes and spray it with N-(1-naphthyl)ethylenediamine hydrochloride/ethanol TS. If necessary, allow it to dry before repeating the spraying and examine the chromatogram in daylight. Any spot obtained with solution A, other than the principal spot, is not more intense than that obtained with solution C.

Assay. Carry out the assay as described under "Nitrite titration" (vol. 1, p. 133), using about 0.5 g, accurately weighed, dissolved in a mixture of 20 ml of hydrochloric acid (~250 g/l) TS and 50 ml of water, and titrate with sodium nitrite (0.1 mol/l) VS. Each ml of sodium nitrite (0.1 mol/l) VS is equivalent to 21.42 mg of $C_8H_{10}N_2O_3S$.

SULFACETAMIDUM NATRICUM

Sulfacetamide sodium

Molecular formula. $C_8H_9N_2NaO_3S,H_2O$

Relative molecular mass. 254.2

Graphic formula.

$$NH_2-\underset{}{\bigcirc}-SO_2NNaCOCH_3 \cdot H_2O$$

Chemical name. *N*-Sulfanilylacetamide monosodium salt monohydrate; *N*-[(4-aminophenyl)sulfonyl]acetamide monosodium salt monohydrate; CAS Reg. No. 6209-17-2 (monohydrate).

Other name. Sulfacylum-natrium.

Description. A white or yellowish white, crystalline powder; odourless.

Solubility. Soluble in 1.5 parts of water; slightly soluble in ethanol ($\sim$750 g/l) TS; practically insoluble in chloroform R and in ether R.

Category. Antiinfective agent.

Storage. Sulfacetamide sodium should be kept in a well-closed container, protected from light.

Additional information. Even in the absence of light, Sulfacetamide sodium is gradually degraded on exposure to a humid atmosphere, the decomposition being faster at higher temperatures.

REQUIREMENTS

General requirement. Sulfacetamide sodium contains not less than 99.0% and not more than 101.0% of $C_8H_9N_2NaO_3S$, calculated with reference to the anhydrous substance.

Identity tests

● Either test A alone or tests B, C and D may be applied.

A. Dissolve 1 g in 10 ml of water and add 2 ml of acetic acid ($\sim$300 g/l) TS; a white precipitate is produced. Collect the precipitate on a filter, wash it with cold water, and dry it at 105 °C. Carry out the examination with the dried residue as described under "Spectrophotometry in the infrared region" (vol. 1, p. 40). The infrared absorption spectrum is concordant with the spectrum obtained from sulfacetamide RS or with the *reference spectrum* of sulfacetamide. Keep the remaining precipitate for tests B and C.

B. Melting temperature of the precipitate obtained in test A, about 183 °C (sulfacetamide).

C. Dissolve 0.1 g of the precipitate obtained in test A in 5 ml of ethanol ($\sim$750 g/l) TS, add about 0.2 ml of sulfuric acid ($\sim$1760 g/l) TS, and heat; ethyl acetate, perceptible by its odour (proceed with caution), is produced.

D. When tested for sodium as described under "General identification tests" (vol. 1, p. 115), yields the characteristic reactions. If reaction B is to be used, ignite 0.5 g and dissolve the residue in acetic acid ($\sim$60 g/l) TS.

Clarity and colour of solution.   A solution of 0.5 g in 10 ml of carbon-dioxide-free water R is clear and not more intensely coloured than standard colour solution Yw1 when compared as described under "Colour of liquids" (vol. 1, p. 50).

Water.   Determine as described under "Determination of water by the Karl Fischer method", Method A (vol. 1, p. 135), using about 0.2 g of the substance; the water content is not less than 60 mg/g and not more than 80 mg/g.

pH value.   pH of a 0.05 g/ml solution in carbon-dioxide-free water R, 8.0–9.5.

Related substances.   Carry out the test as described under "Thin-layer chromatography" (vol. 1, p. 83), using silica gel R6 as the coating substance (a precoated plate from a commercial source is suitable) and a mixture of 50 volumes of 1-butanol R, 25 volumes of dehydrated ethanol R, 25 volumes of water, and 10 volumes of ammonia (~260 g/l) TS as the mobile phase.   Apply separately to the plate 5 µl of each of 3 solutions containing (A) 0.10 g of the test substance per ml, (B) 0.50 mg of sulfanilamide RS per ml, and (C) 0.25 mg of sulfanilamide RS per ml.   After removing the plate from the chromatographic chamber, allow it to dry in air until the solvents have evaporated.   Spray the plate with 4-dimethylaminobenzaldehyde TS5.   Any spot obtained with solution A, other than the principal spot, is not more intense than that obtained with solution B.   Not more than one of any such spots is more intense than the spot obtained with solution C.

Assay.   Carry out the assay as described under "Nitrite titration" (vol. 1, p. 133), using about 0.5 g, accurately weighed, dissolved in a mixture of 50 ml of water and 20 ml of hydrochloric acid (~70 g/l) TS, and titrate with sodium nitrite (0.1 mol/l) VS.   Each ml of sodium nitrite (0.1 mol/l) VS is equivalent to 23.62 mg of $C_8H_9N_2NaO_3S$.

SULFADIMIDINUM

Sulfadimidine

Molecular formula. $C_{12}H_{14}N_4O_2S$

Relative molecular mass.   278.3

Graphic formula.

Chemical name. N^1-(4,6-Dimethyl-2-pyrimidinyl)sulfanilamide; 4-amino-N-(4,6-dimethyl-2-pyrimidinyl)benzenesulfonamide; CAS Reg. No. 57-68-1.

Other names. Sulfadimezinum, sulfamethazine.

Description. A white or creamy white, crystalline powder; odourless or almost odourless.

Solubility. Very slightly soluble in water; slightly soluble in ethanol ($\sim$750 g/l) TS; soluble in acetone R; practically insoluble in ether R.

Category. Antibacterial drug.

Storage. Sulfadimidine should be kept in a well-closed container, protected from light.

REQUIREMENTS

General requirement. Sulfadimidine contains not less than 99.0% and not more than 100.5% of $C_{12}H_{14}N_4O_2S$, calculated with reference to the dried substance.

Identity tests

● Either test A alone or tests B, C and D may be applied.

A.   Carry out the examination as described under "Spectrophotometry in the infrared region" (vol. 1, p. 40). The infrared absorption spectrum is concordant with the spectrum obtained from sulfadimidine RS or with the *reference spectrum* of sulfadimidine.

B.   About 0.05 g yields the reaction described for the identification of primary aromatic amines under "General identification tests" (vol. 1, p. 111), producing an orange precipitate.

C.   Boil gently 0.5 g with 1 ml of sulfuric acid ($\sim$700 g/l) TS until a precipitate is formed (about 2 minutes). Cool, add 15 ml of sodium hydroxide ($\sim$80 g/l) TS and extract the mixture with 20 ml of ether R. Filter the ether extract through a layer of anhydrous sodium sulfate R and evaporate to dryness on a water-bath. Melting temperature, about 153 °C (2-amino-4,6-dimethylpyrimidine).

D.   Melting temperature, about 197 °C with decomposition.

Heavy metals. Use 1.0 g for the preparation of the test solution as described under "Limit test for heavy metals", Procedure 4 (vol. 1, p. 119); determine the heavy metals content according to Method A (vol. 1, p. 119); not more than 20 µg/g.

Sulfated ash. Not more than 1.0 mg/g.

Loss on drying. Dry to constant weight at 105 °C; it loses not more than 5.0 mg/g.

Acidity. Heat 2.0 g with 100 ml of carbon-dioxide-free water R at about 70 °C for 5 minutes, cool and filter. Titrate 25 ml of the filtrate with sodium hydroxide (0.1 mol/l) VS, using bromothymol blue/ethanol TS as indicator; not more than 0.2 ml is required to obtain the midpoint of the indicator (green).

Related substances. Carry out the test as described under "Thin-layer chromatography" (vol. 1, p. 83), using silica gel R3 as the coating substance and a mixture of 15 volumes of 1-butanol R and 3 volumes of ammonia (~17 g/l) TS as the mobile phase. Apply separately to the plate 10 µl of each of 2 solutions in acetone R containing (A) 10 mg of the test substance per ml and (B) 0.050 mg of sulfanilamide RS per ml. After removing the plate from the chromatographic chamber, heat it at 105 °C for 10 minutes and spray it with 4-dimethylaminobenzaldehyde TS3. Any spot obtained with solution A, other than the principal spot, is not more intense than that obtained with solution B.

Assay. Carry out the assay as described under "Nitrite titration" (vol. 1, p. 133), using about 0.5 g, accurately weighed, dissolved in 50 ml of hydrochloric acid (~70 g/l) TS, and titrate with sodium nitrite (0.1 mol/l) VS. Each ml of sodium nitrite (0.1 mol/l) VS is equivalent to 27.83 mg of $C_{12}H_{14}N_4O_2S$.

SULFADIMIDINUM NATRICUM

Sulfadimidine sodium

Molecular formula. $C_{12}H_{13}N_4NaO_2S$

Relative molecular mass. 300.3

Graphic formula.

Chemical name. N^1-(4,6-Dimethyl-2-pyrimidinyl)sulfanilamide monosodium salt; 4-amino-N-(4,6-dimethyl-2-pyrimidinyl)benzenesulfonamide monosodium salt; CAS Reg. No. 1981-58-4.

Description. A white or creamy white, crystalline powder; odourless or almost odourless.

Solubility.   Soluble in 2.5 parts of water and in 60 parts of ethanol ($\sim$750 g/l) TS.

Category.   Antibacterial drug.

Storage.   Sulfadimidine sodium should be kept in a well-closed container, protected from light.

Additional information.   Even in the absence of light, Sulfadimidine sodium is gradually degraded on exposure to a humid atmosphere, the decomposition being faster at higher temperatures.

REQUIREMENTS

General requirement.   Sulfadimidine sodium contains not less than 98.0% and not more than 101.0% of $C_{12}H_{13}N_4NaO_2S$, calculated with reference to the dried substance.

Identity tests

● Either tests A and D or tests B, C and D may be applied.

A.   Dissolve 0.1 g in 10 ml of water, acidify with hydrochloric acid ($\sim$70 g/l) TS, filter, and dry the residue at 105 °C.   Carry out the examination with the dried residue as described under "Spectrophotometry in the infrared region" (vol. 1, p. 40).   The infrared absorption spectrum is concordant with the spectrum obtained from sulfadimidine RS or with the *reference spectrum* of sulfadimidine.

B.   Dissolve 0.1 g in 10 ml of water, add 2 ml of acetic acid ($\sim$300 g/l) TS, separate the precipitate by filtration, and wash with cold water.   It yields the reaction described for the identification of primary aromatic amines under "General identification tests" (vol. 1, p. 111), producing a bright orange-red precipitate.
C.   Boil gently 0.5 g with 1.5 ml of sulfuric acid ($\sim$700 g/l) TS until a precipitate is formed (about 2 minutes).   Cool, add 15 ml of sodium hydroxide ($\sim$80 g/l) TS and extract the mixture with 20 ml of ether R.   Filter the ether extract through a layer of anhydrous sodium sulfate R and evaporate to dryness on a water-bath.   Melting temperature, about 153 °C (2-amino-4,6-dimethylpyrimidine).

D.   When tested for sodium as described under "General identification tests" (vol. 1, p. 115) yields the characteristic reactions.   If reaction B is to be used, ignite a small quantity and dissolve the residue in acetic acid ($\sim$60 g/l) TS.

Heavy metals.   Use 1.0 g for the preparation of the test solution as described under "Limit test for heavy metals", Procedure 4 (vol. 1, p. 119); determine the heavy metals content according to Method A (vol. 1, p. 119); not more than 20 µg/g.

Clarity and colour of solution.   A solution of 3.3 g in 10 ml of carbon-dioxide-free water R is clear and not more intensely coloured than standard colour solution Yw4 when compared as described under "Colour of liquids" (vol. 1, p. 50).

Loss on drying.   Dry to constant weight at 105 °C; it loses not more than 20 mg/g.

pH value.   pH of a 0.10 g/ml solution in carbon-dioxide-free water R, 10.0–11.0.

Related substances.   Carry out the test as described under "Thin-layer chromatography" (vol. 1, p. 83), using silica gel R3 as the coating substance and a mixture of 15 volumes of 1-butanol R and 3 volumes of ammonia (~17 g/l) TS as the mobile phase. Apply separately to the plate 10 µl of each of 2 solutions in a mixture of 9 volumes of ethanol (~750 g/l) TS and 1 volume of ammonia (~260 g/l) TS containing (A) 10 mg of the test substance per ml and (B) 0.050 mg of sulfanilamide RS per ml (for the preparation of solution A, first dissolve the test substance in a little ammonia (~260 g/l) TS, add 9 volumes of ethanol (~750 g/l), and then dilute to the required volume with the ethanol/ammonia mixture). After removing the plate from the chromatographic chamber, heat it at 105 °C for 10 minutes and spray it with 4-dimethylaminobenzaldehyde TS3. Any spot obtained with solution A, other than the principal spot, is not more intense than that obtained with solution B.

Assay.   Carry out the assay as described under "Nitrite titration" (vol. 1, p. 133), using about 0.5 g, accurately weighed, dissolved in a mixture of 75 ml of water and 10 ml of hydrochloric acid (~420 g/l) TS, and titrate with sodium nitrite (0.1 mol/l) VS. Each ml of sodium nitrite (0.1 mol/l) VS is equivalent to 30.03 mg of $C_{12}H_{13}N_4NaO_2S$.

SULFADOXINUM

Sulfadoxine

Molecular formula. $C_{12}H_{14}N_4O_4S$

Relative molecular mass.   310.3

Graphic formula.

CH_3O OCH_3

NH_2—⟨phenyl⟩—SO_2NH—⟨pyrimidine⟩

Chemical name. N^1-(5,6-Dimethoxy-4-pyrimidinyl)sulfanilamide; 4-amino-N-(5,6-dimethoxy-4-pyrimidinyl)benzenesulfonamide; CAS Reg. No. 2447-57-6.

Description. A white or creamy white, crystalline powder; odourless.

Solubility. Very slightly soluble in water; slightly soluble in ethanol ($\sim$750 g/l) TS and in methanol R; practically insoluble in ether R.

Category. Antimalarial drug.

Storage. Sulfadoxine should be kept in a well-closed container, protected from light.

REQUIREMENTS

General requirement. Sulfadoxine contains not less than 99.0% and not more than 101.0% of $C_{12}H_{14}N_4O_4S$, calculated with reference to the dried substance.

Identity tests

• Either test A alone or tests B, C and D may be applied.

A. Carry out the examination as described under "Spectrophotometry in the infrared region" (vol. 1, p. 40). The infrared absorption spectrum is concordant with the spectrum obtained from sulfadoxine RS or with the *reference spectrum* of sulfadoxine.

B. About 0.05 g yields the reaction described for the identification of primary aromatic amines under "General identification tests" (vol. 1, p. 111), producing an orange-red precipitate.

C. Dissolve 50 mg in 3 ml of sodium hydroxide (0.1 mol/l) VS, heating slightly. Cool and add 1.0 ml of copper(II) sulfate (80 g/l) TS; a greenish yellow precipitate is produced, the colour of which changes to blue (distinction from certain other sulfonamides).

D. Melting temperature, about 199 °C.

Heavy metals. Use 1.0 g for the preparation of the test solution as described under "Limit test for heavy metals", Procedure 4 (vol. 1, p. 119); determine the heavy metals content according to Method A (vol. 1, p. 119); not more than 20 µg/g.

Chlorides. For the preparation of the test solution, boil 2.5 g with 30 ml of water, cool and filter. Add 10 ml of nitric acid ($\sim$130 g/l) TS to the filtrate and proceed as described under "Limit test for chlorides" (vol. 1, p. 116); the chloride content is not more than 0.1 mg/g.

Sulfates.   For the preparation of the test solution, boil 2.5 g with 40 ml of water, cool and filter.   Proceed with the filtrate as described under "Limit test for sulfates" (vol. 1, p. 116); the sulfate content is not more than 0.2 mg/g.

Clarity and colour of solution.   A solution of 0.50 g in 10 ml of hydrochloric acid (~70 g/l) TS is clear and not more intensely coloured than standard colour solution Yw3 when compared as described under "Colour of liquids" (vol. 1, p. 50).

Sulfated ash.   Not more than 1.0 mg/g.

Loss on drying.   Dry to constant weight at 105 °C; it loses not more than 5.0 mg/g.

Acidity.   Heat 1.0 g with 50 ml of carbon-dioxide-free water R at about 70 °C for 5 minutes, cool quickly to 20 °C, and filter; titrate 25 ml of the filtrate to pH 7.0 with sodium hydroxide (0.1 mol/l) VS; not more than 0.25 ml is required.

Related substances.   Carry out the test as described under "Thin-layer chromatography" (vol. 1, p. 83), using silica gel R3 as the coating substance and a mixture of 15 volumes of 1-butanol R and 3 volumes of ammonia (~17 g/l) TS as the mobile phase. Apply separately to the plate 10 μl of each of 2 solutions in a mixture of 9 volumes of ethanol (~750 g/l) TS and 1 volume of ammonia (~260 g/l) TS containing (A) 10 mg of the test substance per ml and (B) 0.050 mg of sulfanilamide RS per ml. After removing the plate from the chromatographic chamber, heat it at 105 °C for 10 minutes and spray it with 4-dimethylaminobenzaldehyde TS3. Any spot obtained with solution A, other than the principal spot, is not more intense than that obtained with solution B.

Assay.   Carry out the assay as described under "Nitrite titration" (vol. 1, p. 133), using about 0.5 g, accurately weighed, dissolved in a mixture of 75 ml of water and 10 ml of hydrochloric acid (~250 g/l) TS, and titrate with sodium nitrite (0.1 mol/l) VS. Each ml of sodium nitrite (0.1 mol/l) VS is equivalent to 31.03 mg of $C_{12}N_{14}N_4O_4S$.

SULFASALAZINUM

Sulfasalazine

Molecular formula. $C_{18}H_{14}N_4O_5S$

Relative molecular mass.   398.4

Graphic formula.

Chemical name.   5-[[*p*-(2-Pyridylsulfamoyl)phenyl]azo]salicylic acid; 2-hydroxy-5-[[4-[(2-pyridinylamino)sulfonyl]phenyl]azo]benzoic acid; CAS Reg. No. 599-79-1.

Other name.   Salazosulfapyridine.

Description.   A bright yellow to brownish yellow powder; odourless.

Solubility.   Practically insoluble in water, ether R, and chloroform R; very slightly soluble in ethanol ($\sim$750 g/l) TS; soluble in alkali hydroxides.

Category.   Antibacterial drug.

Storage.   Sulfasalazine should be kept in a tightly closed container, protected from light.

Additional information.   Sulfasalazine melts at about 255 °C with decomposition.

REQUIREMENTS

General requirement.   Sulfasalazine contains not less than 93.0% and not more than 103.0% of $C_{18}H_{14}N_4O_5S$, calculated with reference to the dried substance.

Identity tests

● Either test A or tests B and C may be applied.

A.   Carry out the examination as described under "Spectrophotometry in the infrared region" (vol. 1, p. 40). The infrared absorption spectrum is concordant with the spectrum obtained from sulfasalazine RS or with the *reference spectrum* of sulfasalazine.

B.   The absorption spectrum of the solution as prepared in the assay below, when observed between 230 nm and 600 nm, exhibits maxima and minima at the same wavelengths as does the absorption spectrum of a solution of sulfasalazine RS prepared in a similar manner.

C.   Dissolve 0.10 g in a mixture of 1.0 ml of ethanol ($\sim$750 g/l) TS and 4 ml of hydrochloric acid ($\sim$70 g/l) TS, then add 0.20 g of zinc R powder. Heat on a water-bath for 5 minutes and filter. To 1.0 ml of the filtrate add 0.1 ml of ferric chloride (25 g/l) TS; a red colour is produced. To 1.0 ml of the filtrate add 1.0 ml of sodium nitrite (10 g/l) TS and allow to stand for 1 minute. Then add 2.0 ml of sodium hydroxide ($\sim$80 g/l) TS and 0.1 ml of 2-naphthol TS1; a strong red colour is produced.

Heavy metals.   Use 1.0 g for the preparation of the test solution as described under "Limit test for heavy metals", Procedure 3 (vol. 1, p. 118); determine the heavy metals content according to Method A (vol. 1, p. 119); not more than 20 µg/g.

Chlorides.   Digest 2.0 g with 100 ml of water at 70 °C for 5 minutes. Cool immediately to room temperature and filter. To 25 ml of the filtrate (keep the remaining filtrate for the limit test for sulfates) add 1 ml of nitric acid ($\sim$1000 g/l) TS and allow to stand for 5 minutes. Filter through a fine-texture filter-paper and proceed with the filtrate as described under "Limit test for chlorides" (vol. 1, p. 116); the chloride content is not more than 0.14 mg/g.

Sulfates.   To 25 ml of the filtrate retained from the limit test for chlorides add 1.5 ml of hydrochloric acid (2 mol/l) VS and allow to stand for 5 minutes. Filter through a fine-texture filter-paper and proceed with the filtrate as described under "Limit test for sulfates" (vol. 1, p. 116); the sulfate content is not more than 0.4 mg/g.

Sulfated ash.   Not more than 5.0 mg/g.

Loss on drying.   Dry to constant weight at 105 °C; it loses not more than 10 mg/g.

Assay.   Carry out the test as described under "Thin-layer chromatography" (vol. 1, p. 83) using silica gel R2 as the coating substance and a mixture of 4 volumes of chloroform R, 1 volume of 1-butanol R, 1 volume of acetone R, and 1 volume of formic acid ($\sim$1080 g/l) TS as the mobile phase, allowing the chamber to equilibrate for 18 hours. Apply separately to the plate 10 µl of each of 2 solutions in dimethylformamide R containing (A) 12 mg of the test substance per ml, (B) 12 mg of sulfasalazine RS per ml, and (C) 10 µl of dimethylformamide R to serve as a blank. Dry the spotted plate thoroughly at room temperature to remove traces of dimethylformamide and develop the plate over a distance of 15 cm. After removing the plate from the chromatographic chamber, mark the solvent front and allow the solvent to evaporate.   Locate the spots by examination of the chromatogram in ultraviolet light (254 nm) and mark the sulfasalazine spots at an R_f value of about 0.6, excluding an adjacent impurity band. Remove quantitatively and separately the silica gel mixture containing each of the 3 spots from solutions A, B and C, transferring them to separate glass-stoppered centrifuge tubes. (NOTE: The dimethylformamide R employed in the next step should be obtained from a recently opened bottle and should contain less than 10 mg of water per g. Dimethylformamide dried over alkali pellets is not acceptable.) Add 10.0 ml of dimethylformamide R to each tube, insert the stopper, shake for 10 minutes, and centrifuge until clear. Measure the absorbance of the solutions in a 1-cm layer at the maximum at about 406 nm against a solvent cell containing the blank obtained from solution C. Calculate the amount of $C_{18}H_{14}N_4O_5S$ in the substance being tested (solution A) by comparison with sulfasalazine RS (solution B).

SURAMINUM NATRICUM

Suramin sodium

Molecular formula. $C_{51}H_{34}N_6Na_6O_{23}S_6$

Relative molecular mass.   1429

Graphic formula.

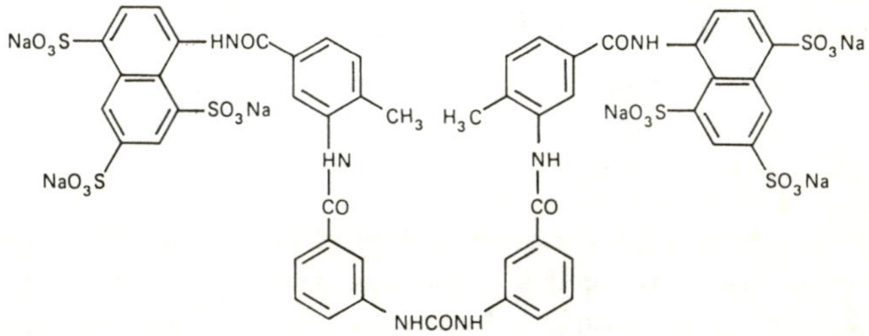

Chemical name.   Hexasodium 8,8′-[ureylenebis[*m*-phenylenecarbonylimino(4-methyl-*m*-phenylene)carbonylimino]]di-1,3,5-naphthalenetrisulfonate; hexasodium 8,8′-[carbonylbis[imino-3,1-phenylenecarbonylimino(4-methyl-3,1-phenylene)carbonylimino]]bis[1,3,5-naphthalenetrisulfonate]; CAS Reg. No. 129-46-4.

Other name.   Nagananinum.

Description.   A white, pinkish white or cream-coloured, crystalline powder; odourless.

Solubility.   Very soluble in water; slightly soluble in ethanol ($\sim$750 g/l) TS; practically insoluble in chloroform R and ether R.

Category.   Antifilarial drug; antitrypanosomal drug.

Storage.   Suramin sodium should be kept in a tightly closed container, protected from light, and stored in a cool place.

Additional information.   Suramin sodium is very hygroscopic and discolours on exposure to light.

REQUIREMENTS

General requirement.   Suramin sodium contains not less than 96.0% and not more than 100.5% of $C_{51}H_{34}N_6Na_6O_{23}S_6$, calculated with reference to the anhydrous substance.

Identity tests

A.   Dissolve 20 mg in 2.0 ml of water, add 1.0 ml of hydrochloric acid ($\sim$70 g/l) TS, and heat on a water-bath for 5 minutes. Cool, add 0.25 ml of sodium nitrite (10 g/l) TS, allow to stand for 1 minute, then add 1.0 ml of sodium hydroxide ($\sim$80 g/l) TS and 0.15 ml of 2-naphthol TS1; a red colour is produced.

B.   In a porcelain crucible, mix 20 mg with 0.10 g of anhydrous sodium carbonate R and heat until the gas evolution has ceased. Cool, dissolve the residue in 4 ml of hydrochloric acid ($\sim$70 g/l) TS, and filter. To 2.0 ml of the filtrate add 0.25 ml of barium chloride (50 g/l) TS; a white precipitate is produced.

C.   Dissolve 0.05 g in 2.0 ml of water and add 0.25 ml of glacial acetic acid R; it yields reaction B characteristic of sodium as described under "General identification tests" (vol. 1, p. 115).

Heavy metals.   Use 1.0 g for the preparation of the test solution as described under "Limit test for heavy metals", Procedure 3 (vol. 1, p. 118); determine the heavy metals content according to Method A (vol. 1, p. 119); not more than 20 µg/g.

Chlorides.   Dissolve 0.5 g in 10 ml of water, add 5 ml of nitric acid ($\sim$130 g/l) TS, 5 ml of silver nitrate (0.1 mol/l) VS, and 3 ml of nitrobenzene R, and shake vigorously. Titrate the excess of silver nitrate with ammonium thiocyanate (0.1 mol/l) VS, using 2 ml of ferric ammonium sulfate (45 g/l) TS as indicator; not less than 3.6 ml of ammonium thiocyanate (0.1 mol/l) VS are required.

Sulfates.   Dissolve 0.50 g in 20 ml of water, add 3 ml of hydrochloric acid ($\sim$250 g/l) TS, and proceed as described under "Limit test for sulfates" (vol. 1, p. 116); the sulfate content is not more than 1 mg/g.

Clarity of solution.   A solution of 0.50 g in 10 ml of carbon-dioxide-free water R is clear.

Water.   Determine as described under "Determination of water by the Karl Fischer method", Method A (vol. 1, p. 135), using about 0.2 g of the substance; the water content is not more than 0.10 g/g.

pH value.   pH of a 10 mg/ml solution in carbon-dioxide-free water R, 5.5 – 7.0.

Free amines.   Dissolve 5 g in 30 ml of water and add 30 ml of hydrochloric acid (1 mol/l) VS. Titrate at a temperature between 15 and 20 °C with sodium nitrite (0.1 mol/l) VS, stirring vigorously, until a blue colour is obtained on starch/iodide paper R. The endpoint of the titration is reached when the blue colour is reproduced after the titrated solution has been allowed to stand for 1 minute. The titration can also be performed electrometrically. Repeat the operation without the substance to be examined. The difference in volume between the two titrations does not exceed 0.4 ml.

Undue toxicity.   Carry out the test as described under "Test for undue toxicity" (vol. 1, p. 154), using 0.5 ml of a solution in saline TS containing a quantity equivalent to 13 mg per ml.

Therapeutic potency.   For therapeutic potency, the sample is tested in mice infected with a strain of *Trypanosoma equiperdum,* or other suitable species of trypanosome sensitive to suramin sodium. The test may be carried out as follows: Inoculate at least 10 mice with the trypanosomes. After forty-eight hours examine the blood of each mouse microscopically and estimate the number of trypanosomes per ml in the blood of each mouse. The number should lie between 1000 and 20 000. The estimate may be made by examining a thin film of the blood in the form of a cover-slip preparation, and counting the trypanosomes in at least 10 microscopic fields with an area of 0.12 mm^2. The presence of 1 to 20 trypanosomes in each of two fields corresponds approximately to a content of 1000 to 20 000 trypanosomes per ml.

Inject into 10 of the infected mice, intravenously, 0.16 ml of a 50 mg/l solution of the sample in freshly distilled water per g of body mass. Examine the blood of each mouse microscopically, using a microscope with a 4-mm objective, on the first and third days after the injection. If no trypanosomes are found in the blood of 5 or more mice when 20 fields are examined on the third day, the sample passes the test. If trypanosomes are found under these conditions in the blood of more than 5 mice, repeat the test. The sample passes the test if no trypanosomes are found under these conditions in the blood of not less than 50% of the total number of mice treated.

Assay.   To about 0.5 g, accurately weighed, add 12 ml of sulfuric acid (~700 g/l) TS, and boil under a reflux condenser for 1 hour; cool, and dilute to about 100 ml with water. Add 1 g of potassium bromide R and titrate at a temperature between 15 and 20 °C with sodium nitrite (0.1 mol/l) VS, stirring vigorously until a blue colour is obtained on starch/iodide paper R. The endpoint of the titration is reached when the blue colour is reproduced after the titrated solution has been allowed to stand for 1 minute. The titration can also be performed electrometrically. Repeat the operation without the substance to be examined. Each ml of sodium nitrite (0.1 mol/l) VS is equivalent to 23.82 mg of $C_{51}H_{34}N_6Na_6O_{23}S_6$.

SUXAMETHONII CHLORIDUM

Suxamethonium chloride

Molecular formula. $C_{14}H_{30}Cl_2N_2O_4,2H_2O$

Relative molecular mass.   397.3

Graphic formula.

$$\begin{bmatrix} COOCH_2CH_2N^+(CH_3)_3 \\ | \\ (CH_2)_2 \\ | \\ COOCH_2CH_2N^+(CH_3)_3 \end{bmatrix} 2Cl^- \cdot 2H_2O$$

Chemical name.   Choline chloride, succinate (2:1), dihydrate; 2,2′-[(1,4-dioxo-1,4-butanediyl)bis(oxy)]bis[*N,N,N*-trimethylethanaminium] dichloride, dihydrate; 2,2′-succinyldioxybis(ethyltrimethylammonium) dichloride, dihydrate; CAS Reg. No. 6101-15-1(dihydrate).

Other name.   Succinylcholine chloride.

Description.   A white or almost white, crystalline powder; odourless or almost odourless.

Solubility.   Soluble in 1 part of water; slightly soluble in ethanol ($\sim$750 g/l) TS; practically insoluble in ether R.

Category.   Muscle relaxant.

Storage.   Suxamethonium chloride should be kept in a tightly closed container, protected from light.

Additional information.   Suxamethonium chloride is hygroscopic. Even in the absence of light, it is gradually degraded on exposure to a humid atmosphere, the decomposition being faster at higher temperatures.

REQUIREMENTS

General requirement.   Suxamethonium chloride contains not less than 98.0% and not more than 101.0% of $C_{14}H_{30}Cl_2N_2O_4$, calculated with reference to the anhydrous substance.

Identity tests

A.   Dissolve 25 mg in 1 ml of water, add 0.1 ml of cobalt(II) chloride (5 g/l) TS and 0.1 ml of potassium ferrocyanide (45 g/l) TS; an emerald green colour is produced.

B.   Dissolve 0.05 g in 10 ml of water, add 10 ml of sulfuric acid ($\sim$100 g/l) TS and 30 ml of ammonium reineckate (10 g/l) TS; a pink precipitate is produced. Allow to stand for 30 minutes, filter and wash with water, then with ethanol ($\sim$750 g/l) TS and with ether R.   Dry the residue at 80 °C; melting temperature, about 183 °C.

C.   A 0.05 g/ml solution yields reaction A described under "General identification tests" as characteristic of chlorides (vol. 1, p. 112).

Clarity and colour of solution.   A solution of 1.0 g in 10 ml of water is clear and colourless.

Sulfated ash.   Not more than 1.0 mg/g.

Water.   Determine as described under "Determination of water by the Karl Fischer method", Method A (vol. 1, p. 135), using about 0.15 g of the substance; not less than 80 mg/g and not more than 100 mg/g.

pH value.   pH of a 10 mg/ml solution, 4.0 – 5.0.

Related substances.   Carry out the test as described under "Thin-layer chromatography" (vol. 1, p. 83), using cellulose R2 as the coating substance and a mixture of 4 volumes of 1-butanol R, 1 volume of acetic acid ($\sim$300 g/l) TS, and 5 volumes of water as the mobile phase.   Apply separately to the plate 10 µl of each of 2 solutions containing (A) 5.0 mg of the test substance per ml and (B) 0.10 mg of the test substance per ml. Develop the plate for $2\frac{1}{2}$ hours.   After removing the plate from the chromatographic chamber, dry it at 90 °C for 15 minutes, allow it to cool, spray it with potassium iodoplatinate TS2 and examine the chromatogram in daylight.   Any spot obtained with solution A, other than the principal spot, is not more intense than that obtained with solution B.

Assay.   Dissolve about 0.3 g, accurately weighed, in 30 ml of glacial acetic acid R1, add 30 ml of acetic anhydride R and 10 ml of mercuric acetate/acetic acid TS, and titrate with perchloric acid (0.1 mol/l) VS as described under "Non-aqueous titration", Method A (vol. 1, p. 131).   Each ml of perchloric acid (0.1 mol/l) VS is equivalent to 18.07 mg of $C_{14}H_{30}Cl_2N_2O_4$.

TESTOSTERONI ENANTAS

Testosterone enantate

Molecular formula. $C_{26}H_{40}O_3$

Relative molecular mass.   400.6

Graphic formula.

OCO(CH$_2$)$_5$CH$_3$
CH$_3$ H
CH$_3$ H
H H
O

Chemical name.   Testosterone, heptanoate; 17β-[(1-oxoheptyl)oxy]androst-4-en-3-one; CAS Reg. No. 315-37-7.

Description.   A white or creamy white, crystalline powder; odourless or almost odourless.

Solubility.   Practically insoluble in water; very soluble in ethanol ($\sim$750 g/l) TS, ether R, and acetone R.

Category.   Androgen.

Storage.   Testosterone enantate should be kept in a tightly closed container, protected from light, and stored at a temperature not exceeding 15 °C.

Additional information.   Testosterone enantate melts at about 37 °C.

REQUIREMENTS

General requirement.   Testosterone enantate contains not less than 97.0% and not more than 103.0% of $C_{26}H_{40}O_3$, calculated with reference to the dried substance.

Identity tests

● Either test A alone or tests B and C may be applied.

A.   Carry out the examination as described under "Spectrophotometry in the infrared region" (vol. 1, p. 40). The infrared absorption spectrum is concordant with the spectrum obtained from testosterone enantate RS or with the *reference spectrum* of testosterone enantate.

B.   Carry out the test as described under "Thin-layer chromatography" (vol. 1, p. 83), using kieselguhr R1 as the coating substance and a mixture of 10 volumes of liquid paraffin R and 90 volumes of light petroleum R to impregnate the plate, dipping it about 5 mm into the liquid.   After the solvent has reached a height of at least 16 cm, remove the plate from the chromatographic chamber and allow it to stand at room temperature until the solvents have completely evaporated. Use the impregnated plate within 2 hours, carrying out the chromatography in the same direction as the impregnation.   Use a mixture of 4 volumes of glacial acetic acid R and 6 volumes of water as the mobile phase.   Apply separately to the plate 2 µl of each of 2 solutions in a mixture of 9 volumes of chloroform R and 1 volume of methanol R containing (A) 1.0 mg of the test substance per ml and (B) 1.0 mg of testosterone enantate RS per ml.   Develop the plate for a distance of 12 cm.   After removing the plate from the chromatographic chamber, allow it to dry in air until the solvents have evaporated, heat it at 120 °C for 5–10 minutes, spray it with 4-toluenesulfonic acid/ethanol TS, and then heat it at 120 °C for 10 minutes. Allow it to cool and examine the chromatogram in daylight and in ultraviolet light (365 nm).   The principal spot obtained with solution A corresponds in position, appearance, and intensity with that obtained with solution B.

C.   Suspend 5 mg in 2.0 ml of a mixture prepared by previously cooling 2 volumes of sulfuric acid (~1760 g/l) TS and 1 volume of ethanol (~750 g/l) TS, then place it in a water-bath; a greenish yellow fluorescence develops that changes to orange, whereas the walls of the tube take on a dichroic blue colour, changing to red below a certain depth.

Specific optical rotation.   Use a 10 mg/ml solution in dioxan R; $[\alpha]_D^{20\,°C} = +77$ to $+83°$.

Loss on drying.   Dry to constant weight at ambient temperature under reduced pressure (not exceeding 0.6 kPa or about 5 mm of mercury) over phosphorus pentoxide R; it loses not more than 5.0 mg/g.

Free heptanoic acid.   Dissolve 0.5 g, accurately weighed, in 10 ml of ethanol (~750 g/l) TS, previously neutralized to bromothymol blue/ethanol TS, and titrate immediately with sodium hydroxide (0.01 mol/l) VS, using bromothymol blue/ethanol TS as indicator; not more than 0.6 ml of sodium hydroxide (0.01 mol/l) VS is required to obtain the midpoint of the indicator (green).

Related substances.   Carry out the test as described under "Thin-layer chromatography" (vol. 1, p. 83), using silica gel R1 as the coating substance and a mixture of 92 volumes of dichloroethane R, 8 volumes of methanol R, and 0.5 volume of water as the mobile phase.   Apply separately to the plate 5 µl of each of 2 solutions in a mixture of 9 volumes of chloroform R and 1 volume of methanol R containing (A) 20 mg of the test substance per ml and (B) 0.20 mg of the test substance per ml. After removing the plate from the chromatographic chamber, allow it to dry in air and heat it at 110 °C for 10 minutes. Spray the hot plate with sulfuric acid/ethanol

TS, again heat it at 110 °C for 10 minutes, and examine the chromatogram in ultraviolet light (365 nm). Any spot obtained with solution A, other than the principal spot, is not more intense than that obtained with solution B.

Assay. Dissolve about 20 mg, accurately weighed, in dehydrated ethanol R to produce 100 ml; dilute 5.0 ml of this solution to 100 ml with the same solvent. Measure the absorbance of a 1-cm layer of the diluted solution at the maximum at about 241 nm. Calculate the amount of $C_{26}H_{40}O_3$ in the substance being tested by comparison with testosterone enantate RS, similarly and concurrently examined. In an adequately calibrated spectrophotometer the absorbance of a 10 µg/ml solution of testosterone enantate RS in dehydrated ethanol R should be 0.42 ± 0.02.

TETRACAINI HYDROCHLORIDUM

Tetracaine hydrochloride

Molecular formula. $C_{15}H_{24}N_2O_2,HCl$

Relative molecular mass. 300.8

Graphic formula.

$$CH_3(CH_2)_3NH-\!\!\!\left\langle\!\!\!\bigcirc\!\!\!\right\rangle\!\!\!-COOCH_2CH_2N(CH_3)_2 \cdot HCl$$

Chemical name. 2-(Dimethylamino)ethyl *p*-(butylamino)benzoate monohydrochloride; 2-(dimethylamino)ethyl 4-(butylamino)benzoate monohydrochloride; CAS Reg. No. 136-47-0.

Other names. Amethocaine hydrochloride; dicainum.

Description. A white, crystalline powder; odourless.

Solubility. Soluble in about 8 parts of water; soluble in ethanol ($\sim$750 g/l) TS; sparingly soluble in chloroform R; practically insoluble in ether R.

Category. Local anaesthetic.

Storage. Tetracaine hydrochloride should be kept in a tightly closed container, protected from light.

Additional information. Tetracaine hydrochloride is hygroscopic; it has a slightly bitter taste and causes local numbness after being placed on the tongue. Even in the absence of light, it is gradually degraded on exposure to a humid atmosphere, the decomposition being faster at higher temperatures.

Tetracaine hydrochloride melts at about 148 °C or may exist in either of the two polymorphic forms, one of which melts at 134 °C and the other at 139 °C. Mixtures of the forms melt within the range 134–147 °C.

REQUIREMENTS

General requirement.   Tetracaine hydrochloride contains not less than 98.0 % and not more than 101.0 % of $C_{15}H_{24}N_2O_2$,HCl, calculated with reference to the dried substance.

Identity tests

A.   Dissolve 0.2 g in 10 ml of water and add 1 ml of ammonium thiocyanate (75 g/l) TS.   Collect the precipitate on a filter, recrystallize from water, and dry it at 80 °C for 2 hours; melting temperature, about 131 °C.

B.   A 20 mg/ml solution yields reaction A described under "General identification tests" as characteristic of chlorides (vol. 1, p. 112).

Clarity and colour of solution.   A solution of 0.20 g in 10 ml of carbon-dioxide-free water R is clear and colourless.

Sulfated ash.   Not more than 1.0 mg/g.

Loss on drying.   Dry to constant weight at 105 °C; it loses not more than 10 mg/g.

pH value.   pH of a 10 mg/ml solution in carbon-dioxide-free water R, 4.5–6.0.

Related substances.   Carry out the test as described under "Thin-layer chromatography" (vol. 1, p. 83), using silica gel R4 as the coating substance and a mixture of 80 volumes of dibutyl ether R, 16 volumes of hexane R, and 4 volumes of glacial acetic acid R as the mobile phase.   Place the plate in the chromatographic chamber, dipping it about 5 mm into the liquid.   After the solvent has reached a height of about 12 cm, remove the plate from the chromatographic chamber and dry it for a few minutes in a current of warm air.   Allow it to cool and apply separately to the plate 5 μl of each of 2 solutions containing (A) 0.10 g of the test substance per ml and (B) 0.050 mg of 4-aminobenzoic acid R per ml.   Allow the solvent front to ascend 10 cm above the line of application.   After removing the plate from the chromatographic chamber, dry it at 105 °C for 10 minutes and examine the chromatogram in ultraviolet light (254 nm).   Any spot obtained with solution A, other than the principal spot, is not more intense than that obtained with solution B.   The principal spot remains on the baseline.

Assay.   Carry out the assay as described under "Nitrite titration" (vol. 1, p. 133), using about 0.5 g, accurately weighed, dissolved in a mixture of 50 ml of water and 5 ml of hydrochloric acid ($\sim$420 g/l) TS, and titrate with sodium nitrite (0.1 mol/l) VS.   Each ml of sodium nitrite (0.1 mol/l) VS is equivalent to 30.08 mg of $C_{15}H_{24}N_2O_2,HCl$.

<hr>

THIAMINI HYDROBROMIDUM

Thiamine hydrobromide

Thiamine hydrobromide, anhydrous
Thiamine hydrobromide hemihydrate

Molecular formula. $C_{12}H_{17}BrN_4OS,HBr$ (anhydrous); $C_{12}H_{17}BrN_4OS,HBr,\frac{1}{2}H_2O$ (hemihydrate).

Relative molecular mass.   426.2 (anhydrous); 435.2 (hemihydrate).

Graphic formula.

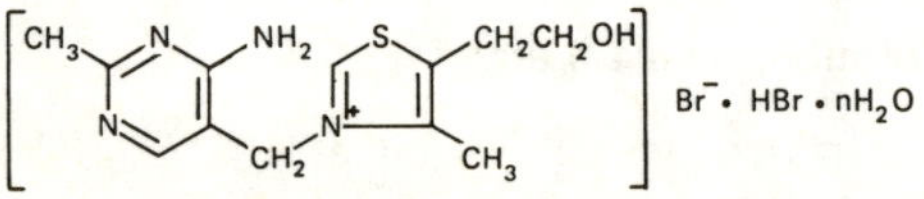

$$n = 0 \text{ (anhydrous)}$$
$$n = 1/2 \text{ (hemihydrate)}$$

Chemical name.   Thiamine bromide, monohydrobromide; 3-[(4-amino-2-methyl-5-pyrimidinyl)methyl]-5-(2-hydroxyethyl)-4-methylthiazolium bromide, monohydrobromide; CAS Reg. No. 4234-86-0 (anhydrous).
Thiamine bromide, monohydrobromide, hemihydrate; 3-[(4-amino-2-methyl-5-pyrimidinyl)methyl]-5-(2-hydroxyethyl)-4-methylthiazolium bromide, monohydrobromide, hemihydrate; CAS Reg. No. 62084-87-1 (hemihydrate).

Description.   A white to yellowish white, crystalline powder; odour, slight and characteristic.

Solubility.   Freely soluble in water and in methanol R; sparingly soluble in ethanol ($\sim$750 g/l) TS; practically insoluble in ether R.

Category.   Component of vitamin B.

Storage.   Thiamine hydrobromide should be kept in a tightly closed, non-metallic container, protected from light.

REQUIREMENTS

General requirement.   Thiamine hydrobromide contains not less than 98.0% and not more than 101.0% of $C_{12}H_{17}BrN_4OS,HBr$, calculated with reference to the dried substance.

Identity tests

A.   Dissolve 10 mg in 1 ml of water, add 1 ml of sodium hydroxide ($\sim$80 g/l) TS, 0.5 ml of potassium ferricyanide (10 g/l) TS; the solution remains pale yellow. Shake with 5 ml of 2-butanol R and allow to stand for 5–10 minutes; in bright daylight or in ultraviolet light (365 nm) the 2-butanol layer shows a blue fluorescence.

B.   Spread a small quantity of the powder on a watch-glass; the odour is slight and characteristic, resembling that of yeast.

C.   A 20 mg/ml solution yields reaction A described under "General identification tests" as characteristic of bromides (vol. 1, p. 112).

Heavy metals.   Use 1.0 g for the preparation of the test solution as described under "Limit test for heavy metals", Procedure 1 (vol. 1, p. 118); determine the heavy metals content according to Method A (vol. 1, p. 119); not more than 20 µg/g.

Clarity and colour of solution.   A solution of 0.6 g in 10 ml of water is clear and colourless.

Sulfated ash.   Not more than 1.0 mg/g.

Loss on drying.   Dry to constant weight at 105 °C.   Anhydrous thiamine hydrobromide loses not more than 5.0 mg/g.   Thiamine hydrobromide hemihydrate loses not more than 25 mg/g.

pH value.   pH of a 0.06 g/ml solution, 2.7–3.4.

Assay.   Dissolve about 0.30 g, accurately weighed, in 30 ml of glacial acetic acid R1, add 10 ml of mercuric acetate/acetic acid TS, and titrate with perchloric acid (0.1 mol/l) VS as described under "Non-aqueous titration".   Method A (vol. 1, p. 131).   Each ml of perchloric acid (0.1 mol/l) VS is equivalent to 21.31 mg of $C_{12}H_{17}BrN_4OS,HBr$.

THIAMINI HYDROCHLORIDUM

Thiamine hydrochloride

Molecular formula. $C_{12}H_{17}ClN_4OS,HCl$

Relative molecular mass.   337.3

Graphic formula.

$$\left[CH_3{-}\text{pyrimidine ring}{-}NH_2 \quad \text{thiazole ring} {-}CH_2CH_2OH \right] \quad Cl^- \cdot HCl$$

Chemical name.   Thiamine chloride, hydrochloride; 3-[(4-amino-2-methyl-5-pyrimidinyl)methyl]-5-(2-hydroxyethyl)-4-methylthiazolium   chloride,   monohydrochloride; CAS Reg. No. 67-03-8.

Description.   Colourless crystals or a white or yellowish white, crystalline powder; odour, slight and characteristic.

Solubility.   Soluble in 1 part of water and in 100 parts of ethanol ($\sim$750 g/l) TS; practically insoluble in acetone R and ether R.

Category.   Component of vitamin B.

Storage.   Thiamine hydrochloride should be kept in a tightly closed, non-metallic container, protected from light.

Additional information.   Even in the absence of light, Thiamine hydrochloride is gradually degraded on exposure to a humid atmosphere, the decomposition being faster at higher temperatures.   When exposed to air, the anhydrous product rapidly absorbs about 4 g of water per 100 g.   Melting temperature, about 248 °C with some decomposition.   In solution at pH 4.0 or less, it loses its activity only very slowly.   Neutral and alkaline solutions deteriorate rapidly, especially in contact with air.

REQUIREMENTS

General requirement.   Thiamine hydrochloride contains not less than 98.0% and not more than 101.0% of $C_{12}H_{17}ClN_4OS,HCl$, calculated with reference to the dried substance.

Identity tests

A.   Dissolve 10 mg in 1 ml of water, add 1 ml of sodium hydroxide ($\sim$80 g/l) TS and 0.5 ml of potassium ferricyanide (10 g/l) TS; the solution remains pale yellow.

Shake with 5 ml of 2-butanol R and allow to stand for 5–10 minutes; in bright daylight or in ultraviolet light (365 nm) the 2-butanol layer shows a blue fluorescence.

B.   Spread a small quantity of the powder on a watch-glass; the odour is slight and characteristic, resembling that of yeast.

C.   A 0.05 g/ml solution yields reaction A described under "General identification tests" as characteristic of chlorides (vol. 1, p. 112).

Heavy metals.   Use 1.0 g for the preparation of the test solution as described under "Limit test for heavy metals", Procedure 1 (vol. 1, p. 118); determine the heavy metals content according to Method A (vol. 1, p. 119); not more than 20 µg/g.

Clarity and colour of solution.   A solution of 2.0 g in 10 ml of water is clear and not more intensely coloured than standard colour solution Yw2 when compared as described under "Colour of liquids" (vol. 1, p. 50).

Sulfated ash.   Not more than 1.0 mg/g.

Loss on drying.   Dry to constant weight at 105 °C; it loses not more than 50 mg/g.

pH value.   pH of a 25 mg/ml solution, 2.7–3.3.

Assay.   Dissolve about 0.25 g, accurately weighed, in 30 ml of glacial acetic acid R1, add 10 ml of mercuric acetate/acetic acid TS, and titrate with perchloric acid (0.1 mol/l) VS as described under "Non-aqueous titration", Method A (vol. 1, p. 131).   Each ml of perchloric acid (0.1 mol/l) VS is equivalent to 16.86 mg of $C_{12}H_{17}ClN_4OS,HCl$.

THIAMINI MONONITRAS

Thiamine mononitrate

Molecular formula. $C_{12}H_{17}N_5O_4S$

Relative molecular mass.   327.4

Graphic formula.

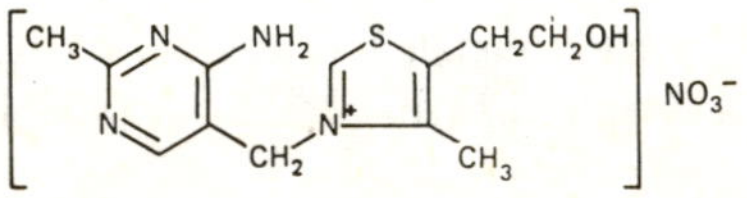

$$\left[CH_3\text{-pyrimidine-}NH_2\text{-}CH_2\text{-}N^+\text{-thiazole-}CH_2CH_2OH,\ CH_3 \right] NO_3^-$$

Chemical name. Thiamine nitrate (salt); 3-[(4-amino-2-methyl-5-pyrimidi-nyl)methyl]-5-(2-hydroxyethyl)-4-methylthiazolium nitrate (salt); CAS Reg. No. 532-43-4.

Description. Colourless crystals or a white, crystalline powder; odour, slight and characteristic.

Solubility. Sparingly soluble in water; very slightly soluble in ethanol ($\sim$750 g/l) TS; practically insoluble in chloroform R.

Category. Component of vitamin B.

Storage. Thiamine mononitrate should be kept in a tightly closed, non-metallic container, protected from light.

Additional information. Even in the absence of light, Thiamine mononitrate is gradually degraded on exposure to a humid atmosphere, the decomposition being faster at higher temperatures.

REQUIREMENTS

General requirement. Thiamine mononitrate contains not less than 98.0% and not more than 101.0% of $C_{12}H_{17}N_5O_4S$, calculated with reference to the dried substance.

Identity tests

A.   Dissolve 10 mg in 1 ml of water, add 1 ml of sodium hydroxide ($\sim$80 g/l) TS and 0.5 ml of potassium ferricyanide (10 g/l) TS; the solution remains pale yellow. Shake with 5 ml of 2-butanol R and allow to stand for 5–10 minutes; in bright daylight or in ultraviolet light (365 nm) the 2-butanol layer shows a blue fluorescence.

B.   Spread a small quantity of the powder on a watch-glass; the odour is slight and characteristic, resembling that of yeast.

C.   To 2 ml of a 0.05 g/ml solution add 2 ml of ferrous sulfate (15 g/l) TS; it yields reaction A described under "General identification tests" as characteristic of nitrates (vol. 1, p. 114).

Heavy metals. Use 1.0 g for the preparation of the test solution as described under "Limit test for heavy metals", Procedure 1 (vol. 1, p. 118); determine the heavy metals content according to Method A (vol. 1, p. 119); not more than 20 µg/g.

Clarity and colour of solution.   A solution of 0.2 g in 10 ml of water is clear and not more intensely coloured than standard colour solution Yw2 when compared as described under "Colour of liquids" (vol. 1, p. 50).

Sulfated ash.   Not more than 1.0 mg/g.

Loss on drying.   Dry to constant weight at 105 °C; it loses not more than 10 mg/g.

pH value.   pH of a 20 mg/ml solution, 6.0–7.5.

Assay.   Dissolve about 0.1 g, accurately weighed, in 30 ml of glacial acetic acid R1, add 0.15 ml of 1-naphtholbenzein/acetic acid TS, and titrate with perchloric acid (0.1 mol/l) VS to a green endpoint, as described under "Non-aqueous titration", Method A (vol. 1, p. 131).   Each ml of perchloric acid (0.1 mol/l) VS is equivalent to 16.37 mg of $C_{12}H_{17}N_5O_4S$.

THIOACETAZONUM

Thioacetazone

Molecular formula. $C_{10}H_{12}N_4OS$

Relative molecular mass.   236.3

Graphic formula.

$$CH=N-NH-CS-NH_2$$

$$NH-CO-CH_3$$

Chemical name.   4′-Formylacetanilide 4′-(thiosemicarbazone); N-[4-[[(amino-thioxomethyl)hydrazono]methyl]phenyl]acetamide; CAS Reg. No. 104-06-3.

Description.   Pale yellow crystals or a yellow, crystalline powder; almost odourless.

Solubility.   Very slightly soluble in water; slightly soluble in ethanol ($\sim$750 g/l) TS and methanol R; soluble in 10 parts of dimethylformamide R.

Category.   Antituberculosis drug.

Storage.   Thioacetazone should be kept in a tightly closed container, protected from light.

REQUIREMENTS

General requirement. Thioacetazone contains not less than 98.0% and not more than 102.0% of $C_{10}H_{12}N_4OS$, calculated with reference to the dried substance.

Identity tests

● Either test A alone or tests B, C and D may be applied.

A. Carry out the examination as described under "Spectrophotometry in the infrared region" (vol. 1, p. 40). The infrared absorption spectrum is concordant with the spectrum obtained from thioacetazone RS or with the *reference spectrum* of thioacetazone.

B. The absorption spectrum of a 3.0 μg/ml solution in dehydrated ethanol R, when observed between 230 nm and 350 nm, exhibits a maximum at about 328 nm; the absorbance of a 1-cm layer at this wavelength is about 0.58.

C. Dissolve 10 mg by heating in 1 ml of sodium hydroxide (5 mol/l) VS, add 0.25 ml of lead acetate (80 g/l) TS and boil for 1 minute; a black precipitate is produced.

D. About 10 mg yields the reaction described for the identification of primary aromatic amines under "General identification tests" (vol. 1, p. 111), producing a red colour.

Heavy metals. Use 1.0 g for the preparation of the test solution as described under "Limit test for heavy metals", Procedure 3 (vol. 1, p. 118); determine the heavy metals content according to Method A (vol. 1, p. 119); not more than 10 μg/g.

Sulfated ash. Not more than 2.0 mg/g.

Loss on drying. Dry to constant weight at 105 °C; it loses not more than 5.0 mg/g.

Related substances. Carry out the test as described under "Thin-layer chromatography" (vol. 1, p. 83), using silica gel R4 as the coating substance and ethyl acetate R as the mobile phase. Apply separately to the plate 10 μl of each of 2 solutions in a mixture of 9 volumes of methanol R and 1 volume of water containing (A) 2.0 mg of the test substance per ml, and (B) 4.0 μg of *p*-acetamidobenzalazine RS per ml. After removing the plate from the chromatographic chamber, allow it to dry in air, spray it evenly with nitric acid (~130 g/l) TS, and examine the chromatogram in ultraviolet light (365 nm). Any spot obtained with solution A, other than the principal spot, is not more intense than that obtained with solution B.

Thiosemicarbazide.   Finely powder the test substance and to about 2 g, accurately weighed, add sufficient water to produce 50 ml. Allow to stand for at least 1 hour, shaking occasionally.   Filter, reject the first few ml of the filtrate, and transfer 25 ml of the filtrate to a 250-ml conical flask. Acidify with sulfuric acid ($\sim$100 g/l) TS and titrate with ceric sulfate (0.1 mol/l) VS, using o-phenanthroline TS as indicator, to a blue endpoint that persists for 1 minute.   Not more than 0.8 ml of ceric sulfate (0.1 mol/l) VS is required (not more than 1.0 mg/g).

Assay.   Dissolve about 0.1 g, accurately weighed, in 60 ml of methanol R by warming to 60 °C on a water-bath. Slowly add 20 ml of hot silver nitrate/methanol TS, maintain the temperature at 60 °C until the formed precipitate congeals and settles, leaving a clear supernatant liquor. Cool and filter through a dried and weighed sintered-glass crucible and wash the precipitate with methanol R until the washings are free from silver. Dry to constant weight at 105 °C, cool and weigh. Each g of precipitate is equivalent to 460.6 mg of $C_{10}H_{12}N_4OS$.

TIABENDAZOLUM

Tiabendazole

Molecular formula. $C_{10}H_7N_3S$

Relative molecular mass.   201.3

Graphic formula.

Chemical name.   2-(4-Thiazolyl)benzimidazole; 2-(4-thiazolyl)-1H-benzimida-zole; CAS Reg. No. 148-79-8.

Description.   A white to almost white powder; odourless or almost odourless.

Solubility.   Practically insoluble in water; soluble in 150 parts of ethanol ($\sim$750 g/l) TS; slightly soluble in chloroform R and ether R.

Category.   Anthelmintic.

Storage.   Tiabendazole should be kept in a well-closed container.

REQUIREMENTS

General requirement.   Tiabendazole contains not less than 98.0% and not more than 101.0% of $C_{10}H_7N_3S$, calculated with reference to the dried substance.

Identity tests

● Either test A alone or tests B and C may be applied.

A.   Carry out the examination as described under "Spectrophotometry in the infrared region" (vol. 1, p. 40). The infrared absorption spectrum is concordant with the spectrum obtained from tiabendazole RS or with the *reference spectrum* of tiabendazole.

B.   The absorption spectrum of a 4.0 μg/ml solution in hydrochloric acid (0.1 mol/l) VS, when observed between 230 nm and 350 nm, exhibits maxima at about 243 nm and 302 nm; the absorbances of a 1-cm layer at these maxima are about 0.23 and 0.49, respectively.

C.   Dissolve 5 mg in 5 ml of hydrochloric acid (0.1 mol/l) VS, add 3 mg of 1,4-phenylenediamine dihydrochloride R, and shake until dissolved. Add 0.1 g of zinc R powder, mix, allow to stand for 2 minutes, and add 10 ml of ferric ammonium sulfate (45 g/l) TS; a deep blue or blue-violet colour is produced.

Sulfated ash.   Not more than 1.0 mg/g.

Loss on drying.   Dry to constant weight at 105 °C; it loses not more than 5.0 mg/g.

Related substances.   Carry out the test as described under "Thin-layer chromatography" (vol. 1, p. 83), using silica gel R4 as the coating substance and a mixture of 50 volumes of toluene R, 20 volumes of glacial acetic acid R, 8 volumes of acetone R, and 2 volumes of water as the mobile phase. Apply separately to the plate 10 μl of each of 2 solutions in methanol R containing (A) 10 mg of the test substance per ml and (B) 0.15 mg of the test substance per ml. After removing the plate from the chromatographic chamber, allow it to dry in air and examine the chromatogram in ultraviolet light (254 nm). Any spot obtained with solution A, other than the principal spot, is not more intense than that obtained with solution B.

Assay.   Dissolve about 0.16 g, accurately weighed, in 30 ml of glacial acetic acid R1 and titrate with perchloric acid (0.1 mol/l) VS as described under "Non-aqueous titration", Method A (vol. 1, p. 131). Each ml of perchloric acid (0.1 mol/l) VS is equivalent to 20.13 g of $C_{10}H_7N_3S$.

TRIHEXYPHENIDYLI HYDROCHLORIDUM

Trihexyphenidyl hydrochloride

Molecular formula. $C_{20}H_{31}NO,HCl$

Relative molecular mass.   337.9

Graphic formula.

Chemical name.   α-Cyclohexyl-α-phenyl-1-piperidinepropanol hydrochloride; CAS Reg. No. 52-49-3.

Other names.   Benzhexol hydrochloride; cyclodolum.

Description.   A white or off-white, crystalline powder; odourless or almost odourless.

Solubility.   Slightly soluble in water; soluble in ethanol (~750 g/l) TS, chloroform R, and methanol R.

Category.   Anticholinergic; antiparkinsonism drug.

Storage.   Trihexyphenidyl hydrochloride should be kept in a tightly closed container.

REQUIREMENTS

General requirement.   Trihexyphenidyl hydrochloride contains not less than 98.0% and not more than 101.0% of $C_{20}H_{31}NO,HCl$, calculated with reference to the dried substance.

Identity tests

● Either tests A and C or tests B and C may be applied.

A.   Carry out the examination as described under "Spectrophotometry in the infrared region" (vol. 1, p. 40). The infrared absorption spectrum is concordant with the spectrum obtained from trihexyphenidyl hydrochloride RS or with the *reference spectrum* of trihexyphenidyl hydrochloride.

B.   Dissolve 0.5 g in 5 ml of warm methanol R and add sufficient sodium hydroxide (~80 g/l) TS to make the solution alkaline to litmus paper R; a white precipitate is formed. Collect the precipitate, wash with a small portion of water, recrystallize from methanol R, and dry under reduced pressure (not exceeding 0.6 kPa or about 5 mm of mercury) over silica gel, desiccant, R for 2 hours; melting temperature, about 115 °C (trihexyphenidyl base).

C.   A 0.05 g/ml solution yields reaction B described under "General identification tests" as characteristic of chlorides (vol. 1, p. 113).

Sulfated ash.   Not more than 1.0 mg/g.

Loss on drying.   Dry to constant weight at 105 °C; it loses not more than 5.0 mg/g.

pH value.   Dissolve 1.0 g in 100 ml of carbon-dioxide-free water R by warming, then cool; pH of this solution, 5.0–6.0.

Piperidylpropiophenone.   Dissolve 0.10 g in a mixture of 40 ml of water and 1 ml of hydrochloric acid (1 mol/l) VS with the aid of heat, cool, and add sufficient water to produce 100 ml. Measure the absorbance of a 1-cm layer at the maximum at about 247 nm; not more than 0.5.

Assay.   Dissolve about 0.5 g, accurately weighed, in 30 ml of glacial acetic acid R1, add 10 ml of mercuric acetate/acetic acid TS and titrate with perchloric acid (0.1 mol/l) VS, as described under "Non-aqueous titration", Method A (vol. 1, p. 131).   Each ml of perchloric acid (0.1 mol/l) VS is equivalent to 33.79 mg of $C_{20}H_{31}NO,HCl$.

TUBOCURARINI CHLORIDUM

Tubocurarine chloride

Molecular formula. $C_{37}H_{41}ClN_2O_6,HCl,5H_2O$

Relative molecular mass.   771.7

Graphic formula.

Chemical name.   (+)-Tubocurarine chloride hydrochloride, pentahydrate; 7′,12′-dihydroxy-6,6′-dimethoxy-2,2′,2′-trimethyltubocuraranium chloride hydrochloride pentahydrate; CAS Reg. No. 6989-98-6 (pentahydrate).

Description.   A white to yellowish white, crystalline powder; odourless.

Solubility.   Soluble in 20 parts of water and 30 parts of ethanol ($\sim$750 g/l) TS; practically insoluble in acetone R, chloroform R, and ether R.

Category.   Muscle relaxant.

Storage.   Tubocurarine chloride should be kept in a tightly closed container.

Additional information.   Tubocurarine chloride melts at about 270 °C with decomposition.

REQUIREMENTS

General requirement.   Tubocurarine chloride contains not less than 98.0% and not more than 102.0% of $C_{37}H_{41}ClN_2O_6,HCl$, calculated with reference to the dried substance.

Identity tests

A.   Dissolve 10 mg in 1 ml of water and add 1 ml of mercuric nitrate TS; a cherry red colour is slowly produced.

B.   Dissolve 10 mg in 1 ml of water and add 0.1 ml of ferric chloride (25 g/l) TS; a green colour is produced, which becomes brown on warming on a water-bath.

C.   A 20 mg/ml solution yields reaction A described under "General identification tests" as characteristic of chlorides (vol. 1, p. 113).

Specific optical rotation.   Use a 10 mg/ml solution, which has been allowed to stand for 3 hours, and calculate with reference to the dried substance;
$[\alpha]_D^{20\,°C} = +210$ to $+220°$.

Chloroform-soluble substances.   Dissolve 0.25 g in 150 ml of water, add 5 ml of a saturated solution of sodium hydrogen carbonate R, and extract with 3 quantities, each of 20 ml, of chloroform R. Wash the combined chloroform extracts with 10 ml of water, filter the chloroform solution into a beaker, wash the filter with 2 successive quantities, each of 5 ml, of chloroform R, and add the washings to the filtrate. Evaporate the combined filtrate and washings on a water-bath and dry the residue at 105 °C for 1 hour; the weight of the residue is not more than 5 mg (2.0%). Add 10 ml of water to the residue; the residue does not dissolve. Then add 1 ml of hydrochloric acid ($\sim$70 g/l) TS; the residue dissolves.

Sulfated ash.   Not more than 2.5 mg/g.

Loss on drying.   Dry to constant weight at 100 °C under reduced pressure (not exceeding 0.6 kPa or about 5 mm of mercury); it loses not less than 90 mg/g and not more than 120 mg/g.

pH value.   pH of a 10 mg/ml solution, 4.0–6.0.

Assay.   Dissolve about 0.5 g, accurately weighed, in 20 ml of glacial acetic acid R1 by warming on a water-bath, cool, and add 60 ml of acetic anhydride R and 10 ml of mercuric acetate/acetic acid TS.   Titrate with perchloric acid (0.1 mol/l) VS, determining the endpoint potentiometrically as described under "Non-aqueous titration", Method A (vol. 1, p. 131).   Each ml of perchloric acid (0.1 mol/l) VS is equivalent to 34.08 mg of $C_{37}H_{41}ClN_2O_6,HCl$.

VERAPAMILI HYDROCHLORIDUM

Verapamil hydrochloride

Molecular formula. $C_{27}H_{38}N_2O_4,HCl$

Relative molecular mass.   491.1

Graphic formula.

Chemical name.   5-[(3,4-Dimethoxyphenethyl)methylamino]-2-(3,4-dimethoxyphenyl)-2-isopropylvaleronitrile hydrochloride; α-[3-[[2-(3,4-dimethoxyphenyl)-ethyl]methylamino]propyl]-3,4-dimethoxy-α-(1-methylethyl)benzeneacetonitrile monohydrochloride; CAS Reg. No. 152-11-4.

Description.   A white or almost white, crystalline powder; odourless or almost odourless.

Solubility.   Soluble in 20 parts of water; sparingly soluble in ethanol (~750 g/l) TS; freely soluble in chloroform R.

Category.   Antianginal drug.

Storage.   Verapamil hydrochloride should be kept in a well-closed container, protected from light.

REQUIREMENTS

General requirement.   Verapamil hydrochloride contains not less than 99.0% and not more than 101.0% of $C_{27}H_{38}N_2O_4,HCl$, calculated with reference to the dried substance.

Identity tests

• Either tests A and D or tests B, C, D and E may be applied.

A.   Carry out the examination as described under "Spectrophotometry in the infrared region" (vol. 1, p. 40). The infrared absorption spectrum is concordant with the spectrum obtained from verapamil hydrochloride RS or with the *reference spectrum* of verapamil hydrochloride.

B.   The absorption spectrum of a 20 µg/ml solution in hydrochloric acid (0.01 mol/l) VS, when observed between 220 nm and 350 nm, exhibits maxima at about 229 nm and 278 nm; the absorbances of a 1-cm layer at these maxima are about 0.63 and 0.24, respectively.

C.   Dissolve 20 mg in 2.5 ml of water, add 0.5 ml of sulfuric acid ($\sim$570 g/l) TS and 0.2 ml of potassium permanganate (10 g/l) TS; a violet precipitate is produced, which quickly dissolves to produce a very pale yellow solution.

D.   A 20 mg/ml solution yields reaction A described under "General identification tests" as characteristic of chlorides (vol. 1, p. 113).

E.   Melting temperature, about 143 °C.

Clarity and colour of solution.   A solution of 0.50 g in 10 ml of carbon-dioxide-free water R is clear and colourless.

Readily carbonizable substances.   Dissolve 0.10 g in 5 ml of sulfuric acid ($\sim$1760 g/l) TS. After 5 minutes the solution is clear and not more intensely coloured than standard colour solution Yw2 when compared as described under "Colour of liquids" (vol. 1, p. 50).

Sulfated ash.   Not more than 1.0 mg/g.

Loss on drying.   Dry to constant weight at 105 °C; it loses not more than 5.0 mg/g.

pH value.   pH of a 0.05 g/ml solution in carbon-dioxide-free water R, 4.5–6.5.

Related substances

A.   Carry out the test as described under "Thin-layer chromatography" (vol. 1, p. 83), using silica gel R5 as the coating substance (a precoated plate from a commercial source is suitable) and a mixture of 85 volumes of cyclohexane R and 15 volumes of diethylamine R as the mobile phase. Apply separately to the plate 10 μl of each of 3 solutions in chloroform R containing (A) 50 mg of the test substance per ml, (B) 25 μg of the test substance per ml, and (C) 50 μg of the test substance per ml. After removing the plate from the chromatographic chamber, allow it to dry at room temperature for 10 minutes and develop the plate a second time. Remove the plate, heat it at 110 °C for 1 hour, allow it to cool, and spray it with a solution prepared by dissolving 5 g of ferric chloride R and 2 g of iodine R in 50 ml of tartaric acid (200 g/l) TS, applying a total of 15–20 ml of the reagent. Examine the plate immediately in daylight disregarding any spot on the line of application. Up to 3 secondary spots may be more intense than the spot obtained with solution B but they must be less intense than the spot obtained with solution C. Any other secondary spots in the chromatogram obtained with solution A must be less intense than the spot obtained with solution B.

B.   Carry out test A once more using a mixture of 70 volumes of toluene R, 20 volumes of methanol R, 5 volumes of acetone R, and 5 volumes of glacial acetic acid R as the mobile phase. The result is the same as that with test A.

Assay.   Dissolve about 0.5 g, accurately weighed, in 30 ml of glacial acetic acid R1, add 10 ml of mercuric acetate/acetic acid TS followed by 0.15 ml of 1-naphtholbenzein/acetic acid TS as indicator, and titrate with perchloric acid (0.1 mol/l) VS as described under "Non-aqueous titration", Method A (vol. 1, p. 131). Each ml of perchloric acid (0.1 mol/l) VS is equivalent to 49.11 mg of $C_{27}H_{38}N_2O_4,HCl$.

VINCRISTINI SULFAS

Vincristine sulfate

Molecular formula. $C_{46}H_{56}N_4O_{10},H_2SO_4$

Relative molecular mass.   923.0

Graphic formula.

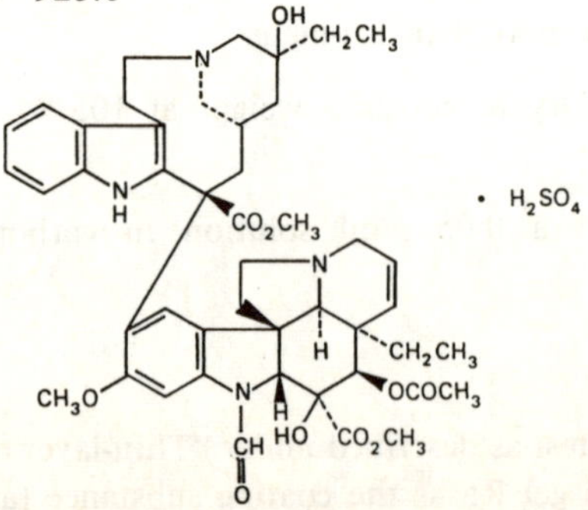

Chemical name.   Leurocristine sulfate (1 : 1) (salt); 22-oxovincaleukoblastine sulfate (1 : 1) (salt); CAS Reg. No. 2068-78-2.

Description.   A white to slightly yellow, amorphous or crystalline powder; odourless.

Solubility.   Freely soluble in water; slightly soluble in ethanol (~750 g/l) TS; practically insoluble in ether R.

Category.   Cytotoxic drug.

Storage.   Vincristine sulfate should be kept in a tightly closed container, protected from light, and stored at a temperature between 2 and 10 °C.

Additional information.   Vincristine sulfate is hygroscopic and very toxic. CAUTION: Vincristine sulfate must be handled with care, avoiding contact with the skin and inhalation of airborne particles.

REQUIREMENTS

General requirement.   Vincristine sulfate contains not less than 95.0 % and not more than 105.0 % of $C_{46}H_{56}N_4O_{10},H_2SO_4$, calculated with reference to the dried substance.

Identity tests

● Either tests A and D or tests B, C and D may be applied.

A.   Carry out the examination as described under "Spectrophotometry in the infrared region" (vol. 1, p. 40). The infrared absorption spectrum of the substance dried under reduced pressure for 16 hours at 40 °C is concordant with the spectrum obtained from vincristine sulfate RS similarly prepared or with the *reference spectrum* of vincristine sulfate.

B.   See the test described below under "Related substances". The principal spot obtained with solution A corresponds in position, appearance, and intensity with that obtained with solution C.

C.   To about 1 mg add 0.2 ml of vanillin/hydrochloric acid TS and allow to stand for approximately 1 minute; an orange colour is produced (distinction from vinblastine sulfate).

D.   A 20 mg/ml solution yields reaction A described under "General identification tests" as characteristic of sulfates (vol. 1, p. 115).

Loss on drying.   Dry at 40 °C under reduced pressure (not exceeding 0.6 kPa or about 5 mm of mercury) for 16 hours; it loses not more than 120 mg/g.

pH value.   pH of 1.0 g/ml solution, 3.5–4.5.

Related substances. Carry out the test as described under "Thin-layer chromatography" (vol. 1, p. 83), using silica gel R2 as the coating substance and a mixture of 40 volumes of toluene R, 20 volumes of chloroform R, and 3 volumes of diethylamine R as the mobile phase. Apply separately to the plate 5 µl of each of 3 solutions in methanol R containing (A) 10 mg of the test substance per ml, (B) 0.20 mg of the test substance per ml, and (C) 10 mg of vincristine sulfate RS per ml. After removing the plate from the chromatographic chamber, allow it to dry in air, and examine the chromatogram in ultraviolet light (254 nm). Any spot obtained with solution A, other than the principal spot, is not more intense than that obtained with solution B.

Assay. Dissolve about 10 mg, accurately weighed, in sufficient methanol R to produce 500 ml. Measure the absorbance of this solution in a 1-cm layer at the maximum at about 297 nm and calculate the content of $C_{46}H_{56}N_4O_{10},H_2SO_4$, using the absorptivity value of 17.7 ($A_{1\ cm}^{1\ \%} = 177$).

WARFARINUM NATRICUM

Warfarin sodium

Molecular formula. $C_{19}H_{15}NaO_4$; $C_{19}H_{15}NaO_4,C_3H_8O,H_2O$ (hyclate).

Relative molecular mass. 330.3; 408.4 (hyclate).

Graphic formula.

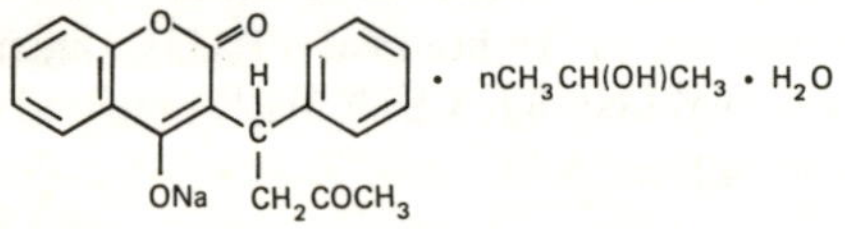

Chemical name. 3-(α-Acetonylbenzyl)-4-hydroxycoumarin sodium salt; 4-hydroxy-3-(3-oxo-1-phenylbutyl)-2*H*-1-benzopyran-2-one sodium salt; CAS Reg. No. 129-06-6.
3-(α-Acetonylbenzyl)-4-hydroxycoumarin sodium salt compound with 2-propanol monohydrate; 4-hydroxy-3-(3-oxo-1-phenylbutyl)-2*H*-benzopyran-2-one sodium salt 2-propanol monohydrate.

Description. A white, amorphous or crystalline powder; odourless.

Solubility. Soluble in less than 1 part of water and in ethanol ($\sim$750 g/l) TS; slightly soluble in chloroform R and in ether R.

Category. Anticoagulant.

Storage.   Warfarin sodium should be kept in a well-closed container, protected from light.

Labelling.   The designation on the container of Warfarin sodium should state whether the substance is in the amorphous or the crystalline, clathrate form.

Additional information.   Warfarin sodium is discoloured by light. Even in the absence of light, it is gradually degraded on exposure to a humid atmosphere, the decomposition being faster at higher temperatures.

REQUIREMENTS

General requirement.   Warfarin sodium contains not less than 98.0% and not more than 102.0% of $C_{19}H_{15}NaO_4$, calculated with reference to the anhydrous and 2-propanol-free substance.

Identity tests

A.   Dissolve 0.1 g in 25 ml of water, add 0.1 ml of hydrochloric acid ($\sim$70 g/l) TS, collect the precipitate on a filter (keep the filtrate for test C), wash with water, and dry the residue at 105 °C. Melting temperature, about 162 °C (warfarin). (Keep the residue for test B).

B.   Carry out the examination of the residue obtained in test A as described under "Spectrophotometry in the infrared region" (vol. 1, p. 40). The infrared absorption spectrum is concordant with the spectrum obtained from warfarin RS or with the *reference spectrum* of warfarin.

C.   The filtrate obtained in test A yields reaction B described under "General identification tests" as characteristic of sodium (vol. 1, p. 115).

D.   Dissolve 1 g in 10 ml of water, add 5 ml of nitric acid ($\sim$1000 g/l) TS, and filter. To the filtrate add 2 ml of potassium dichromate (0.0167 mol/l) VS and shake for 5 minutes; only the clathrate yields a light greenish blue solution.

Clarity of solution.   The opalescence of a solution of 0.50 g in 10 ml of carbon-dioxide-free water R is not more intense than that of opalescence standard TS2.

Water.   Determine as described under "Determination of water by the Karl Fischer method", Method A (vol. 1, p. 135), using about 0.4 g of the substance; the water content is not more than 45 mg/g.

pH value.   pH of a 10 mg/ml solution in carbon-dioxide-free water R, 7.2–8.3.

Related substances.   Carry out the test as described under "Thin-layer chromatography" (vol. 1, p. 83), using silica gel R4 as the coating substance and a mixture

of 5 volumes of chloroform R, 5 volumes of cyclohexane R, and 2 volumes of glacial acetic acid R as the mobile phase. Apply separately to the plate 20 µl of each of 2 solutions in acetone R containing (A) 20 mg of the test substance per ml and (B) 0.020 mg of the test substance per ml. After removing the plate from the chromatographic chamber, allow it to dry in air and immediately examine the chromatogram in ultraviolet light (254 nm). Any spot obtained with solution A, other than the principal spot, is not more intense than that obtained with solution B.

Absorbance in alkaline solution.   Dissolve 1.25 g, accurately weighed, in 10 ml of sodium hydroxide (50 g/l) TS, filter through a membrane filter, and, within 15 minutes, measure the absorbance of a 1-cm layer at the maximum at about 385 nm against a solvent cell containing sodium hydroxide (50 g/l) TS; not more than 0.3.

2-Propanol content.   Dissolve about 0.8 g, accurately weighed, in 25.0 ml of water. Add 25.0 ml of sulfuric acid (0.125 mol/l) VS while swirling, filter, and transfer 10 ml of the clear filtrate to a 250-ml flask containing 40 ml of water. Add some boiling chips, then 30 ml of potassium dichromate TS3, and connect the flask to a condenser by means of a 75° connecting tube. Distil 60 ml, collecting the distillate in 20 ml of sodium hydroxide ($\sim$80 g/l) TS contained in a 250-ml iodine flask immersed in an ice-bath. Add, with swirling, 20.0 ml of iodine (0.1 mol/l) VS, insert the stopper in the flask, and allow to stand for 30 minutes. Add 5 ml of hydrochloric acid ($\sim$420 g/l) TS through the well in the flask, rinse the well and the neck of the flask with water, swirl to mix, remove the stopper, and titrate the excess iodine with sodium thiosulfate (0.1 mol/l) VS, adding 3 ml of starch TS towards the end of the titration. Each ml of iodine (0.1 mol/l) VS is equivalent to 1.001 mg of 2-propanol. The amorphous substance contains not more than 3 mg per g and the crystalline clathrate contains between 43 and 83 mg of 2-propanol per g.

Assay.   Dissolve about 0.1 g, accurately weighed, in sufficient sodium hydroxide (0.01 mol/l) VS to produce 100 ml and dilute 10 ml to 1000 ml with sodium hydroxide (0.01 mol/l) VS. Measure the absorbance of a 1-cm layer of the diluted solution at the maximum at about 308 nm. Calculate the amount of $C_{19}H_{15}NaO_4$ in the substance being tested by comparison with warfarin RS, similarly and concurrently examined, taking into account that each mg of warfarin RS is equivalent to 1.071 mg of $C_{19}H_{15}NaO_4$. In an adequately calibrated spectrophotometer the absorbance of the reference solution should be 0.47 $\pm$ 0.03.

ZINCI OXYDUM

Zinc oxide

Molecular formula.   ZnO

Relative molecular mass.   81.38

Chemical name.   Zinc oxide; CAS Reg. No. 1314-13-2.

Description.   A white or faintly yellowish white, very fine, amorphous powder, free from grittiness; odourless.

Solubility.   Practically insoluble in water and ethanol ($\sim$750 g/l) TS; soluble in hydrochloric acid ($\sim$70 g/l) TS.

Category.   Mild astringent used topically as a protective.

Storage.   Zinc oxide should be kept in a well-closed container.

Additional information.   Zinc oxide gradually absorbs carbon dioxide from the air.

REQUIREMENTS

General requirement.   Zinc oxide contains not less than 99.0% and not more than 100.5% of ZnO, calculated with reference to the freshly ignited substance.

Identity tests

A.   Heat strongly a small amount of the substance; it assumes a yellow colour, which disappears on cooling.

B.   Dissolve 20 mg in 2.0 ml of hydrochloric acid ($\sim$70 g/l) TS, add 0.15 ml of potassium ferrocyanide (45 g/l) TS; a greenish white precipitate is formed.

Arsenic.   Use a solution of 1.6 g in 35 ml of hydrochloric acid ($\sim$70 g/l) TS and proceed as described under "Limit test for arsenic" (vol. 1, p. 122); the arsenic content is not more than 6 μg/g.

Carbonates and acid-insoluble substances.   Mix 2.0 g with 10 ml of water, add 30 ml of sulfuric acid ($\sim$100 g/l) TS, and heat on a water-bath with constant stirring; no effervescence occurs and the resulting solution is clear and colourless.

Iron.   Dissolve 0.20 g in 5 ml of hydrochloric acid ($\sim$250 g/l) TS and 30 ml of water. Treat the solution as described under "Limit test for iron" (vol. 1, p. 121); not more than 200 μg/g.

Lead.   Add 2 g to 20 ml of water, stir well, add 5 ml of glacial acetic acid R, and warm on a water-bath until solution is effected. Then add 0.25 ml of potassium chromate (100 g/l) TS; no turbidity or precipitate is produced.

Loss on ignition.   Ignite 1.0 g at 500 °C to constant weight; it loses not more than 10 mg/g.

Alkalinity.   Mix 1 g with 10 ml of hot water, add 0.1 ml of phenolphthalein/ethanol TS and filter; if the filtrate is red, not more than 0.3 ml of hydrochloric acid (0.1 mol/l) VS is required to discharge the colour.

Assay.   Dissolve about 0.15 g, accurately weighed, in 10 ml of acetic acid (~120 g/l) TS and proceed with the titration as described under "Complexometric titrations" for zinc (vol. 1, p. 129). Each ml of disodium edetate (0.05 mol/l) VS is equivalent to 4.069 mg of ZnO.

LIST OF REAGENTS, TEST SOLUTIONS, AND VOLUMETRIC SOLUTIONS

LIST OF REAGENTS, TEST SOLUTIONS, AND VOLUMETRIC SOLUTIONS

Attention is drawn to the notes at the head of the "List of reagents, test solutions, and volumetric solutions" published in volume 2. These contain explanations of the various abbreviations used.

Acacia R. The dried gummy exudate from the stems and branches of *Acacia senegal* (L.) Willd. and of other species of *Acacia* of African origin.

Description. Rounded or ovoid tears of varying diameters from about 1 cm to 3 cm; yellowish white or pale amber; odourless.

Solubility. Very slowly soluble in twice its weight of water, leaving only a very small residue of vegetable particles; practically insoluble in ethanol ($\sim$750 g/l) TS and ether R.

Ash. Not more than 50 mg/g.

Acid-insoluble ash. Not more than 5.0 mg/g.

Insoluble matter. Mix 5 g of powdered or finely ground material with 100 ml of water and 10 ml of hydrochloric acid ($\sim$70 g/l) TS and boil gently for 15 minutes, stirring frequently. Filter while hot through a sintered glass crucible, wash the residue with hot water, and dry to constant weight at 105 °C; not more than 5 mg/g.

Tannin. Dissolve 1 g in 10 ml of water and add 0.1 ml of ferric chloride (25 g/l) TS; no bluish black colour or blackish precipitate is produced.

Acacia (5 g/l) TS. A solution in water containing about 5 g of acacia R per litre.

p-**Acetamidobenzalazine RS.** International Chemical Reference Substance.

Acetate buffer, pH 4.5, TS.
Procedure. Dissolve 10.9 g of sodium acetate R in 100 ml of water, add 8 ml of glacial acetic acid R, mix, and dilute to 1000 ml with water.

Acetate buffer, pH 4.7, TS.
Procedure. Dissolve 8.4 g of sodium acetate R in 100 ml of water, add 3.35 ml of glacial acetic acid R, mix, and dilute to 1000 ml with water.

Acetate buffer, pH 5.0, TS.
Procedure. Dissolve 13.6 g of sodium acetate R in 100 ml of water, add 6 ml of glacial acetic acid R, mix, and dilute to 1000 ml with water.

Acetate buffer, pH 5.5, TS.
Procedure. Dissolve 54.4 g of sodium acetate R in 50 ml of water, heating to 35 °C, if necessary. After cooling, slowly add 10 ml of glacial acetic acid R. Shake and dilute to 1000 ml with water.

Acetic acid (~120 g/l) TS. Acetic acid (~300 g/l) TS, diluted with water to contain 120 g of $C_2H_4O_2$ per litre (approximately 2 mol/l); d~1.016.

Acetic acid (~90 g/l) TS. Acetic acid (~300 g/l) TS, diluted with water to contain about 90 g of $C_2H_4O_2$ per litre (approximately 1.5 mol/l).

Acetic acid (5.0 g/l) TS. Acetic acid (~300 g/l) TS, diluted with water to contain about 5.0 g of $C_2H_4O_2$ per litre; d~1.0007.

Amiloride hydrochloride RS. International Chemical Reference Substance.

4-Aminoantipyrine R. $C_{11}H_{13}N_3O$. 4-Amino-2,3-dimethyl-1-phenyl-3-pyrazolin-5-one; ampyrone; aminopyrazolone.
Description. Pale yellow crystals or powder.
Solubility. Sparingly soluble in water; freely soluble in ethanol (~750 g/l) TS; very slightly soluble in ether R.
Melting temperature. About 108 °C.

4-Aminoantipyrine TS1.
Procedure. Dissolve 0.125 g of 4-aminoantipyrine R in 25 ml of methanol R containing 0.25 ml of hydrochloric acid (~420 g/l) TS.

4-Aminoantipyrine TS2.
Procedure. Dissolve about 0.1 g of 4-aminoantipyrine R in 30 ml of water and add a mixture of 10 ml of sodium carbonate (200 g/l) TS and 2 ml of sodium hydroxide (1 mol/l) VS; dilute with sufficient water to produce 100 ml.
Note: 4-Aminoantipyrine TS2 must be freshly prepared.

2-Amino-5-nitrothiazole R. $C_3H_3N_3O_2S$.
Description. Greenish yellow to orange-yellow, fluffy powder.
Solubility. Very slightly soluble in water; soluble in dilute mineral acids; slightly soluble in ethanol (~750 g/l) TS and ether R; practically insoluble in chloroform R.
Melting temperature. About 198 °C with decomposition.

4-Aminophenol R. C_6H_7NO.
Description. A white or almost white, crystalline powder.
Melting temperature. About 184 °C with decomposition.

Ammonia (~50 g/l) TS. Ammonia (~260 g/l) TS, diluted with water to contain about 50 g of NH_3 per litre (approximately 3 mol/l); d~0.977.

Ammonia buffer TS2.
Procedure. Dissolve 67.5 g of ammonium chloride R in 650 ml of ammonia (~260 g/l) TS and dilute with water to produce 1000 ml.

Ammonium acetate (100 g/l) TS. A solution of ammonium acetate R containing 100 g of $C_2H_7NO_2$ per litre.

Ammonium acetate (40 g/l) TS. A solution of ammonium acetate R containing about 38.5 g of $C_2H_7NO_2$ per litre (approximately 0.5 mol/l).
Note: Ammonium acetate (40 g/l) TS must be freshly prepared.

Ammonium acetate (2 g/l) TS. A solution of ammonium acetate R containing about 2 g of $C_2H_7NO_2$ per litre.
Note: Ammonium acetate (2 g/l) TS must be freshly prepared.

Ammonium acetate buffer, pH 4.62, TS.
Procedure. Adjust the pH of ammonium acetate (100 g/l) TS to 4.62 using acetic acid (~60 g/l) TS.

Ammonium mercurithiocyanate TS.
Procedure. Dissolve 30 g of ammonium thiocyanate R and 27 g of mercuric chloride R in sufficient water to produce 1000 ml.

Ammonium molybdate/sulfuric acid TS.
Procedure. Dissolve 0.5 g of ammonium molybdate R in sufficient sulfuric acid (~1760 g/l) TS to produce 10 ml.

Ammonium molybdate/vanadate TS.
Procedure. Shake 4 g of finely powdered ammonium molybdate R and 0.1 g of finely powdered ammonium vanadate R with 70 ml of water. Add 20 ml of nitric acid (~1000 g/l) TS and dilute to 100 ml with water.

Ammonium persulfate R. $(NH_4)_2S_2O_8$ (SRIP, 1963, p. 37).

Ammonium persulfate/phosphate buffer TS.
Procedure. Dissolve 10 g of ammonium persulfate R in sufficient phosphate buffer, pH 7.4, TS to produce 100 ml.

Ammonium reineckate R. $NH_4[Cr(NH_3)_2(SCN)_4],H_2O$ (SRIP, 1963, p. 39).

Ammonium reineckate (10 g/l) TS.   A solution of ammonium reineckate R containing about 10 g of $NH_4[Cr(NH_3)_2(SCN)_4]$ per litre.

Ammonium sulfamate (50 g/l) TS.   A solution of ammonium sulfamate R containing 50 g of $NH_4OSO_2NH_2$ per litre.

Ammonium sulfide TS.
Procedure.   Prepare a saturated solution of hydrogen sulfide R in ammonia ($\sim$100 g/l) TS.   To 25 ml of this solution add 50 ml of ammonia ($\sim$100 g/l) TS.

Ammonium thiocyanate/cobalt(II) nitrate TS.
Procedure.   Dissolve 20 g of ammonium thiocyanate R and 5 g of cobalt(II) nitrate R in 100 ml of water.   Add sufficient sodium chloride R to saturate the solution.

Ammonium vanadate R. NH_4VO_3.
Description.   A white to slightly yellowish, crystalline powder.
Solubility.   Slightly soluble in water; soluble in ammonia ($\sim$100 g/l) TS.

Amodiaquine hydrochloride RS.   International Chemical Reference Substance.

Amphotericin B RS.   International Chemical Reference Substance (containing the declared content of tetraenes).

Anthrone R. $C_{14}H_{10}O$.
Description.   A pale yellow, crystalline powder.
Solubility.   Practically insoluble in water; slightly soluble in ethanol ($\sim$750 g/l) TS and in sulfuric acid ($\sim$100 g/l) TS.
Solubility in carbon tetrachloride R.   Add 0.5 g to 10 ml of carbon tetrachloride R; a clear, non-fluorescent solution is produced.
Melting range.   154–156 °C.

Anthrone TS.
Procedure.   Dissolve 35 mg of anthrone R in 100 ml of sulfuric acid ($\sim$1760 g/l) TS.

Azathioprine RS.   International Chemical Reference Substance.

Bacitracin zinc RS.   International Chemical Reference Substance.

Beclometasone dipropionate RS.   International Chemical Reference Substance.

Benzyl alcohol R. C_7H_8O.

Description.   A colourless liquid; almost odourless.

Miscibility.   Miscible with 25 parts of water; miscible with ethanol ($\sim 750\,g/l$) TS, chloroform R, and ether R.

Boiling temperature.   About 204 °C.

Mass density. ρ_{20} = about 1.05 kg/l.

Betamethasone valerate RS.   International Chemical Reference Substance.

Biperiden RS.   International Chemical Reference Substance.

Biperiden hydrochloride RS.   International Chemical Reference Substance.

2-Butanol R. $C_4H_{10}O$ (SRIP, 1963, p. 53).

Butyl acetate R. $C_6H_{12}O_2$.

Description.   A clear, colourless, flammable liquid; odour, characteristic.

Miscibility.   Slightly miscible with water; miscible with ethanol ($\sim 750\ g/l$) TS.

Mass density. ρ_{20} = about 0.88 kg/l.

Butylated hydroxytoluene R.   2,6-Di-*tert*-butyl-4-methylphenol, $C_{15}H_{24}O$.

Description.   Colourless crystals, or a white, crystalline powder.

Solubility.   Practically insoluble in water; freely soluble in ethanol ($\sim 750\ g/l$) TS; very soluble in ether R.

Melting temperature.   About 70 °C.

Sulfated ash.   Not more than 1.0 mg/g.

Calcium folinate RS.   International Chemical Reference Substance.

Calcium standard (100 µg/ml Ca), ethanolic, TS.

Procedure.   Dilute 100.0 ml of solution A, described under calcium standard (10 µg/ml Ca) TS, with sufficient ethanol ($\sim 750\ g/l$) TS to produce 1000 ml.

Calcium standard (10 µg/ml Ca) TS.

Procedure.   Dissolve 2.50 g of dried calcium carbonate R2 in 15 ml of acetic acid ($\sim 300\ g/l$) TS and dilute with water to 1000 ml (solution A). Dilute 10.0 ml of this solution with water to produce 1000 ml.

Calcium sulfate R. $CaSO_4,2H_2O$ (SRIP, 1963, p. 62).

Calcium sulfate, hemihydrate R.   Plaster of Paris, $CaSO_4,\tfrac{1}{2}H_2O$.

Description.   A white powder which, when mixed with half its weight of water, rapidly solidifies to a hard and porous mass.

Calcium sulfate TS.
Procedure.   Shake 5 g of calcium sulfate hemihydrate R for 1 hour with 100 ml of water and filter.

Carbamazepine RS.   International Chemical Reference Substance.

Carbidopa RS.   International Chemical Reference Substance.

Carboxymethylcellulose R.   A suitable grade for column chromatography.

Cephaëline hydrochloride R. $C_{28}H_{38}N_2O_4,2HCl,7H_2O$.
Description.   A white, crystalline powder.
Specific optical rotation.   Use a 20 mg/ml solution; $[\alpha]_D^{20\,°C} = +25°$.

Ceric sulfate (0.1 mol/l) VS.
Procedure.   Dissolve ceric sulfate R, equivalent to 33.23 g of $Ce(SO_4)$, in a mixture of 28 ml of sulfuric acid ($\sim$1760 g/l) TS and 500 ml of water, dilute to 1000 ml and mix. Allow the solution to stand for 48 hours and filter through a sintered glass filter.
Method of standardization.   Ascertain the exact concentration of the 0.1 mol/l solution in the following manner: Place about 25 ml, accurately measured, in a glass-stoppered flask, dilute with 80 ml of water, add 10 ml of phosphoric acid ($\sim$105 g/l) TS and 2.5 g of potassium iodide R, and allow the solution to stand for 15 minutes. Add 1 g of sodium carbonate R and titrate with sodium thiosulfate (0.1 mol/l) VS, using starch TS as indicator.

Chloramphenicol palmitate RS.   International Chemical Reference Substance.

Chloraniline R.   4-Chloroaniline, C_6H_6ClN.
Description.   White or faintly coloured crystals.
Melting temperature.   About 70 °C.

4-Chloroacetanilide R. C_8H_8ClNO.
Description.   Colourless, needle-shaped crystals or a white to pale yellow, crystalline powder.
Solubility.   Practically insoluble in water; soluble in ethanol ($\sim$750 g/l) TS and ether R.
Melting temperature.   About 180 °C.

Cimetidine RS.   International Chemical Reference Substance.

Cinchonine R. $C_{19}H_{22}N_2O$ (SRIP, 1963, p. 69).

Citric acid PbR.   Citric acid R free of lead.

Clofazimine RS.   International Chemical Reference Substance.

Clomifene citrate RS.   International Chemical Reference Substance.

Clomifene citrate Z-isomer RS.   International Chemical Reference Substance.

Cobalt(II) chloride R.   Cobaltous chloride; $CoCl_2,6H_2O$ (SRIP, 1963, p. 70).
The present text supersedes that published in volume 1, p. 174.

Cobalt(II) chloride (30 g/l) TS.   A solution of cobalt(II) chloride R containing about 30 g of $CoCl_2$ per litre.

Cobalt(II) chloride (5 g/l) TS.   A solution of cobalt(II) chloride R containing about 5 g of $CoCl_2$ per litre.

Cobalt(II) chloride TS.
  Procedure.   Dissolve 6.5 g of cobalt(II) chloride R in a sufficient quantity of a mixture of 2.5 ml of hydrochloric acid ($\sim$250 g/l) TS and 97.5 ml of water to produce 100 ml.
The present text supersedes that published in volume 2, p. 290.

Cobalt(II) nitrate R. $Co(NO_3)_2,6H_2O$.
Description.   Small red crystals.
Solubility.   Very soluble in water.

Cobalt(II) nitrate (100 g/l) TS.   A solution of cobalt(II) nitrate R containing about 100 g of $Co(NO_3)_2$ per litre.

Cobalt(II) nitrate (10 g/l) TS.
Procedure.   Dissolve about 1.6 g of cobalt(II) nitrate R in sufficient water to produce 100 ml.

Colchicine RS.   International Chemical Reference Substance.

Copper(II) acetate (45 g/l) TS.   A solution of copper(II) acetate R containing about 50 g of $C_4H_6CuO_4,H_2O$ per litre.

Copper(II) chloride R. $CuCl_2,2H_2O$.
Description.   Bluish green, deliquescent crystals.
Solubility.   Freely soluble in water; soluble in ethanol ($\sim$750 g/l) TS; slightly soluble in ether R.

Copper(II) chloride/ammonia TS.
Procedure.   Dissolve 22.5 g of copper(II) chloride R in 200 ml of water and add 100 ml of ammonia ($\sim$260 g/l) TS.

Copper standard (10 µg/ml Cu) TS.
Procedure. Dissolve 0.393 g of copper(II) sulfate R in sufficient water to produce 100 ml and dilute 10.0 ml of this solution to produce 1000 ml

Copper standard TS1.
Procedure. Dissolve 1.965 g of copper(II) sulfate R, accurately weighed, in sufficient hydrochloric acid (0.1 mol/l) VS to produce 1000 ml.

Copper standard TS2.
Procedure. Transfer 3.0 ml of copper standard TS1 to a 1000-ml flask and dilute with hydrochloric acid (0.1 mol/l) VS to produce 1000 ml. This solution contains 1.5 µg of Cu per ml.

Copper(II) sulfate (1 g/l) TS. A solution of copper(II) sulfate R containing 1 g of $CuSO_4$ per litre.

Cresol red R. $C_{21}H_{18}O_5S$.
Description. A red-brown powder.
Solubility. Slightly soluble in water; soluble in ethanol ($\sim$750 g/l) TS and in dilute solutions of alkali hydroxides.

Cresol red/ethanol TS.
Procedure. Warm 0.05 g of cresol red R with 2.65 ml of sodium hydroxide (0.05 mol/l) VS and 5 ml of ethanol ($\sim$710 g/l) TS; after solution has been effected, add sufficient ethanol ($\sim$150 g/l) TS to produce 250 ml.

Culture medium Cm8
Procedure. Dissolve 10 g of dried peptone R, 10 g of beef extract R, 10 g of glycerol R, 3.0 g of sodium chloride R, and 17 g of agar R in sufficient water to produce 1000 ml. Adjust the pH with sodium hydroxide (0.05 mol/l) VS to 6.9–7.1, and sterilize in an autoclave at 121 °C for 18–20 minutes.

Culture medium Cm9.
Procedure. Dissolve 10 g of dried peptone R, 10 g of beef extract R, 10 g of glycerol R, and 3.0 g of sodium chloride R in sufficient water to produce 1000 ml. Adjust the pH with sodium hydroxide (0.05 mol/l) VS to 6.9–7.1, and sterilize in an autoclave at 121 °C for 18–20 minutes.

Culture medium Cm10.
Procedure. Dissolve 1 g of water-soluble yeast extract R, 5 g of ammonium nitrate R, 5 g of sodium dihydrogen phosphate R, 5 g of anhydrous glucose R, and 14 g of agar R in sufficient water to produce 1000 ml.

Culture medium Cm11.

Procedure.   Dissolve 10 g of dried peptone R, 6 g of beef extract R, and 15 g of agar R in sufficient water to produce 1000 ml. Adjust the pH of the solution with sodium hydroxide (1 mol/l) VS, if necessary, so that the pH of the final and sterilized medium will be 7.8. Filter, if necessary to clarify, distribute the solution into suitable vessels and sterilize in an autoclave at 121 °C for 18–20 minutes.

Cytarabine RS.   International Chemical Reference Substance.

Dexamethasone sodium phosphate RS.   International Chemical Reference Substance.

Dextromethorphan hydrobromide RS.   International Chemical Reference Substance.

Diatomaceous support R.

Description.   White granules of silica consisting chiefly of the skeletons of diatoms. The material is flux-calcined to sequester coloured metallic oxides in a colourless form, and is supplied commercially in various forms, such as: acid-washed, silanized, and alkali-washed.

Dichlorofluorescein R. $C_{20}H_{10}Cl_2O_5$.

Description.   A light orange-coloured, crystalline powder.

Solubility.   Sparingly soluble in water; soluble in ethanol (~750 g/l) TS.

Dichlorofluorescein TS.

Procedure.   Dissolve 0.2 g of dichlorofluorescein R in 100 ml of methanol R.

Dicloxacillin sodium RS.   International Chemical Reference Substance.

Diethylaminoethylcellulose R.   A suitable grade for column chromatography.

Diethyl phthalate R. $C_{12}H_{14}O_4$.

Mass density. ρ_{20} = about 1.117 kg/l.

Refractive index. n_D^{20} = 1.500–1.505.

Diloxanide furoate RS.   International Chemical Reference Substance.

Dimethylacetamide R. C_4H_9NO.

Description.   A colourless liquid.

Boiling temperature.   About 165 °C.

Mass density. ρ_{20} = 0.94 kg/l.

4-Dimethylaminobenzaldehyde TS5.

Procedure. Dissolve without heating 2 g of 4-dimethylaminobenzaldehyde R in a mixture of 45 ml of water and 55 ml of hydrochloric acid ($\sim$420 g/l) TS.

4-Dimethylaminobenzaldehyde TS6.

Procedure. Dissolve 0.2 g of 4-dimethylaminobenzaldehyde R in 20 ml of ethanol ($\sim$750 g/l) TS and add 0.5 ml of hydrochloric acid ($\sim$420 g/l) TS. Shake the solution with charcoal R and filter. The colour of this test solution is less intense than that of iodine (0.0001 mol/l) VS.

Note: 4-Dimethylaminobenzaldehyde TS6 must be freshly prepared.

N,N-**Dimethylaniline R.** $C_8H_{11}N$.

Description. A colourless liquid darkening on storage.

Miscibility. Practically immiscible with water, miscible with ethanol ($\sim$750 g/l) TS, chloroform R, and ether R.

Boiling point. About 193 °C.

Mass density. ρ_{20} = 0.96 kg/l.

Dimethyl sulfoxide R. C_2H_6OS.

Description. A colourless liquid; odourless or with a slight, but unpleasant odour.

Mass density. ρ_{20} = 1.10 kg/l.

2,4-Dinitrochlorobenzene R. $C_6H_4ClN_2O_4$ (SRIP, 1963, p. 80).

Diphenoxylate hydrochloride RS. International Chemical Reference Substance.

Diphenylamine/sulfuric acid TS.

Procedure. Dissolve 1.0 g of diphenylamine R in 100 ml of sulfuric acid ($\sim$1760 g/l) TS.

Storage. Diphenylamine/sulfuric acid TS must be colourless and should be kept protected from light.

1,5-Diphenylcarbazide R. $C_{13}H_{14}N_4O$.

Description. A white, crystalline powder, gradually turning pink on exposure to air.

Melting point. About 174 °C.

Diphenylcarbazide TS.

Procedure. Dissolve 0.2 g of 1,5-diphenylcarbazide R in a mixture of 10 ml of glacial acetic acid R and 90 ml of ethanol ($\sim$710 g/l) TS.

Sensitivity test to chromate. Dilute 0.5 ml of potassium dichromate (0.0167 mol/l) VS with water to 1000 ml. Dilute 5 ml of this solution to 50 ml with water, add 0.2 ml of hydrochloric acid (2 mol/l) VS and 0.5 ml of diphenylcarbazide TS; a reddish violet colour is produced.

Disodium edetate (20 g/l) TS. A solution of disodium edetate R containing about 20 g of $C_{10}H_{14}N_2Na_2O_8$ per litre.

Disodium edetate (10 g/l) TS. A solution of disodium edetate R containing about 10 g of $C_{10}H_{14}N_2Na_2O_8$ per litre.

Disodium edetate (0.01 mol/l) VS. Disodium edetate R, dissolved in water to contain 3.342 g of $C_{10}H_{14}N_2Na_2O_8$ in 1000 ml.
Method of standardization. Ascertain the exact concentration of the solution following an appropriate method, e.g., as described under disodium edetate (0.05 mol/l) VS in volume 1, p. 179.

Disodium hydrogen phosphate (100 g/l) TS. A solution of disodium hydrogen phosphate R containing about 100 g of Na_2HPO_4 per litre.

Disodium hydrogen phosphate (28.4 g/l) TS. A solution of anhydrous disodium hydrogen phosphate R containing 28.4 g of Na_2HPO_4 per litre.

Dithizone standard TS.
Procedure. Dissolve 10 mg of dithizone R in 1000 ml of chloroform R.
Storage. Store the solution in a glass-stoppered, lead-free bottle, protected from light, and kept at a temperature not exceeding 4 °C.

Dithizone TS.
Procedure. Dissolve 0.10 g of dithizone R in sufficient ethanol (~750 g/l) TS to produce 100 ml.

Dopamine hydrochloride RS. International Chemical Reference Substance.

Doxorubicin hydrochloride RS. International Chemical Reference Substance.

Emetine hydrochloride RS. International Chemical Reference Substance.

Eosin Y R. Sodium tetrabromofluorescein; $C_{20}H_6Br_4N_2O_5$.
Description. Red to brownish lumps or a powder.
Solubility. Freely soluble in water; sparingly soluble in ethanol (~750 g/l) TS.

Eosin Y (5 g/l) TS. A solution of eosin Y R containing about 5 g of $C_{20}H_6Br_4Na_2O_5$ per litre.

Ergocalciferol RS. International Chemical Reference Substance.

Ergosterol R. Provitamin D_2; ergosta-5,7,22-trien-3-ol; $C_{28}H_{44}O$. Contains not less than 95.0% of $C_{28}H_{44}O$.
Description. White or almost white needles or a crystalline powder.
Melting temperature. About 163 °C.
Specific optical rotation. Use a 20 mg/ml solution in chloroform R; $[\alpha]_D^{20\,°C} = -133°$.

Erythromycin RS. International Chemical Reference Substance.

Erythromycin ethylsuccinate RS. International Chemical Reference Substance.

Erythromycin stearate RS. International Chemical Reference Substance.

Ethionamide RS. International Chemical Reference Substance.

Ethylene glycol monomethyl ether R. 2-Methoxyethanol; $C_3H_8O_2$.
Description. A colourless liquid.
Boiling temperature. About 125 °C.
Mass density. ρ_{20} = about 0.96 kg/l.

Ferric ammonium sulfate (0.1 mol/l) VS. Ferric ammonium sulfate R, dissolved in a mixture of sulfuric acid ($\sim$1760 g/l) TS and water to contain 48.22 g of $FeNH_4(SO_4)_2,12H_2O$ in 1000 ml.
Procedure. Dissolve 50 g of ferric ammonium sulfate R in a mixture of 300 ml of water and 6 ml of sulfuric acid ($\sim$1760 g/l) TS. Dilute with sufficient water to produce 1000 ml.
Method of standardization. Ascertain the exact concentration of the 0.1 mol/l solution in the following manner: Transfer 25 ml to a glass-stoppered flask and add 3 ml of hydrochloric acid ($\sim$420 g/l) TS and 2 g of potassium iodide R. Allow the solution to stand for 10 minutes and titrate the liberated iodine with sodium thiosulfate (0.1 mol/l) VS, using starch TS as indicator. Perform a blank determination and make any necessary corrections.
Storage. Store this solution in a tightly closed container, protected from light.

Ferric chloride (65 g/l) TS. A solution of ferric chloride R containing about 65 g of $FeCl_3$ per litre.

Ferric chloride (50 g/l) TS.   A solution of ferric chloride R containing about 50 g of $FeCl_3$ per litre.

Ferric chloride/ferricyanide/arsenite TS.
Procedure.   Prepare 3 separate solutions:
(1)   Dissolve 2.7 g of ferric chloride R in 100 ml of hydrochloric acid ($\sim$70 g/l) TS.
(2)   Dissolve 3.5 g of potassium ferricyanide R in 100 ml of water. This solution should be freshly prepared.
(3)   Dissolve 3.8 g of arsenic trioxide R in 25 ml of hot sodium hydroxide ($\sim$80 g/l) TS. Allow to cool, add 50 ml of sulfuric acid ($\sim$100 g/l) TS, and dilute to 100 ml with water.
Immediately before use mix 5 volumes of solution (1), 5 volumes of solution (2), and 1 volume of solution (3).

Ferric chloride/potassium ferricyanide TS.
Procedure.   Dissolve 2 g of ferric chloride R and 0.10 g of potassium ferricyanide R in sufficient water to produce 20 ml.
Note.   Ferric chloride/potassium ferricyanide TS must be freshly prepared.

Ferricyanide standard (50 µg/ml) TS
Procedure.   Prepare a solution of potassium ferricyanide R in water to contain 7.8 g of $K_3Fe(CN)_6$ per 100 ml. Dilute 1.0 ml of this solution with sufficient water to produce 1000 ml.
Note.   Ferricyanide standard (50 µg/ml) TS must be freshly prepared.

Ferrocyanide standard (100 µg/ml) TS.
Procedure.   Prepare a solution of potassium ferrocyanide R in water to contain 2.0 g of $K_4Fe(CN)_6,3H_2O$ per 100 ml. Dilute 1.0 ml of this solution with sufficient water to produce 100.0 ml.
Note.   Ferrocyanide standard (100 µg/ml) TS must be freshly prepared.

Flucytosine RS.   International Chemical Reference Substance.

Fludrocortisone acetate RS.   International Chemical Reference Substance.

Fluorouracil RS.   International Chemical Reference Substance.

3-Formylrifamycin SV RS.   International Chemical Reference Substance.

Fuchsin, decolorized, TS.
Procedure.   Dissolve 1 g of basic fuchsin R in 600 ml of water and cool in an ice-bath; add 20 g of sodium sulfite R dissolved in 100 ml of water; cool in an ice-bath and add slowly, with constant stirring, 10 ml of hydrochloric acid

($\sim$250 g/l) TS; dilute with water to 1000 ml. If the resulting solution is turbid, it should be filtered and, if brown in colour, it should be shaken with sufficient charcoal R (0.2–0.3 g) to render it colourless, and then filtered immediately. Occasionally, it is necessary to add 2–3 ml of hydrochloric acid ($\sim$250 g/l) TS, followed by shaking, to remove a little residual pink colour. The solution resulting from any of the foregoing modifications should be allowed to stand overnight before use. Decolorized fuchsin TS should be protected from light.

Gallamine triethiodide RS. International Chemical Reference Substance.

Gentamicin sulfate RS. International Chemical Reference Substance.

Glibenclamide RS. International Chemical Reference Substance.

Glucose, anhydrous, R. $C_6H_{12}O_6$. Use anhydrous glucose as described in the monograph in volume 2, p. 135.

Heptane R. C_7H_{16} (SRIP, 1963, p. 94).

Hexamethyldisilazane R. $C_6H_{19}NSi_2$.
Description. A clear, colourless liquid, having a characteristic odour.
Mass density. ρ_{20} = about 0.77 kg/l.

Hydrazine sulfate R. $(NH_4)_2,H_2SO_4$.
Description. Colourless crystals or a white, crystalline powder.
Solubility. Soluble in about 40 parts of water; practically insoluble in ethanol ($\sim$750 g/l) TS.
Arsenic. Use a solution of 10 g in 35 ml of boiling water and proceed as described under "Limit test for arsenic" (vol. 1, p. 122); not more than 1 µg/g.
Sulfated ash. Not more than 1.0 mg/g.

Hydrochloric acid ($\sim$330 g/l) TS. A solution of hydrochloric acid ($\sim$420 g/l) TS in water, containing approximately 330 g of HCl per litre; $d\sim$1.15 (about 9 mol/l).

Hydrochloric acid (0.05 mol/l) VS. Hydrochloric acid ($\sim$250 g/l) TS, diluted with water to contain 1.824 g of HCl in 1000 ml.
Method of standardization. Ascertain the exact concentration of the solution following the method described under hydrochloric acid (1 mol/l) VS, volume 1, p. 184.

Hydrochloric acid (0.005 mol/l) VS.   Hydrochloric acid ($\sim$250 g/l) TS, diluted with water to contain 0.1824 g of HCl in 1000 ml.
Method of standardization.   Ascertain the exact concentration of the solution following the method described under hydrochloric acid (1 mol/l) VS, volume 1, p. 184.

Hydrochloric acid (0.0001 mol/l) VS.   Hydrochloric acid ($\sim$250 g/l) TS, diluted with water to contain 3.647 mg of HCl in 1000 ml.
Method of standardization.   Ascertain the exact concentration of the solution following the method described under hydrochloric acid (1 mol/l) VS, volume 1, p. 184.

Hydrochloric acid/methanol (0.01 mol/l) VS.   Hydrochloric acid ($\sim$250 g/l) TS, diluted with methanol R to contain 0.3647 g of HCl in 1000 ml of methanol R.
Method of standardization.   Ascertain the exact concentration of the solution following the method described under hydrochloric acid (1 mol/l) VS, volume 1, p. 184.

Hydrocortisone sodium succinate RS.   International Chemical Reference Substance.

Hydroquinone R. $C_6H_4(OH)_2$.
Description.   Colourless or almost colourless crystals or a crystalline powder.
Solubility.   Soluble in water, ethanol ($\sim$750 g/l) TS, and ether R.
Melting temperature.   About 173 °C.
Note.   Hydroquinone R darkens on exposure to air and light.

Hydroxylamine hydrochloride (200 g/l) TS.   A solution of hydroxylamine hydrochloride R containing about 200 g of NH_2OH,HCl per litre.

(–)-3-(4-Hydroxy-3-methoxyphenyl)-2-hydrazino-2-methylalanine RS.   International Chemical Reference Substance.

Iminodibenzyl R.   10,11-Dihydro-5*H*-dibenz[*b,f*]azepine; $C_{14}H_{13}N$.
Description.   A pale yellow, crystalline powder.
Melting temperature.   About 106 °C.

pH-Indicator paper R.   A paper impregnated with a suitable mixture of colour indicators such that the changes in colour permit estimation of the pH of a solution with an adequate sensitivity (usually 1 pH unit), at least in the pH range 1–10.

Iodine/chloroform TS.
Procedure.   Dissolve 5.0 g of iodine R in sufficient chloroform R to produce 100 ml.

Iodine (0.05 mol/l) VS.   Iodine R and potassium iodide R, dissolved in water to contain 12.69 g of I and 18.0 g of KI in 1000 ml.
Method of standardization.   Ascertain the exact concentration of the solution following the method described under iodine (0.1 mol/l) VS, volume 1, p. 185.

Iodine (0.005 mol/l) VS.   Iodine R and potassium iodide R, dissolved in water to contain 1.269 g of I and 1.80 g of KI in 1000 ml.
Method of standardization.   Ascertain the exact concentration of the solution following the method described under iodine (0.1 mol/l) VS, volume 1, p. 185.

Iodine (0.0001 mol/l) VS.   Iodine R and potassium iodide R, dissolved in water to contain 25.38 mg of I and 0.36 mg of KI in 1000 ml.
Method of standardization.   Ascertain the exact concentration of the solution following the method described under iodine (0.1 mol/l) VS, volume 1, p. 185.

Iron salicylate TS.
Procedure.   Dissolve 0.5 g of ferric ammonium sulfate R in 250 ml of water containing 10 ml of sulfuric acid ($\sim$100 g/l) TS and dilute with sufficient water to produce 500 ml. To 100 ml of this solution add 50 ml of sodium salicylate (11.5 g/l) TS, 20 ml of acetic acid ($\sim$60 g/l) TS and 80 ml of sodium acetate (150 g/l) TS, and dilute with water to 500 ml.
Storage.   Store in a well-closed container, protected from light.
Note.   Iron salicylate must be freshly prepared.

Isopropylamine R. C_3H_9N.
Description.   A colourless, volatile liquid with an ammoniacal odour.
Boiling point.   About 33 °C.
Mass density. ρ_{20} = about 0.69 kg/l.

Lead acetate paper R.
Procedure.   Dip white filter-paper into a mixture of 10 volumes of lead acetate (80 g/l) TS and 1 volume of acetic acid ($\sim$60 g/l) TS. Allow to dry and cut the paper into strips measuring 15 mm $\times$ 40 mm.
Storage.   Lead acetate paper R should be kept in a well-closed container.

Lead nitrate (100 g/l) TS.   A solution of lead nitrate R containing 100 g of $Pb(NO_3)_2$ per litre.

Lead(IV) oxide R. PbO_2 (SRIP, 1963, p. 105).

Levonorgestrel RS.   International Chemical Reference Substance.

Levothyroxine sodium RS.   International Chemical Reference Substance.

Liothyronine RS.   International Chemical Reference Substance.

Lithium carbonate R. Li_2CO_3.
Description.   A white, granular powder; odourless.
Solubility.   Sparingly soluble in water; very slightly soluble in ethanol
($\sim$750 g/l) TS.

Lithium carbonate/trinitrophenol TS.
Procedure.   Dissolve 0.25 g of lithium carbonate R and 0.5 g of trinitrophenol
R in sufficient water to produce 100 ml.

Lithium chloride R.   LiCl.
Description.   White, deliquescent crystals or granules.
Solubility.   Freely soluble in water; soluble in acetone R, ethanol ($\sim$750 g/l)
TS, and ether R.
Storage.   Store in a tightly closed container.

Lithium chloride (10 g/l) TS.   A solution of lithium chloride R containing about
10 g of LiCl per litre.

Loperamide hydrochloride RS.   International Chemical Reference Substance.

Macrogol 1000 R.
Description.   A white, waxy mass.
Viscosity.   At 100 °C, about 17.3 mm^{2}s^{-1}.

Macrogol *p*-isooctylphenyl ether R. $C_{34}H_{62}O_{11}$, *p-tert*-octylphenoxy polyethoxy-
ethanol. Use a suitable grade for the "Sterility testing of antibiotics".

Magnesium acetate R. $C_4H_6MgO_4,4H_2O$.
Description.   Colourless crystals. Deliquescent.
Solubility.   Freely soluble in water and ethanol ($\sim$750 g/l) TS.

Magnesium chloride R. $MgCl_2,6H_2O$ (SRIP, 1963, p. 110).

Magnesium chloride (0.1 mol/l) VS.
Procedure.   Dissolve 20.5 g of magnesium chloride R in sufficient water to
produce 1000 ml.

Method of standardization. Ascertain the exact concentration of the 0.1 mol/l solution, carrying out the complexometric titration of magnesium (vol. 1, p. 129) using 25 ml of magnesium chloride solution. Each ml of disodium edetate (0.1 mol/l) VS is equivalent to 20.33 mg of $MgCl_2,6H_2O$.

Magnesium (0.1 mg/ml Mg) TS.
Procedure. Dissolve 1.014 g of magnesium sulfate R in water, add 5 ml of sulfuric acid ($\sim$100 g/l) TS and dilute with water to 1000 ml.

Magnesium standard (10 µg/ml Mg) TS.
Procedure. Dilute 10 ml of magnesium (0.1 mg/ml) TS with sufficient water to produce 100 ml.

Magnesium sulfate/sulfuric acid TS.
Procedure. Dissolve 25 g of magnesium sulfate R in sufficient sulfuric acid ($\sim$100 g/l) TS to produce 100 ml.

Mebendazole RS. International Chemical Reference Substance.

Menadione R. 2-Methyl-1,4-naphthoquinone, $C_{11}H_8O_2$.
Description. Bright yellow crystals.
Melting temperature. About 106 °C.

Mercuric chloride/ethanol TS.
Procedure. Dissolve 2 g of mercuric chloride R in sufficient ethanol ($\sim$375 g/l) TS to produce 100 ml.

Mercuric nitrate TS.
Procedure. Dissolve 40 g of yellow mercuric oxide R in a mixture of 32 ml of nitric acid ($\sim$1000 g/l) TS and 15 ml of water.
Storage. Keep in a container protected from light.

Mercuric nitrate (0.02 mol/l) VS.
Procedure. Weigh accurately about 6.85 g of mercuric nitrate R, dissolve in a mixture of 10 ml of nitric acid ($\sim$130 g/l) TS and 500 ml of water, and dilute with water to 1000 ml.
Method of standardization. Ascertain the exact concentration of the 0.02 mol/l solution following the method described under mercuric nitrate (0.01 mol/l) VS, volume 1, p. 190.

Mercury/nitric acid TS.
Procedure. Dissolve 3 ml of mercury R in 27 ml of cold fuming nitric acid R and dilute the solution with an equal volume of water.
Storage. The solution should be stored, protected from light, and for not more than 2 months.

Methotrexate RS.   International Chemical Reference Substance.

Metoclopramide hydrochloride RS.   International Chemical Reference Substance.

Miconazole nitrate RS.   International Chemical Reference Substance.

Molybdenum trioxide R. MoO_3 (SRIP, 1963, p. 120).

Monoethanolamine R. C_2H_7NO.
Description.   A clear, colourless to faintly yellow, viscous liquid; odour, ammoniacal.
Miscibility.   Miscible with water, methanol R, and acetone R.
Boiling temperature.   About 170 °C.
Mass density. $\rho_{20} = 1.01$ kg/l.
Refractive index. $n_D^{20} = 1.453–1.455$.

Naloxone hydrochloride RS.   International Chemical Reference Substance.

Neamine RS.   International Chemical Reference Substance.

Neomycin B sulfate RS.   International Chemical Reference Substance.

Neostigmine metilsulfate RS.   International Chemical Reference Substance.

Neutral red R.   C.I. 50040; C.I. Basic Red; $C_{15}H_{17}ClN_4$ (SRIP, 1963, p. 124).

Neutral red/ethanol TS.
Procedure.   Dissolve 0.1 g of neutral red R in sufficient ethanol (~375 g/l) TS to produce 100 ml.

Nifurtimox RS.   International Chemical Reference Substance.

Niridazole RS.   International Chemical Reference Substance.

Niridazole-chlorethylcarboxamide RS.   International Chemical Reference Substance.

Nitrofurantoin RS.   International Chemical Reference Substance.

Nitromethane R. CH_3NO_2.
Description.   A colourless, oily liquid.
Miscibility.   Miscible with water, ethanol (~750 g/l) TS, ether R, and dimethylformamide R.

Mass density. ρ_{20} = about 1.13 kg/l.
Refractive index. n_D^{22}= about 1.380.
Boiling temperature.   About 101 °C.

Noroxymorphone hydrochloride RS.   (−)-4,5α-Epoxy-3,14-dihydroxymorphinan-6-one hydrochloride. International Chemical Reference Substance.

Noscapine RS.   International Chemical Reference Substance.

Nystatin RS.   International Chemical Reference Substance.

Octanoic acid R.   Caprylic acid, $C_8H_{16}O_2$.
Description.   A colourless, oily liquid.
Boiling temperature.   About 237 °C.
Mass density. ρ_{20} = about 0.92 kg/l.

Oracet blue B R.   Solvent blue 19; a mixture of 1-methylamino-4-anilinoanthra-quinone ($C_{21}H_{16}N_2O_2$) and 1-amino-4-anilinoanthraquinine ($C_{20}H_{14}N_2O_2$).

Oracet blue B/acetic acid TS.
Procedure.   Dissolve 0.5 g of oracet blue B R in sufficient glacial acetic acid R1 to produce 100 ml.

Oxalic acid R. $C_2H_2O_4,2H_2O$ (SRIP, 1963, p. 131).

Oxalic acid (0.05 g/l) TS.   A solution of oxalic acid R containing 0.05 g of $C_2H_2O_4$ in 1000 ml.
Procedure.   Dissolve 0.07 g of oxalic acid R in sufficient water to produce 1000 ml.

Oxamniquine RS.   International Chemical Reference Substance.

Oxytetracycline dihydrate RS.   International Chemical Reference Substance.

Paracetamol, 4-aminophenol-free, R.   Paracetamol as described in the monograph, p. 237, or paracetamol recrystallized from water until it complies with the following test:
Dissolve 5 g of the dried material in a mixture of equal volumes of methanol R and water and dilute to 100 ml with this solvent mixture. Add 1.0 ml of alkaline sodium nitroprusside TS, mix, and allow to stand for 30 minutes; no blue or green colour is produced.

Paraformaldehyde R. $(CH_2O)_n$.
Description.   A white, crystalline powder; odour, characteristic of formal-dehyde.

Solubility. Slowly soluble in cold water, freely soluble in hot water, with evolution of formaldehyde; practically insoluble in ethanol ($\sim$750 g/l) TS and ether R.

Solubility in ammonia. Dissolve 1 g in 10 ml of ammonia ($\sim$100 g/l) TS; a practically clear and colourless solution is produced.

Sulfated ash. Not more than 1.0 mg/g.

Acidity or alkalinity. Shake 1 g with 20 ml of water for 1 minute and filter; the filtrate is neutral to litmus paper R.

Paromomycin sulfate RS. International Chemical Reference Substance.

1-Pentanesulfonic acid sodium salt R. $C_5H_{11}NaO_3S,H_2O$.

Description. A white, crystalline powder.

Solubility. Soluble in water.

Clarity and colour of solution. A solution of 1 g in 25 ml of water is clear and colourless.

Water. Determined by the Karl Fischer method; not more than 20 mg/g.

1-Pentanesulfonic acid TS.

Procedure. Dissolve 0.960 g of 1-pentanesulfonic acid sodium salt R in 1000 ml of deaerated acetic acid (5.0 g/l) TS and adjust the pH to 4.3 with ammonia ($\sim$260 g/l) TS. Filter and deaerate before use.

Perchloric acid/dioxan (0.1 mol/l) VS.

Procedure. Mix 8.5 ml of perchloric acid ($\sim$1170 g/l) TS with sufficient dioxan R, which has been especially purified by adsorption, to produce 1000 ml.

Method of standardization. Ascertain the exact concentration of the solution by titrating 0.7 g of potassium hydrogen phthalate R, accurately weighed and previously dried at 120 °C for 2 hours, using Method A, as described under "Non-aqueous titration" (vol. 1, p. 131). Each ml of perchloric acid/dioxan (0.1 mol/l) VS is equivalent to 20.42 mg of $C_8H_5KO_4$.

Perchloric acid (0.02 mol/l) VS.

Procedure. Dilute 20 ml of perchloric acid (0.1 mol/l) VS with sufficient glacial acetic acid R1 to produce 100 ml.

Water and method of standardization. Immediately before use determine the content of water and ascertain the exact concentration of the solution following the methods described under perchloric acid (0.1 mol/l) VS, volume 1, p. 194.

1,4-Phenylenediamine dihydrochloride R. $C_6H_8N_2,2HCl$.

Description. A white to pale tan, crystalline powder, turning pink on exposure to air.

Solubility. Freely soluble in water; slightly soluble in ethanol ($\sim$750 g/l) TS and ether R.

Storage. Keep in a well-closed container, protected from light.

Phenylhydrazine/hydrochloric acid TS.
Procedure. Dissolve 0.75 g of phenylhydrazine hydrochloride R in 50 ml of water and shake with 2 g of charcoal R. Filter, add 25 ml of hydrochloric acid ($\sim$420 g/l) TS and sufficient water to produce 200 ml.

Phenylhydrazine hydrochloride (10 g/l) TS. A solution of phenylhydrazine hydrochloride R containing 10 g of $C_6H_8N_2,HCl$ in 1000 ml.

Phenyl/methylpolysiloxane R. A suitable grade of a mixture to be used in gas chromatography composed of 5 g of phenylpolysiloxane and 95 g of methyl-polysiloxane per 100 g.

Phosphate buffer, pH 7.4, TS.
Procedure. Dissolve 6.8 g of potassium dihydrogen phosphate R in 250 ml of water and add 393.4 ml of sodium hydroxide (0.1 mol/l) VS.

Phosphate buffer, pH 7.6, TS.
Procedure. Place 1.36 g of potassium dihydrogen phosphate R in a 200-ml volumetric flask, dissolve it in water, add 42.4 ml of sodium hydroxide (0.2 mol/l) VS, and dilute to volume with water.

Phosphate buffer, pH 8.0, TS.
Procedure. Dissolve 8.95 g of anhydrous disodium hydrogen phosphate R and 0.50 g of potassium dihydrogen phosphate R in sufficient water to produce 1000 ml.

Phosphate buffer, sterile, pH 7.8, TS.
Procedure. Dissolve 6.8 g of potassium dihydrogen phosphate R in water, add 45.2 ml of sodium hydroxide (1 mol/l) VS and sufficient water to produce 1000 ml. If necessary, adjust the pH to 7.8 with phosphoric acid ($\sim$1440 g/l) TS or potassium hydroxide ($\sim$110 g/l) TS and then sterilize the solution for 20 minutes in an autoclave at 120 °C.

Phosphate buffer, sterile, pH 10.5, TS1.
Procedure. Dissolve 35.0 g of dipotassium hydrogen phosphate R in water, add 20 ml of sodium hydroxide (1 mol/l) VS and sufficient water to produce 1000 ml. If necessary, adjust the pH to 10.5 with phosphoric acid ($\sim$1440 g/l) TS or potassium hydroxide ($\sim$110 g/l) TS and then sterilize the solution for 20 minutes in an autoclave at 120 °C.

Phosphate/citrate buffer pH 6.0, TS.
Procedure. Dissolve 4.52 g of disodium hydrogen phosphate R in 60 ml of water, add 35 ml of citric acid (20 g/l) TS, and, if necessary, adjust the pH of the solution to 6.0.

Phosphate standard (5 µg/ml) TS.
Procedure. Dissolve 0.716 g of potassium dihydrogen phosphate R in sufficient water to produce 1000 ml. Immediately before use dilute 1 ml to 100 ml with water.

Phosphoric acid ($\sim$105 g/l) TS.
Procedure. Mix about 115 g of phosphoric acid ($\sim$1440 g/l) TS with 885 g of water.

Phosphotungstic acid TS.
Procedure. Dissolve 25 g of sodium tungstate R in 175 ml of water and add 18.75 ml of phosphoric acid ($\sim$1440 g/l) TS. Heat under a reflux condenser for 6 hours, filter, and add sufficient water to produce 250 ml.
Storage. Store at a temperature between 2 and 8 °C, protected from light.

Piperidine R. $C_5H_{11}N$.
Description. A colourless to yellowish liquid; odour, characteristic.
Miscibility. Miscible with water and ethanol ($\sim$750 g/l) TS.
Mass density. ρ_{20} = about 0.86 kg/l.
Refractive index. n_D^{20} = about 1.454.
Boiling temperature. About 106 °C.
Congealing temperature. Between 12 and 15 °C.

Potassium antimonate R. $KSbO_3$ (SRIP, 1963, p. 145).

Potassium antimonate TS.
Procedure. Boil 2 g of potassium antimonate R with 95 ml of water until it has dissolved. Cool rapidly and add 50 ml of potassium hydroxide (1 mol/l) VS and 5 ml of sodium hydroxide (1 mol/l) VS. Allow to stand for 24 hours and dilute with sufficient water to produce 150 ml.
Sensitivity to sodium. To 10 ml add 7 ml of sodium hydroxide (0.1 mol/l) VS; a white, crystalline precipitate is formed within 15 minutes.
Note. Potassium antimonate TS must be freshly prepared.

Potassium bromate (0.00833 mol/l) VS. Potassium bromate R, dissolved in water to contain 1.392 g of $KBrO_3$ in 1000 ml.

Potassium carbonate R. $K_2CO_3, 1\tfrac{1}{2}H_2O$.
Description. Small granular crystals.

Solubility.   Very soluble in water; practically insoluble in ethanol (~750 g/l) TS.

Potassium carbonate, anhydrous, R. K_2CO_3.
Description.   Granules or a granular powder; hygroscopic.
Solubility.   Soluble in 1 part of water; practically insoluble in ethanol (~750 g/l) TS.

Potassium chloride (100 g/l) TS.   A solution of potassium chloride R containing about 100 g of KCl per litre.

Potassium cyanide PbTS.
Procedure.   Dissolve 10 g of potassium cyanide R in 90 ml of water, add 2 ml of hydrogen peroxide (~60 g/l) TS, allow to stand for 24 hours, dilute with water to 100 ml, and filter.

Potassium dichromate TS2.
Procedure.   Dissolve 1 g of potassium dichromate R in 60 ml of water and cautiously add 7.5 ml of sulfuric acid (~1760 g/l) TS.

Potassium dichromate TS3.
Procedure.   Dissolve 0.5 g of potassium dichromate R in sufficient sulfuric acid (~100 g/l) TS to produce 100 ml.

Potassium dihydrogen phosphate (100 g/l) TS.   A solution of potassium dihydrogen phosphate R containing about 100 g of KH_2PO_4 per litre.

Potassium dihydrogen phosphate (27.2 g/l) TS.   A solution of potassium dihydrogen phosphate R containing 27.2 g of KH_2PO_4 per litre (0.2 mol/l).

Potassium dihydrogen phosphate (13.6 g/l) TS.   A solution of potassium dihydrogen phosphate R containing 13.6 g of KH_2PO_4 per litre (0.1 mol/l).

Potassium iodate (3.6 mg/l) TS.   A freshly prepared solution of potassium iodate R containing 3.6 mg of KIO_3 per litre.

Potassium iodide (100 g/l) TS.   A solution of potassium iodide R containing about 100 g of KI per litre.

Potassium iodoplatinate TS2.
Procedure.   Dissolve 0.25 g of platinic chloride R in 2.5 ml of water, add 45 ml of potassium iodide (100 g/l) TS, and dilute with sufficient acetone R to produce 100 ml.

Potassium permanganate (25 g/l) TS. A solution of potassium permanganate R containing about 25 g of $KMnO_4$ per litre.

Potassium thiocyanate (200 g/l) TS. A solution of potassium thiocyanate R containing 200 g of KCNS per litre.

Praziquantel RS. International Chemical Reference Substance.

Prednisolone acetate RS. International Chemical Reference Substance.

Prednisolone sodium phosphate RS. International Chemical Reference Substance.

Probenecid RS. International Chemical Reference Substance.

Procarbazine hydrochloride RS. International Chemical Reference Substance.

Protionamide RS. International Chemical Reference Substance.

Pyrantel embonate RS. International Chemical Reference Substance.

Pyrazinamide RS. International Chemical Reference Substance.

Pyrimethamine RS. International Chemical Reference Substance.

Rifampicin quinone RS. International Chemical Reference Substance.

Rifampicin RS. International Chemical Reference Substance.

Salbutamol RS. International Chemical Reference Substance.

Salbutamol sulfate RS. International Chemical Reference Substance.

Salicylaldehyde R. $C_7H_6O_2$.
Description. A clear, colourless, oily liquid; odour, bitter, almond-like.
Solubility. Slightly soluble in water; soluble in ethanol ($\sim$750 g/l) TS and ether R.
Relative density. $d_4^{20} = 1.17$.

Salicylaldehyde TS.
Procedure. Mix 2 g of salicylaldehyde R with 100 ml of methanol R and add 0.1 ml of hydrocloric acid ($\sim$420 g/l) TS.

Silica gel R6. Silica gel 60 (UV 254).

Description.   A white, homogeneous powder.

Average pore size.   6 nm.

Composition.   Silica gel (average particle size 15 μm) containing a fluorescent indicator having an optimal intensity at 254 nm (about 15 g/kg).

Silver nitrate (100 g/l) TS.   A solution of silver nitrate R containing 100 g of $AgNO_3$ per litre.

Silver nitrate (0.01 mol/l) VS.   Silver nitrate R, dissolved in water to contain 1.699 g of $AgNO_3$ in 1000 ml.

Method of standardization.   Ascertain the exact concentration of the solution following the method described under silver nitrate (0.1 mol/l) VS, vol. 1, p. 202.

Silver nitrate/methanol TS.

Procedure.   Prepare a saturated solution of silver nitrate R in methanol R.

Sodium acetate/glacial acetic acid (0.1 mol/l) VS.

Procedure.   Dissolve 5.3 g of anhydrous sodium carbonate R in small portions in 100 ml of glacial acetic acid R1, stirring well after each addition, and add sufficient glacial acetic acid R1 to produce 1000 ml.

Method of standardization.   Ascertain the exact concentration of the solution in the following manner: Titrate the solution against 15.0 ml of perchloric acid (0.1 mol/l) VS using 2–3 drops of crystal violet/acetic acid TS. Each ml of perchloric acid (0.1 mol/l) VS is equivalent to 8.203 mg of $C_2H_3NaO_2$.

Sodium alizarinsulfonate (10 g/l) TS.   A solution of sodium alizarinsulfonate R containing about 10 g of $C_{14}H_7NaO_7S$ per litre.

Sodium chloride (400 g/l) TS.   A saturated solution of sodium chloride R containing about 400 g of NaCl per litre.

Sodium chloride (10 g/l) TS.   A solution of sodium chloride R containing about 10 g of NaCl per litre.

Sodium cromoglicate RS.   International Chemical Reference Substance.

Sodium dihydrogen phosphate (275 g/l) TS.   A solution of sodium dihydrogen phosphate R containing about 275 g of NaH_2PO_4 per litre.

Sodium formate R. $CHNaO_2$.

Description.   White, deliquescent granules or a crystalline powder; slight odour of formic acid.

Melting temperature.   About 253 °C.

Sodium hydroxide/ethanol TS.
Procedure. Dissolve 50 g of sodium hydroxide R in sufficient ethanol (~750 g/l) TS to produce 1000 ml.

Sodium hydroxide (50 g/l) TS. A solution of sodium hydroxide R containing about 50 g of NaOH per litre.

Sodium nitrite (35 g/l) TS. A solution of sodium nitrite R containing about 35 g of $NaNO_2$ per litre (approximately 0.5 mol/l).

Sodium nitroprusside (8.5 g/l) TS. A solution of sodium nitroprusside R containing about 8.5 g of $Na_2Fe(NO)(CN)_5$ per litre.

Sodium nitroprusside, alkaline, TS.
Procedure. Dissolve 1 g of sodium nitroprusside R and 1 g of sodium carbonate R in sufficient water to produce 100 ml.

Sodium peroxide R. Na_2O_2 (SRIP, 1963, p. 191).

Sodium salicyclate R. $C_7H_5NaO_3$. Use sodium salicylate as described in the monograph in volume 2, p. 193.

Sodium salicylate (11.5 g/l) TS. A solution of sodium salicylate R containing about 11.5 g of $C_7H_5NaO_3$ per litre.

Sodium sulfite R. $Na_2SO_3,7H_2O$ (SRIP, 1963, p. 196).

Spectinomycin hydrochloride RS. International Chemical Reference Substance.

Spironolactone RS. International Chemical Reference Substance.

Squalane R. 2,6,10,15,19,23-Hexamethyltetracosane; $C_{30}H_{62}$.
Description. A colourless, oily liquid.
Solubility. Freely soluble in ether R and chloroform R; slightly soluble in acetone R and ethanol (~750 g/l) TS.
Relative density. $d_{20}^{20} = 0.811 - 0.813$.
Refractive index. $n_D^{20} = 1.451 - 1.453$.

Sudan red G R. 1-(4-Phenylazophenylazo)-2-naphthol; Sudan III; Solvent red 23; C.I. 26100; $C_{22}H_{16}N_4O$.
Description. A reddish brown powder.
Solubility. Practically insoluble in water; soluble in chloroform R.

Sudan red TS.
Procedure. Dissolve 0.5 g of sudan red G R in 100 ml of glacial acetic acid R1.

Sulfacetamide RS. International Chemical Reference Substance.

Sulfadimidine RS. International Chemical Reference Substance.

Sulfadoxine RS. International Chemical Reference Substance.

Sulfamic acid (5 g/l) TS. A solution of sulfamic acid R containing about 5 g of H_3NO_3S per litre.

Sulfanilic acid, diazotized, TS.
Procedure. Dissolve 0.2 g of sulfanilic acid R in 20 ml of hydrochloric acid (1 mol/l) VS with warming, cool in ice, add drop by drop and with continuous stirring 2.5 ml of sodium nitrite (35 g/l) TS, allow to stand in ice for 10 minutes and then add 1 ml of sulfamic acid (50 g/l) TS.

Sulfasalazine RS. International Chemical Reference Substance.

Sulfuric acid/methanol TS.
Procedure. Cool separately 10 ml of sulfuric acid ($\sim$1760 g/l) TS and 90 ml of methanol R. Carefully add the acid to the methanol, keeping the solution as cool as possible, and mix gently.

Sulfuric acid (0.125 mol/l) VS. Sulfuric acid ($\sim$1760 g/l) TS, diluted with water to contain 12.52 g of H_2SO_4 in 1000 ml.
Method of standardization. Ascertain the exact concentration of the solution following the method described under sulfuric acid (0.5 mol/l) VS, volume 1, p. 209.

Tannic acid R. $C_{76}H_{52}O_{46}$ (SRIP, 1963, p. 205).

Tannic acid (50 g/l) TS. A solution of tannic acid R containing about 50 g of $C_{76}H_{52}O_{46}$ per litre.

Tartaric acid (200 g/l) TS. A solution of tartaric acid R containing about 200 g of $C_4H_6O_6$ per litre.

Testosterone enantate RS. International Chemical Reference Substance.

Tetrabutylammonium hydroxide/methanol TS.
Procedure. Dilute a sufficient volume of tetrabutylammonium hydroxide TS

with methanol R to obtain a solution containing 0.25 g of $C_{16}H_{37}NO$ per ml.

Tetrabutylammonium hydroxide TS. $C_{16}H_{37}NO$. A solution in water containing about 400 g of $C_{16}H_{37}NO$ per litre ($\sim$1.5 mol/l).

Tetrahydrofuran R. C_4H_8O.
Description. A colourless liquid; odour, characteristic, pungent.
Boiling point. About 66 °C.
Mass density. ρ_{20} = 0.884–0.886 kg/l.
Storage. Store in small, well-filled containers, protected from light.
Labelling. The name and concentration of any suitable preservative, not exceeding 0.1%, shoud be stated on the label.

Thioacetazone RS. International Chemical Reference Substance.

Tiabendazole RS. International Chemical Reference Substance.

Titanium trichloride R. A solution ot titanium trichloride containing about 15% of $TiCl_3$ (SRIP, 1963, p. 208).
Mass density. ρ_{20} = $\sim$1.2 kg/l.

Titanium trichloride (0.1 mol/l) VS.
Procedure. Dilute 100 ml of titanium trichloride R with 200 ml of hydrochloric acid ($\sim$250 g/l) TS and add sufficient carbon-dioxide-free water R to produce 1000 ml.
Method of standardization. Ascertain the exact concentration immediately before use. With the solution titrate 25 ml of ferric ammonium sulfate (0.1 mol/l) VS acidified with sulfuric acid ($\sim$100 g/l) TS in an atmosphere of carbon dioxide R, adding ammonium thiocyanate (75 g/l) TS just before the endpoint as indicator. Each ml of ferric ammonium sulfate (0.1 mol/l) VS is equivalent to 15.43 mg of $TiCl_3$.

Titan yellow R. $C_{28}H_{19}N_5Na_2O_6S_4$ (SRIP, 1963, p. 208).

Titan yellow TS.
Procedure. Dissolve 0.05 g of titan yellow R in sufficient water to produce 100 ml.

Trihexyphenidyl hydrochloride RS. International Chemical Reference Substance.

Triketohydrindene/butanol TS.
Procedure. Dissolve 0.1 g of triketohydrindene hydrate R in sufficient 1-butanol R previously saturated with water to produce 100 ml.

Triketohydrindene hydrate (1 g/l) TS.   A solution of triketohydrindene hydrate R containing about 1 g of $C_9H_4O_3$ per litre.

Triketohydrindene/methanol TS.
Procedure.   Dissolve 1.0 g of triketohydrindene hydrate R in sufficient methanol R to produce 100 ml.
Note.   Triketohydrindene/methanol TS must be freshly prepared.

Triketohydrindene/pyridine/acetone TS.
Procedure.   Dissolve 0.25 g of triketohydrindene hydrate R in 100 ml of a mixture of equal volumes of pyridine R and acetone R.

Triketohydrindene/pyridine/butanol TS.
Procedure.   Dissolve 1 g of triketohydrindene hydrate R in 1 ml of pyridine R and dilute with sufficient 1-butanol R to produce 100 ml.
Note: It should be freshly prepared.

Triketohydrindene/stannous chloride TS.
Procedure.   Dissolve 4 g of triketohydrindene hydrate R in 100 ml of ethylene glycol monomethyl ether R.   Shake gently with 1 g of cation exchange resin (300 µm – 840 µm) and filter (solution A).   Dissolve 0.16 g of stannous chloride R in 100 ml of acetate buffer, pH 5.5, TS (solution B).   Immediately before use, mix equal volumes of the two solutions.

2,2,4-Trimethylpentane R.   *iso*-Octane; C_8H_{18} (SRIP, 1963, p. 129).

Triphenylantimony R. $C_{18}H_{15}Sb$.
Melting temperature.   About 55 °C.

Trisodium orthophosphate R. $Na_3PO_4,12H_2O$.
Description.   Colourless crystals or a white, crystalline powder.
Solubility.   Freely soluble in water; practically insoluble in ethanol ($\sim$ 750 g/l) TS and carbon disulfide R.

Trisodium orthophosphate (2 g/l) TS.   A solution of trisodium orthophosphate R containing about 2 g of Na_3PO_4 per litre.

Uridine R.   1-β-D-Ribofuranosyluracil; $C_9H_{12}N_2O_6$.
Solubility.   Soluble in water.
Melting temperature.   About 165 °C.
Storage.   Store in a cool place.

Valproic acid RS.   International Chemical Reference Substance.

Vanadium pentoxide R. V_2O_5.

Description.   A yellow-brown to rust-brown powder.

Solubility.   Slightly soluble in water; soluble in concentrated acids and alkalis; practically insoluble in ethanol ($\sim$750 g/l) TS.

Vanadium/sulfuric acid TS.

Procedure.   Dissolve 0.20 g of vanadium pentoxide R in 4 ml of sulfuric acid ($\sim$1760 g/l) TS and dilute carefully with water to 100 ml.

Vanillin/hydrochloric acid TS.

Procedure.   Dissolve 0.1 g of vanillin R in sufficient hydrochloric acid ($\sim$250 g/l) TS to produce 100 ml.

Note.   Vanillin/hydrochloric acid TS must be freshly prepared.

Verapamil hydrochloride RS.   International Chemical Reference Substance.

Vincristine sulfate RS.   International Chemical Reference Substance.

Warfarin RS.   International Chemical Reference Substance.

Xanthydrol R. $C_{13}H_{10}O_2$ (SRIP, 1963, p. 210).

Xanthydrol TS.

Procedure.   Dissolve 20 mg of xanthydrol R in 1 ml of hydrochloric acid ($\sim$420 g/l) TS and 99 ml of acetic acid ($\sim$300 g/l) TS.

Zinc bis(dibenzyldithiocarbamate) R. $Zn(C_5H_{10}NS_2)_2$.

Description.   A white, crystalline powder.

Solubility.   Soluble in chloroform R.

Melting range.   178–180 °C.

Zinc bis(dibenzyldithiocarbamate) TS.

Procedure.   Dissolve 10.0 mg of zinc bis(dibenzyldithiocarbamate) R in sufficient carbon tetrachloride R to produce 100 ml.

AMENDMENTS AND CORRIGENDA
TO VOLUMES 1 AND 2

AMENDMENTS AND CORRIGENDA
TO VOLUMES 1 AND 2

Volume 1. General methods of analysis

Page 84

Replace the last sentence in the first paragraph with the following:

Allow the mobile phase to ascend, usually 10–15 cm, remove the plate, mark the position of the solvent front and dry as specified in the monograph.

Page 88

High Performance Liquid Chromatography[1]

Replace the text with the following expanded version:

This most recently introduced method of chromatography has brought column chromatography, the oldest form of the art, back into prominence. The essential development that has made the technique possible has been the availability of highly pressure-resistant particles of uniform diameters of less than 50 μm. The earlier types of particles have a solid centre, for example, of glass, and a thin porous outer layer, for example, of silica; the small particle size and high surface area so obtained confer a very high efficiency for use in adsorption chromatography. When these particles are coated with a suitable stationary phase, high performance liquid chromatography may be used as a partition technique.

More recently, silica beads having a uniform diameter of about 5 μm (or 3 μm) have become available; they are porous throughout and may have surface areas as high as 300 m^2/g. Consequently, they give more effective separations than the 30–50-μm packing. For column preparation it is possible to dry pack the larger particles, but for the 5-μm (or 3-μm) diameter materials it is essential to use a slurrying technique.

---

[1] Title has been modified to conform to recent trends in analytical terminology.

To ensure stability of the prepared column the stationary phases are frequently chemically bonded (usually by an ester or an ether linkage) to the support. The ether bond affords a more stable product than the ester bond, which may be hydrolysed by polar solvents; for example, in octadecylsilane-coated beads the hydrocarbon chain is bonded by an ether linkage to glass beads coated with a thin layer of silica and these provide a very efficient reverse phase system that is highly stable in use. For chromatography, these particles are packed into narrow-bore (usually 2–4 mm internal diameter) columns; it is clear that such fine material packed into long columns will provide considerable resistance to the flow of the mobile phase and it is for this reason that high pressures must be employed. Typical lengths of columns are 20–30 cm and conditions for quantitative analysis might be a flow rate of about 1–3 ml per minute and a pressure of up to 28 000 kPa (4000 lbf/in^2).

In addition to the adsorption and partition modes referred to above, the principle of the high performance technique is applicable to ion-exchange chromatography provided that suitable resins are available as sufficiently small pressure-resistant particles.

With such high pressures it is obvious that specialized equipment is necessary. The essential features of the apparatus are a suitable pump to deliver the mobile phase from an enclosed solvent reservoir to the column, a means of introducing the test solution on to the column (usually a form of injection valve designed to work at high pressure), the column itself (often at ambient temperature but sometimes maintained at higher temperatures), an appropriate detector system, and an amplifier connected to a suitable recording device, such as a strip-chart recorder, where signals may be plotted against time, or an electronic integrator.

As detectors, the most commonly employed are the ones based on ultraviolet spectrophotometry or on measurements of refractive index or on fluorescence measurements. For pharmaceutical work, the ultraviolet spectrophotometer is the most suitable because of its sensitivity (the lower limit of detectability may be of the order of 1 or 2 ng for materials having good light-absorbing properties) and its stability (particularly its low sensitivity to controlled changes in solvent composition and flow irregularities); naturally, such a detector fails completely when materials exhibiting no significant absorption in ultraviolet light are eluted. The refractometer responds to differences in refractive index between the pure mobile phase and mobile phase containing an eluted material; it is a more generally applicable method than ultraviolet absorption spectrophotometry but lacks sensitivity and is seriously affected by small changes in solvent composition, flow rate, and temperature.

The capacity factor k' of a substance being chromatographed is defined as follows:

$$k' = \frac{\text{amount of substance in stationary phase}}{\text{amount of substance in mobile phase}}$$

This factor determines the retention times of the various substances on the chromatogram and can be computed experimentally by the following formula:

$$k' = \frac{t - t_{\mathrm{o}}}{t_{\mathrm{o}}}$$

where t = retention time of the substance

$\quad t_{\mathrm{o}}$ = retention time of non-retarded component.

For some applications, particularly in experiments designed to determine optimum solvent composition for a method that is subsequently to be used in a routine fashion, the technique of gradient elution is useful. The composition of the solvent mixture constituting the mobile phase is continuously varied at a predetermined rate during chromatography and this enables a single chromatogram to deal with complex mixtures of substances having greatly differing capacity factors.

By using methods of computation similar to those referred to under gas chromatography, the high performance technique is capable of great precision and is thus very suitable for quantitative purposes. It is a rapid procedure and has been used to effect many efficient separations. It requires highly specialized apparatus, however, and, for many applications, expensive column packing materials. A potential advantage over gas chromatography is that volatility and thermostability, so important in gas chromatography, are of no concern. A disadvantage is that no universally applicable detector system is yet available.

RECOMMENDED PROCEDURE

Use the chromatographic system and condition specified in the monograph for the determination. Solvents are filtered through suitable membrane filters of 2 μm or smaller pore size. They are then manually mixed according to the mobile phase composition specified or are pumped through individual pumps or proportionating valves of the liquid chromatograph and mixed according to the desired proportion. Solvents must be degassed (outgassed) before pumping.

The retention time of the test substance can be varied if necessary by changing the relative proportion of solvents in the mobile phase. Generally, an increase in the proportion of a more polar solvent will lead to a shorter retention time on a normal phase column (such as a silica column) and a longer retention time on a reversed phase column (such as an octadecylsilane bonded phase). Other chromatographic parameters such as flow rate, column length, pH, ionic strength, and temperature may also be varied to improve the chromatogram.

The resolution factor is calculated as in gas chromatography. A system suitability test which specifies the minimum resolution required for the determination is sometimes given in the monograph to ensure adequate separation and valid results. Where necessary, resolution may be improved by suitably varying some of the chromatographic parameters.

The peak symmetry factor is calculated as in gas chromatography and an unduly large symmetry factor would indicate an unsuitable column; in which case, the column should be regenerated or replaced.

Unless otherwise specified, solutions of test substance and reference substance should be prepared in a solvent with the same composition as the mobile phase. Distorted peak shapes or even split peaks can occur in the chromatogram if an unsuitable solvent is used to prepare the solutions.

Method

With the specified mobile phase in place, allow about 30 minutes continuous flow for the column to equilibrate with the mobile phase. A stable baseline response should be obtained. Inject solution A and adjust detector attenuation to produce adequate responses. Where a system suitability test is prescribed in the monograph, this should be applied.

Before proceeding to the determination, ensure that resolution and peak symmetry are adequate and that the criteria of any system suitability test specified in the monograph are satisfied. In a stable system, the retention times and peak responses (areas or heights) of replicate injections should vary within reasonable limits. Inject the solutions specified in the monograph and measure the peak responses. Where an internal standard method of quantification is used, one of the solutions to be injected is a solution of the test substance (solution B). This is to ensure that no interfering peak occurs at the same retention time as the internal standard used and to enable an allowance to be made for the quantity present if there is a coincident peak. Calculate the content of the test substance from the relevant peak response ratios between the peak due to the test substance or the peak due to the reference substance and that due to the internal standard. On the other hand, if an external standard method of quantification is used, calculate the content based on a comparison of the peak response of the test substance and that of the reference substance in separate injections. In determining the component composition of a complex mixture, a "normalization" procedure based on the calculation of individual peak areas as percentages of the total peak areas may be used.

If gradient development or elution is specified in the monograph, an instrument equipped with a special pumping system capable of delivering a mobile phase of a continuously varied composition is needed. The mobile phase composition is varied from an initial composition to a final composition within a fixed period of time, as specified in the monograph. Where the mobile phase composition is varied at a linear rate, the procedure is known as a linear gradient development procedure. For determination based on gradient development, carry out a blank run by injecting the solvent specified for preparing the test solutions into the chromatograph so as to establish that the baseline is within scale throughout the entire range of the gradient and that no spurious peaks that would interfere with the analysis occur in the chromatogram. Allow sufficient time for equilibrium to be reestablished when the mobile phase is reset to the initial composition for the next injection.

MICROBIOLOGICAL ASSAY OF ANTIBIOTICS

TABLE 4.   TEST ORGANISMS AND CONDITIONS OF ASSAY OF INDIVIDUAL ANTIBIOTICS

Page 149

Neomycin

delete	*replace by*
Staphylococcus aureus	*Staphylococcus aureus*
ATCC 6538-P	ATCC *29737*

LIST OF REAGENTS, TEST SOLUTIONS AND VOLUMETRIC SOLUTIONS

Page 179

Disodium edetate (0.05 mol/l) VS.

delete	*replace by*
16.81 g of $C_{10}H_{14}N_2Na_2O_8$	*16.71* g of $C_{10}H_{14}N_2Na_2O_8$

Page 185

Iodine TS.

delete	*replace by*
(approximately 0.2 mol/l)	(approximately *0.1* mol/l)

Page 185

Iodine (0.1 mol/l) VS.

delete	*replace by*
12.69 g of I and 18.0 g of KI	*25.38* g of I and *36.0* g of KI

Page 185

Iodine (0.02 mol/l) VS.

delete	*replace by*
2.538 g of I and 3.6 g of KI	*5.076* g of I and *7.2* g of KI

Page 185

Iodine (0.01 mol/l) VS.

delete	*replace by*
1.269 g of I	*2.538* g of I

Page 194

Perchloric acid (0.1 mol/l) VS.

Method of standardization

Replace the text with the following:

Ascertain the exact concentration by titrating 0.5 g, accurately weighed, of potassium hydrogen phthalate R, previously dried at 120 °C for 2 hours, using *method A, as described under "Non-aqueous titration",* see p. *131.* Each ml of perchloric acid (0.1 mol/l) VS is equivalent to 20.42 mg of $C_8H_5KO_4$. Record the temperature at which the standardization is carried out.

Pages 195–197

All sterile phosphate buffers

The adjustment of the pH, if necessary, should be effected before sterilization of the solution.

Page 201

Red stock standard TS.

delete	*replace by*
40.4 ml of cobalt colour TS	*40.5* ml of cobalt colour TS

Volume 2. Quality specifications

ACIDUM ASCORBICUM

Page 22, paragraph 7. *Replace the text with the following:*

Assay. Dissolve about 0.20 g, accurately weighed, in a mixture of 25 ml of carbon-dioxide-free water R and 25 ml of sulfuric acid ($\sim$100 g/l) TS. Titrate the solution at once with iodine (*0.05 mol/l*) VS using starch TS as indicator, added towards the end of the titration, until a persistent blue colour is obtained. Each ml of iodine (*0.05 mol/l*) VS is equivalent to 8.806 mg of $C_6H_8O_6$.

AMPICILLINUM NATRICUM

Page 41, last paragraph. *Replace the text with the following:*

Iodine-absorbing compounds. Dissolve 0.25 g in sufficient water to produce 100 ml. To 10 ml of this solution add 0.5 ml of hydrochloric acid (1 mol/l) VS and 10 ml of iodine (*0.01 mol/l*) VS and titrate with sodium thiosulfate (0.02 mol/l) VS, using starch TS as indicator, added towards the end of the titration. Repeat the operation without the substance being examined; the difference between the titrations represents the amount of iodine-absorbing compounds. Calculate as a percentage the amount of these compounds in the examined substance, taking into account that each ml of sodium thiosulfate (0.02 mol/l) VS is equivalent to 0.7368 mg of iodine-absorbing compounds expressed as $C_{16}H_{19}N_3O_4S$.

BENZYLPENICILLINUM KALICUM

Page 50, paragraph 2. *Replace the text with the following:*

Light-absorbing impurities   Using a freshly prepared 1.9 mg/ml solution in water, measure the absorbances *of a 1-cm layer* at 280 nm and at 325 nm; the absorbance at each of these wavelengths does not exceed 0.10.

BENZYLPENICILLINUM NATRICUM

Page 52, paragraph 9. *Replace the text with the following:*

Light-absorbing impurities. Using a freshly prepared 1.8 mg/ml solution in water, measure the absorbances *of a 1-cm layer* at 280 nm and at 325 nm; the absorbance at each of these wavelengths does not exceed 0.10.

CALCII GLUCONAS

Page 61, last paragraph. *Replace the text with the following:*

Assay. Dissolve about 0.5 g, accurately weighed, in 20 ml of hot water containing 2 ml of hydrochloric acid ($\sim$70 g/l) TS, allow to cool and dilute to 100 ml with water. Proceed with the titration as described under "Complexometric titrations" *for calcium* (vol. 1, p. 128). Each ml of disodium edetate (0.05 mol/l) VS is equivalent to 22.42 mg of $(C_6H_{11}O_7)_2Ca,H_2O$.

CARBO ACTIVATUS

Page 64, paragraph 2. *Replace the text with the following:*

Adsorbing power

B.   To each of two glass-stoppered 100-ml flasks transfer 50 ml of methylthioninium chloride (1 g/l) TS. To one of the flasks add 0.25 g, accurately weighed, of the test substance, insert the stopper in the flask and shake for 5 minutes. Filter the contents of each flask, rejecting the first 20 ml of each filtrate. Transfer 25-ml portions of the filtrates to two 250-ml volumetric flasks. Add to each flask 50 ml of sodium acetate (60 g/l) TS, mix, and add from a burette 35.0 ml of iodine (*0.05 mol/l*) VS, swirling the mixture during the addition. Stopper the flasks and allow them to stand for 50 minutes, shaking them vigorously at 10-minute intervals. Dilute each mixture with water to volume, mix, allow to stand for 10 minutes, and filter, rejecting the first 30 ml of each filtrate. Titrate the excess iodine in a 100-ml aliquot of each filtrate with sodium thiosulfate (0.1 mol/l) VS, adding 3 ml of starch TS towards the end of the titration. Calculate the number of ml of iodine (*0.05 mol/l*) VS consumed in each titration; the difference between the two volumes is not less than 0.7 ml.

DEXAMETHASONI ACETAS

Page 93, paragraphs 2 and 3. *Replace the text and graphic formula with the following:*

Relative molecular mass.   434.5 *(anhydrous); 452.5 (monohydrate).*

Graphic formula.

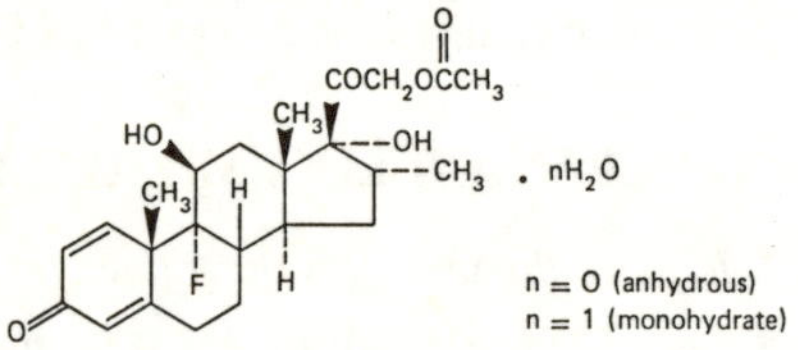

EPINEPHRINI HYDROGENOTARTRAS

Page 110. *Replace the graphic formula with the following:*

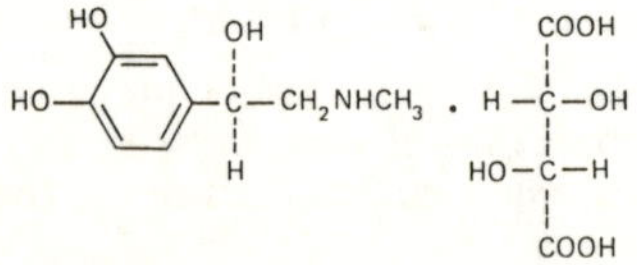

Page 111, paragraph 2. *Replace the text with the following:*

Identity tests

B.   Dissolve 10 mg in 10 ml of water and transfer 1 ml to a flask containing 10 ml of buffer phthalate, pH 3.4, TS; another buffer having the same pH may also be used. Add *0.5 ml* of iodine (0.1 mol/l) VS, and allow to stand for 5 minutes. Add 2 ml of sodium thiosulfate (0.1 mol/l) VS, and allow to stand for 1 minute; a strong red colour is produced (distinction from levarterenol, which gives a clear solution with a pink tinge).

EPINEPHRINUM

Page 112. *Replace the graphic formula with the following:*

Page 113, paragraph 4. *Replace the text with the following:*

Identity tests

B.   Dissolve 10 mg in 10 ml of hydrochloric acid (0.01 mol/l) VS and transfer 1 ml to a flask containing 10 ml of buffer phthalate, pH 3.4, TS; another buffer having the same pH may also be used. Add *0.5 ml* of iodine (0.1 mol/l) VS and allow to stand for 5 minutes. Add 2 ml of sodium thiosulfate (0.1 mol/l) VS, and allow to stand for 1 minute; a strong red colour is produced (distinction from levarterenol, which gives a clear solution with a pink tinge).

Page 114, paragraph 2. *Replace the text with the following:*

Assay.   Dissolve about 0.35 g, accurately weighed, in 30 ml of glacial acetic acid R1, and titrate with perchloric acid (0.1 mol/l) VS as described under "Non-aqueous titration", Method A (vol. 1, p. 131).   Each ml of perchloric acid (0.1 mol/l) VS is equivalent to 18.32 mg of $C_9H_{13}NO_3$.

ERGOTAMINI TARTRAS

Page 118, paragraph 3.*Replace the text with the following:*

Loss on drying.   *Weigh the substance as rapidly as possible and* dry to constant weight at 95 °C under reduced pressure (not exceeding 0.6 kPa or about 5 mm of mercury); it loses not more than 50 mg/g.

ETHOSUXIMIDUM

Page 123. *Replace the graphic formula with the following:*

GLUCOSUM

Page 137, paragraph 1. *Replace the text with the following:*

Assay.   Dissolve about 0.10 g, accurately weighed, in 50 ml of water, add 25.0 ml of iodine (*0.05 mol/l*) VS and 10 ml of sodium carbonate (50 g/l) TS. Allow to stand for 20 minutes in the dark and add 15 ml of sulfuric acid (~100 g/l) TS. Titrate the excess of iodine with sodium thiosulfate (0.1 mol/l) VS, using starch TS as indicator. Repeat the operation without the substance being examined and make any necessary corrections. Each ml of iodine (*0.05 mol/l*) VS is equivalent to 9.008 mg of $C_6H_{12}O_6$.

ISOPRENALINI HYDROCHLORIDUM

Page 160, paragraph 4. *Replace the text with the following:*

Identity tests

B.   Add 1 ml of a 1.0 mg/ml solution to each of two flasks, one containing 10 ml of buffer phthalate, pH 3.4, TS, the other containing 10 ml of buffer phosphate, pH 6.4, TS; other buffers having the same pH may also be used. Add *0.5 ml* of iodine (0.1 mol/l) VS, allow to stand for 5 minutes and add 2 ml of sodium thiosulfate (0.1 mol/l) VS. In the solution of pH 3.4, a strong red colour is produced; in the solution of pH 6.4, a strong red-violet colour is produced (distinction from levarterenol).

ISOPRENALINI SULFAS

Page 162, paragraph 1. *Replace the text with the following:*

Identity tests

B.   Add 1 ml of a 1.0 mg/ml solution to each of two flasks, one containing 10 ml of buffer phthalate, pH 3.4, TS, the other containing 10 ml of buffer phosphate, pH 6.4, TS; other buffers having the same pH may also be used. Add *0.5 ml* of iodine (0.1 mol/l) VS, allow to stand for 5 minutes and add 2 ml of sodium thiosulfate (0.1 mol/l) VS. In the solution of pH 3.4, a strong red colour is produced; in the solution of pH 6.4, a strong red-violet colour is produced (distinction from levarterenol).

KALII CHLORIDUM

Page 164, paragraph 3. *Replace the text with the following:*

Arsenic.   Use a solution of *3.3 g* in 35 ml of water and proceed as described under "Limit test for arsenic" (vol. 1, p. 122); the arsenic content is not more than 3 µg/g.

KALII IODIDUM

Page 166, paragraph 6. *Replace the text with the following:*

Thiosulfates.   Dissolve 1.0 g in 10 ml of carbon-dioxide-free water R and add 0.1 ml of starch TS; not more than *0.05 ml* of iodine (0.01 mol/l) VS is required to produce a blue colour.

LINDANUM

Page 174, paragraph 4. *Replace the text with the following:*

Congealing temperature.   Not *below* 112.0 °C.

MANNITOLUM

Page 178, last paragraph. *Replace the text with the following:*

Assay.   Dissolve about 0.4 g, accurately weighed, in sufficient water to produce 100 ml. Transfer 10 ml to a stoppered flask, add 20.0 ml of a 21.4 g/l solution of sodium metaperiodate R and 2 ml of sulfuric acid ($\sim$100 g/l) TS and heat on a water-bath for 15 minutes. Cool, add 3 g of sodium hydrogen carbonate R, 25 ml of sodium arsenite (*0.05 mol/l*) VS, and 5 ml of a 200 g/l solution of potassium iodide R; allow to stand for 15 minutes, and titrate with iodine (*0.05 mol/l*) VS until the first trace of yellow colour appears. Repeat the procedure without the test substance and determine the difference in volume of iodine (*0.05 mol/l*) VS required for the titration. Each ml of iodine (*0.05 mol/l*) VS is equivalent to 1.822 mg of $C_6H_{14}O_6$.

NATRII SALICYLAS

Page 194, paragraph 6. *Replace the text with the following:*

Sulfites and thiosulfates.   Dissolve 1.0 g in 20 ml of water, add 1 ml of hydrochloric acid ($\sim$250 g/l) TS, and filter. Titrate the filtrate with iodine (*0.05 mol/l*) VS; not more than 0.15 ml of titrant is required to produce a yellow colour.

PHENOBARBITALUM NATRICUM

Page 208. *Replace the graphic formula with the following:*

C_2H_5 H   ONa   O   N   O

PROPRANOLOLI HYDROCHLORIDUM

Page 240. *Replace the CAS Reg. No. with the following:*

318–98–9.

PYRIDOSTIGMINI BROMIDUM

Page 245, paragraph 7. *Replace the text with the following:*

Related substances.   Carry out the test as described under "Thin-layer chromatography" (vol. 1, p. 83) using silica gel R1 as the coating substance and a mixture of 67 volumes of water, 30 volumes of methanol R, and 3 volumes of diethylamine R as the mobile phase. Apply separately to the plate 10 µl of each of 3 solutions containing (A) 20 mg of the test substance per ml, (B) 0.10 mg of the test substance per ml, and (C) 0.10 mg of pyridostigmine bromide RS per ml. After removing the plate from the chromatographic chamber, allow it to dry in a current of warm air, spray it with *4*-nitroaniline TS2 and then with sodium hydroxide (0.1 mol/l) VS. Dry the plate again in a current of warm air, spray it with potassium iodobismuthate TS2 and examine the chromatogram in daylight. Any spot obtained with solution A, other than the principal spot, is not more intense than that obtained with solution B.

QUININI HYDROCHLORIDUM

Page 248, paragraph 10. *Replace the text with the following:*

General requirement.   Quinine hydrochloride contains not less than 98.5% and not more than 101.0% *of total alkaloids, calculated as* $C_{20}H_{24}N_2O_2$,HCl and with reference to the dried substance.

Page 249, last paragraph. *Replace the text the following:*

Limit of dihydroquinine.   Dissolve about 0.2 g, accurately weighed, in 20 ml of water. Add 0.5 g of potassium *bromide* R, *15 ml* of hydrochloric acid (~70 g/l) TS and *0.1 ml* of methyl red/ethanol TS.   Titrate with potassium bromate (0.0167 mol/l) VS until *a yellow colour is produced.* Add 0.5 g of potassium iodide R *in 200 ml of water,* stopper the flask, and allow to stand *in the dark* for 5 minutes. Titrate the iodine *liberated by excess potassium bromate in the solution* with sodium thiosulfate (0.1 mol/l) VS, adding 2 ml of starch TS when the solution has reached a light yellow coloration. Each ml of potassium bromate (0.0167 mol/l) VS is equivalent to 18.04 mg of $C_{20}H_{24}N_2O_2$,HCl. Express the results of both the above determination and the assay in percentages, *calculated with reference to the dried substance.* The difference between the two is not more than 10%.

QUININI SULFAS

Page 251, paragraph 1. *Replace the text with the following:*

General requirement.   Quinine sulfate contains not less than 99.0% and not more than 101.0% *of total alkaloids, calculated as* $(C_{20}H_{24}N_2O_2)_2$,H_2SO_4 and with reference to the dried substance.

Page 251, last paragraph. *Replace the text with the following:*

Limit of dihydroquinine.   Dissolve about 0.2 g, accurately weighed, in 20 ml of water. Add 0.5 g of potassium *bromide R, 15 ml* of hydrochloric acid (~70 g/l) TS and *0.1 ml* of methyl red/ethanol TS.   Titrate with potassium bromate (0.0167 mol/l) VS until *a yellow colour is produced.* Add 0.5 g of potassium iodide R *in 200 ml of water,* stopper the flask, and allow to stand *in the dark* for 5 minutes. Titrate the iodine *liberated by excess potassium bromate in the solution with* sodium thiosulfate (0.1 mol/l) VS, adding 2 ml of starch TS when the solution has reached a light yellow coloration. Each ml of potassium bromate (0.0167 mol/l) VS is equivalent to 24.90 mg of $(C_{20}H_{24}N_2O_2)_2$,H_2SO_4. Express the results of both the above determination and the assay in percentages, *calculated with reference to the dried substance.* The difference between the two is not more than 10%.

RESERPINUM

Page 254. **Assay.** *Replace the absorbance in the last sentence by:* 0.42.

TESTOSTERONI PROPIONAS

Page 263. *Replace the graphic formula with the following:*

TRIMETHADIONUM

Page 273, last paragraph. *Replace the text with the following:*

Assay.   Carry out the assay as described under "Gas chromatography" (vol. 1, p. 94).   As an internal standard use 2-phenylethanol TS.   Use the following 3 solutions: (1) to *0.10 g* of trimethadione RS add 5 ml of 2-phenylethanol TS and sufficient methanol R to produce 10 ml, (2) dissolve 0.20 g of the substance being examined in sufficient methanol R to produce 10 ml, and (3) to 0.20 g of the substance being examined add 5 ml of 2-phenylethanol TS and sufficient methanol R to produce 10 ml.   For the procedure use a glass column 1.5 m long and 0.4 cm in internal diameter packed with an adequate quantity of an adsorbent composed of 10 g of diethylene glycol succinate R supported on 90 g of acid-washed, silanized kieselguhr R4.   Maintain the column at 105 °C, use nitrogen R as the carrier gas and a flame ionization detector.   Prepare chromatograms A, B, and C from solutions 1, 2 and 3, respectively.   Measure the appropriate peak areas in chromatograms A, B, and C, and calculate the content of $C_6H_9NO_3$, using the data obtained from chromatograms A and C, introducing if necessary the correction resulting from chromatogram B.

LIST OF REAGENTS, TEST SOLUTIONS, AND VOLUMETRIC SOLUTIONS

Page 296

Disodium edetate (0.1 mol/l) VS.

delete	*replace by*
33.62 g of $C_{10}H_{14}N_2Na_2O_8$	*33.42 g* of $C_{10}H_{14}N_2Na_2O_8$

Page 303

Levarterenol hydrogen tartrate R.

Specific optical rotation.

delete	*replace by*
−10 to −13 °C	−10 to −13°

Lithium methoxide (0.1 mol/l) VS.

Page 304. *Replace the text with the following:*

Procedure.   Dissolve 0.694 g of lithium R *in 150 ml of methanol R* and add sufficient toluene R to produce 1000 ml.

Page 312

Potassium thiocyanate R.

Other sulfur compounds.

Replace the text with the following:

Dissolve 1.0 g in 50 ml of water, add 2 ml of hydrochloric acid ($\sim$70 g/l) TS, and titrate with iodine (*0.05 mol/l*) VS; not more than 0.5 ml of iodine (*0.05 mol/l*) VS is required.

Page 316

Sodium arsenite (0.05 mol/l) VS.

Method of standardization.

Replace the text with the following:

Ascertain the exact concentration of the 0.05 mol/l solution in the following manner; dilute 25 ml with 50 ml of water, add 5 g of sodium hydrogen carbonate R, and titrate with iodine (*0.05 mol/l*) VS, using starch TS as indicator.

Page 325

Tosylchloramide sodium R.

delete	*replace by*
$C_7H_7CINNaO_2S,3H_2O$	$C_7H_7ClNNaO_2S,3H_2O$

INDEX

INDEX

For the convenience of users of volume 3, the reagents, test solutions, and volumetric solutions described in volumes 1 and 2 are also listed in this index. The numbers printed in bold type, preceding the page numbers, indicate the volume in which the indexed item is to be found.

A

Abbreviations, for reagents, test solutions and volumetric solutions, **1**, 13, 167; **2**, 279; **3**, 339

Acacia R, (5 g/l) TS, **3**, 339

p-Acetamidobenzalazine RS, **3**, 339

Acetaminophen, *see* Paracetamol

Acetate buffer, pH 3.0, TS, **1**, 167; pH 4.5, TS, pH 4.7, TS, **3**, 339; pH 5.0, TS, pH 5.5, TS, **3**, 340

Acetate standard buffer, TS, **2**, 279

Acetazolamide, **2**, 17

Acetazolamide RS, **2**, 279

Acetazolamidum, **2**, 17

Acetic acid, glacial, R, **1**, 168; R1, **2**, 279

Acetic acid (~330 g/l) TS, (~60 g/l) TS, (~60 g/l) PbTS, **1**, 168; (~120 g/l) TS, (~90 g/l) TS, (5.0 g/l) TS, **3**, 340

Acetic anhydride/dioxan TS, **2**, 280

Acetic anhydride R, **1**, 168

Acetone R, **1**, 168

Acetonitrile R, (400 g/l) TS, **1**, 168

Acetyl chloride R, **2**, 280

Acetylsalicylic acid, **2**, 19

Acids, *see under name of acid*

Acidum acetylsalicylicum, **2**, 19

Acidum ascorbicum, **2**, 21; **3**, 379

Acidum benzoicum, **2**, 22

Acidum folicum, **2**, 24

Acidum nicotinicum, **2**, 26

Acidum salicylicum, **2**, 28

Activated charcoal, **2**, 62; **3**, 380

Adrenalin, *see* Epinephrine

Adrenalin tartrate, *see* Epinephrine hydrogen tartrate

Adriamycin, *see* Doxorubicin hydrochloride

Agar R, **1**, 168

Alcohol, ethyl, *see* Ethanol
isopropyl, *see* 2-Propanol
methyl, *see* Methanol

Alizarin Red S, *see* Sodium alizarinsulfonate R

Allopurinol, **2**, 30

Allopurinol RS, **2**, 280

Allopurinolum, **2**, 30

Aluminii hydroxidum, **3**, 15

Aluminium chloride R, TS, **2**, 280

Aluminium hydroxide, **3**, 15

Aluminium hydroxide R, **1**, 168

Aluminium R, **2**, 280

Amethocaine hydrochloride, *see* Tetracaine hydrochloride

Amikacin, **3**, 17

Amikacin sulfate, **3**, 18

Amikacini sulfas, **3**, 18

Amikacinum, **3**, 17

Amiloride hydrochloride, **3**, 21

Amiloride hydrochloride RS, **3**, 340

Amiloridi hydrochloridum, **3**, 21

4-Aminoantipyrine R, TS1, TS2, **3**, 340

4-Aminobenzoic acid R, **2**, 280

4-Aminobutanol R, **2**, 281

4-Amino-6-chloro-1,3-benzenedisulfon-amide R, **2**, 281

2-Amino-5-nitrothiazole R, **3**, 340

4-Aminophenol-free paracetamol R, **3**, 358

4-Aminophenol R, **3**, 341

Aminophylline, **2**, 31

Aminophyllinum, **2**, 31

Aminopyrazole-4-carboxamide hemisulfate RS **2**, 281

Aminopyrazolone, *see* 4-Aminoantipyrine

Amitriptyline hydrochloride, **2**, 34

Amitriptylini hydrochloridum, **2**, 34

Ammonia (∼ 260 g/l) TS, (∼ 100 g/l) TS, (∼ 100 g/l) PbTS, **1**, 168; (∼ 35 g/l) TS, (∼ 17 g/l) TS, **2**, 282; (∼ 100 g/l) FeTS, **2**, 281; (∼ 50 g/l) TS, **3**, 341

Ammonia buffer TS, **1**, 169

Ammonia, strong R, *see* Ammonia (∼ 260 g/l) TS

Ammonium acetate R, (80 g/l) TS, **1**, 169; (100 g/l) TS, (40 g/l) TS, (2 g/l) TS, **3**, 341

Ammonium acetate buffer, pH 4.62, TS, **3**, 341

Ammonium carbonate, R, **1**, 169

Ammonium chloride R (10 μg/ml NH₄) TS, **1**, 169; (100 g/l) TS, **2**, 282

Ammonium chloride buffer, pH 10.0, TS, **1**, 169

Ammonium hydroxide, *see* Ammonia

Ammonium mercurithiocyanate TS, **3**, 341

Ammonium molybdate/nitric acid TS, **2**, 282

Ammonium molybdate R, (95 g/l) TS, **1**, 169; (45 g/l) TS, **2**, 282

Ammonium molybdate/sulfuric acid TS, **3**, 341

Ammonium molybdate/vanadate TS, **3**, 341

Ammonium nitrate R, (50 g/l) TS, **2**, 282

Ammonium oxalate R, (25 g/l) TS, **1**, 169; (50 g/l) TS, **2**, 282

Ammonium persulfate R, **3**, 341

Ammonium persulfate/phosphate buffer TS, **3**, 341

Ammonium phosphate R, *see* Diammonium hydrogen phosphate R

Ammonium reineckate R, (10 g/l) TS, **3**, 342

Ammonium sulfamate R, (25 g/l) TS, (5 g/l) TS, **2**, 282; (50 g/l) TS, **3**, 342

Ammonium sulfate R, **2**, 282

Ammonium sulfide TS, **3**, 342

Ammonium thiocyanate R, (75 g/l) TS, (0.1 mol/l) VS, **1**, 169; (0.01 mol/l) VS, **1**, 170

Ammonium thiocyanate/cobalt(II) nitrate TS, **3**, 342

Ammonium vanadate R, **3**, 342

Amodiaquine, **3**, 23

Amodiaquine hydrochloride, **2**, 35

Amodiaquine hydrochloride RS, **3**, 342

Amodiaquini hydrochloridum, **2**, 35

Amodiaquinum, **3**, 23

Amphotericin B, **3**, 25

Amphotericin B RS, **3**, 342

Amphotericinum B, **3**, 25

Ampicillin, **2**, 37

Ampicillin RS, **2**, 282

Ampicillin sodium, **2**, 40; **3**, 379

Ampicillin sodium RS, **2**, 282

Ampicillin trihydrate RS, **2**, 282

Ampicillinum, **2**, 37

Ampicillinum natricum, **2**, 40; **3**, 379

Ampyrone, *see* 4-Aminoantipyrine R

Amyl alcohol R, **2**, 282

Anaesthetic Ether, **3**, 128

Anhydrotetracycline hydrochloride RS, **2**, 282

Anhydrous calcium chloride R, **1**, 172

Anhydrous disodium hydrogen phosphate R, **1**, 179

Anhydrous glucose R, **3**, 352

Anhydrous potassium carbonate, **3**, 362

Anhydrous pyridine R, **1**, 201

Anhydrous sodium carbonate R, **1**, 203

Anhydrous sodium sulfate, **3**, 205

Anhydrous sodium sulfate R, **1**, 206

Aniline R, (25 g/l) TS, **2**, 283

Anthrone R, TS, **3**, 342

Antimony sodium tartrate, **3**, 293

Antimony sodium tartrate R, (50 g/l) TS, **1**, 170

Antimony trichloride R, TS, **2**, 283

Apressinum, *see* Hydralazine hydrochloride

Argenti nitras, **3**, 28

Arsenic, dilute, AsTS, strong, AsTS, **1**, 170

Arsenic trioxide R, **1**, 170; R1, **2**, 283

Ascorbic acid, **2**, 21; **3**, 379

Atropine sulfate, **2**, 43

Atropine sulfate RS, **2**, 283

Atropini sulfas, **2**, 43

Azathioprine, **3**, 29

Azathioprine RS, **3**, 342

Azathioprinum, **3**, 29

Azo violet R, **2**, 283; TS, **2**, 284

B

Bacitracin, **3**, 31

Bacitracin zinc, **3**, 33

Bacitracin zinc RS, **3**, 342

Bacitracinum, **3**, 31

Bacitracinum zincum, **3**, 33

Barii sulfas, **3**, 35

Barium chloride R, (50 g/l) TS, (0.5 mol/l) VS, **1**, 170

Barium hydroxide R, (15 g/l) TS, **2**, 284

Barium nitrate R, (0.01 mol/l) VS, **1**, 170
Barium oxide R, **1**, 171
Barium sulfate, **3**, 35
Barium sulfate suspension TS, **1**, 171
Beclometasone dipropionate, **3**, 37
Beclometasone dipropionate RS, **3**, 342
Beclometasoni dipropionas, **3**, 37
Beef extract R, **1**, 171
Benzalkonium chloride TS, TS1, **2**, 284
Benzathine benzylpenicillin, **3**, 39
Benzathini benzylpenicillinum, **3**, 39
Benzene R, **2**, 284
Benzhexol hydrochloride,
   see Trihexyphenidyl hydrochloride
Benzocaine, **2**, 45
Benzocainum, **2**, 45
Benzoic acid, **2**, 22
Benzoic acid R, **2**, 284
Benzoyl chloride R, **2**, 285
Benzyl alcohol R, **3**, 343
Benzyl benzoate, **2**, 46
Benzylis benzoas, **2**, 46
Benzylpenicillin potassium, **2**, 48; **3**, 379
Benzylpenicillin potassium RS, **2**, 285
Benzylpenicillin sodium, **2**, 51; **3**, 379
Benzylpenicillin sodium R, TS, **1**, 171; RS, **2**, 285
Benzylpenicillinum kalicum, **2**, 48; **3**, 379
Benzylpenicillinum natricum, **2**, 51; **3**, 379
Bephenii hydroxynaphthoas, **2**, 53
Bephenium hydroxynaphthoate, **2**, 53
Bephenium hydroxynaphthoate RS, **2**, 285
Betamethasone, **2**, 55
Betamethasone RS, **2**, 285
Betamethasone valerate, **3**, 42
Betamethasone valerate RS, **3**, 343
Betamethasoni valeras, **3**, 42
Betamethasonum, **2**, 55
Biperiden, **3**, 45
Biperiden hydrochloride, **3**, 46
Biperiden hydrochloride RS, **3**, 343
Biperiden RS, **3**, 343
Biperideni hydrochloridum, **3**, 46
Biperidenum, **3**, 45
Bismuth oxynitrate R, **2**, 285
Bleomycin hydrochloride, **3**, 48
Bleomycin sulfate, **3**, 52
Bleomycini hydrochloridum, **3**, 48
Bleomycini sulfas, **3**, 52
Blue tetrazolium/ethanol TS, **2**, 286
Blue tetrazolium R, **2**, 285
Blue tetrazolium/sodium hydroxide TS, **2**, 286

Borax, *see* Sodium tetraborate
Boric acid R, (50 g/l) TS, **1**, 171
Bromine R, TS1, AsTS, **1**, 172
Bromocresol green/ethanol TS, **2**, 286
Bromocresol green R, **2**, 286
Breomocresol purple/ethanol TS, **2**, 286
Breomocresol purple R, **2**, 286
Bromophenol blue/ethanol TS, **1**, 172
Bromophenol blue R, **1**, 172
Bromothymol blue/dimethylformamide TS, **2**, 286
Bromothymol blue/ethanol TS, **1**, 172
Bromothymol blue R, **1**, 172
Brown stock standard TS, **1**, 172
Buffer borate, pH 8.0, TS, pH 9.0, TS, pH 9.6, TS, **2**, 286
Buffer phosphate, pH 6.4, TS, pH 6.9, TS, **2**, 287
Buffer phthalate, pH 3.4, TS, pH 3.5, TS, **2**, 287
Buffer solutions, *see under name of buffer*
Bupivacaine hydrochloride, **2**, 58
Bupivacaine hydrochloride RS, **2**, 287
Bupivacaini hydrochloridum, **2**, 58
Busulfan, **3**, 55
Busulfanum, **3**, 55
1-Butanol R, **2**, 287
2-Butanol R, **3**, 343
tert-Butanol R, **2**, 287
Butyl acetate R, **3**, 343
1-Butylamine R, **2**, 287
Butylated hydroxytoluene R, **3**, 343

C

Cadmium acetate R, **2**, 288
Caffeine, **2**, 85
Caffeine RS, **2**, 288
Calciferol, *see* Ergocalciferol
Calcii carbonas, **3**, 57
Calcii folinas, **3**, 59
Calcii gluconas, **2**, 60; **3**, 379
Calcium carbonate, **3**, 57
Calcium carbonate R1, R2, **1**, 172
Calcium chloride R, *see* Calcium chloride, anhydrous, R
Calcium chloride, anhydrous, R, hydrated, (55 g/l) TS, **1**, 172
Calcium folinate, **3**, 59
Calcium folinate RS, **3**, 343
Calcium gluconate, **2**, 60; **3**, 379
Calcium hydroxide R, TS, **2**, 288
Calcium standard 100 µg/ml Ca), ethanolic, TS, **3**, 343

Calcium standard (10 µg/ml Ca) TS, **3**, 343
Calcium sulfate R, hemihydrate R, **3**, 343;
    TS, **3**, 344
Calcon carboxylic acid R, **1**, 173
Calcon carboxylic acid indicator mixture R,
    1, 173
Calcon indicator mixture R, **1**, 173
Calcon R, **1**, 172
Calculation of results, **1**, 11
Caprylic acid, *see* Octanoic acid
Carbamazepine, **3**, 61
Carbamazepine RS, **3**, 344
Carbamazepinum, **3**, 61
Carbidopa, **3**, 63
Carbidopa RS, **3**, 344
Carbidopum, **3**, 63
Carbo activatus, **2**, 62; **3**, 380
Carbomer R, **2**, 288
Carbonate-free sodium hydroxide (1 mol/1)
    VS, (0.5 mol/1) VS, (0.2 mol/1) VS,
    (0.1 mol/1) VS, **1**, 205; (0.02 mol/1) VS,
    (0.01 mol/1) VS, **1**, 206
Carbon-dioxide-free water R, **1**, 211
Carbon dioxide R, **1**, 173
Carbon disulfide R, IR, **1**, 173
Carbon tetrachloride R, **1**, 173
Carboxymethylcellulose R, **3**, 344
Category, **2**, 13
Cellulose R1, R2, R3, **2**, 288
Cephaëline hydrochloride R, **3**, 344
Ceric ammonium nitrate R, TS, **1**, 173
Ceric ammonium sulfate/nitric acid TS, **2**,
    289
Ceric ammonium sulfate R, (0.1 mol/1) VS,
    2, 289
Ceric sulfate R, (35 g/1) TS, **1**, 174;
    (0.1 mol/1) VS, **3**, 344
Ceruleum methylenum, *see* Methylthioni-
    nium chloride
Charcoal, activated, **2**, 62; **3**, 380
Charcoal R, **1**, 174
Chemical formulas, **2**, 10
Chemical names, **2**, 10
Chloralose R, **1**, 144
Chlorambucil, **3**, 65
Chlorambucilum, **3**, 65
Chloramphenicol, **2**, 64
Chloramphenicol palmitate, **3**, 67
Chloramphenicol palmitate RS, **3**, 344
Chloramphenicol RS, **2**, 289
Chloramphenicoli palmitas, **3**, 67
Chloramphenicolum, **2**, 64
Chloraniline R, **3**, 344

Chlorbutinum, *see* Chlorambucilum
Chlorhexidini diacetate, **3**, 69
Chlorhexidini dihydrochloride, **3**, 71
Chlorhexidini diacetas, **3**, 69
Chlorhexidini dihydrochloridum, **3**, 71
Chlorine R, TS, **1**, 174
Chlormethine hydrochloride, **2**, 66
Chlormethini hydrochloridum, **2**, 66
4-Chloroacetanilide R, **3**, 344
Chloroform R, **1**, 174
    ethanol-free, R, **2**, 289
5-Chloro-2-methylaminobenzophenone RS,
    2, 289
2-Chloro-4-nitroaniline R, **2**, 289
Chloroquine phosphate, **2**, 68
Chloroquine sulfate, **2**, 70
Chloroquini phosphas, **2**, 68
Chloroquini sulfas, **2**, 70
2-(4-Chloro-3-sulfamoyl)benzoic acid RS, **2**,
    290
Chlorphenamine hydrogen maleate, **2**, 72
Chlorphenamine hydrogen maleate RS, **2**,
    290
Chlorphenamini hydrogenomaleas, **2**, 72
Chlorpheniramine hydrogen maleate, *see*
    Chlorphenamine hydrogen maleate
Chlorpromazine hydrochloride, **2**, 74
Chlorpromazine hydrochloride RS, **2**, 290
Chlorpromazini hydrochloridum, **2**, 74
Chlortalidone, **2**, 76
Chlortalidone RS, **2**, 290
Chlortalidonum, **2**, 76
Chlortetracycline hydrochloride, **3**, 73
Chlortetracycline hydrochloride RS, **2**, 290
Chlortetracycline hydrochloridum, **3**, 73
Cholecalciferol, *see* Colecalciferol
Chromic acid TS, **2**, 290
Chromium trioxide R, **2**, 290
Chromotropic acid sodium salt R,
    see Disodium chromotropate R
C.I. 14645, *see* Mordant Black 11 R
C.I. 15705, *see* Calcon R
C.I. 50040, *see* Neutral red R
C.I. Basic Red, *see* Neutral red R
Cimetidine, **3**, 76
Cimetidine RS, **3**, 344
Cimetidinum, **3**, 76
C.I. Mordant Black 11, *see* Mordant Black 11
    R
C.I. Mordant Black 17, *see* Calcon R
Cinchonidine R, **2**, 290
Cinchonine R, **3**, 344
Citrate buffer, pH 5.4, TS, **2**, 290

Citric acid, copper-free, R, **2**, 290
Citric acid R, FeR, (180 g/l) FeTS, **1**, 174; (20 g/l) TS, **2**, 290; PbR, **3**, 344
Clarity of solution, **2**, 11
Clofazimine, **3**, 78
Clofazimine RS, **3**, 345
Clofaziminum, **3**, 78
Clomifene citrate, **3**, 80
Clomifene citrate RS, **3**, 345
Clomifene citrate Z-isomer RS, **3**, 345
Clomifeni citras, **3**, 80
Cloxacillin sodium, **2**, 78
Cloxacillin sodium RS, **2**, 290
Cloxacillinum natricum, **2**, 78
Coal tar, **3**, 251
Cobalt(II) chloride R, (30 g/l) TS, (5 g/l) TS, TS, **3**, 345
Cobalt colour, strong, TS, **1**, 174, TS, **1**, 174
Cobalt(II) nitrate R, (100 g/l) TS, (10 g/l) TS, **3**, 345
Cobaltous thiocyanate TS, **2**, 291
Codeine monohydrate, **2**, 80
Codeine phosphate, **2**, 82
Codeine R, **2**, 291
Codeini phosphas, **2**, 82
Codeinum monohydricum, **2**, 80
Coffeinum, **2**, 85
Colchicine, **3**, 82
Colchicine RS, **3**, 345
Colchicinum, **3**, 82
Colecalciferol, **2**, 87
Colecalciferol RS, **2**, 291
Colecalciferolum, **2**, 87
Colourless solution, **2**, 12
Congo red paper R, **1**, 175
Constant weight, **1**, 12
Containers, **1**, 12; **2**, 12
  hermetically closed, definition of, **2**, 12
  tightly closed, definition of, **1**, 12
  well closed, definition of, **1**, 12
Copper(II) acetate R, **2**, 291; (45 g/l) TS, **3**, 345
Copper(II) chloride R, **3**, 345
Copper(II) chloride/ammonia TS, **3**, 345
Copper colour, strong, TS, **1**, 175, TS, **1**, 175
Copper edetate TS, **2**, 291
Copper-free citric acid R, **2**, 290
Copper standard (10 μg/ml Cu) TS, **3**, 346
Copper standard TS1, TS2, **3**, 346
Copper(II) sulfate/ammonia TS, **2**, 291
Copper(II) sulfate/pyridine TS, **2**, 291

Copper(II) sulfate R, (160 g/l) TS, **1**, 175; (80 g/l) TS, **2**, 291; (1 g/l) TS, **3**, 346
Corn starch R, *see* Starch R
Cortisol, *see* Hydrocortisone
Cortisol acetate, *see* Hydrocortisone acetate
o-Cresol R, **2**, 291
Cresol red R, **3**, 346
Cresol red/ethanol TS, **3**, 346
Crystal violet/acetic acid TS, **1**, 175
Crystal violet R, **1**, 175
Culture medium Cm1, Cm2, Cm3, **1**, 175; Cm4, Cm5, Cm6, **1**, 176; Cm7, **1**, 177; Cm8, Cm9, Cm10, **3**, 346; Cm11, **3**, 347
Cyanide/oxalate/thiosulfate TS, **2**, 292
Cyanocobalamin, **2**, 89
Cyanocobalaminum, **2**, 89
Cyanoethylmethyl silicone gum R, **2**, 292
Cyanogen bromide TS, **2**, 292
Cyclodolum, *see* Trihexyphenidyli hydrochloridum
Cyclohexane R, **1**, 177; R1, **2**, 292
Cyclophosphamide, **3**, 84
Cyclophosphamidum, **3**, 84
Cyclophosphanum, *see* Cyclophosphamidum
L-Cystine R, **1**, 177
Cytarabine, **3**, 86
Cytarabine, RS, **3**, 347
Cytarabinum, **3**, 86

D

Dapsone, **2**, 91
Dapsone RS, **2**, 292
Dapsonum, **2**, 91
Deferoxamine mesilate, **3**, 88
Deferoxamini mesilas, **3**, 88
Dehydrated ethanol R, **1**, 179
Dehydrated methanol R, **1**, 191
Dehydroemetine dihydrochloride, **3**, 90
Dehydroemetini dihydrochloridum, **3**, 90
Desferrioxamine mesylate, *see* Deferoxamine mesilate
Dexamethasone, **2**, 95
Dexamethasone acetate, **2**, 93; **3**, 380
Dexamethasone acetate RS, **2**, 292
Dexamethasone RS, **2**, 292
Dexamethasone sodium phosphate, **3**, 91
Dexamethasone sodium phosphate RS, **3**, 347
Dexamethasoni acetas, **2**, 93; **3**, 380
Dexamethasoni natrii phosphas, **3**, 347

Dexamethasonum, **2**, 95
Dextromethorphan hydrobromide, **3**, 94
Dextromethorphan hydrobromide RS, **3**, 347
Dextromethorphani hydrobromidum, **3**, 94
Dextrose, *see* Glucose
Diammonium hydrogen phosphate R, (100 g/l) TS, **2**, 292
Diatomaceous support R, **3**, 347
Diazepam, **2**, 98
Diazepam RS, **2**, 292
Diazepamum, **2**, 98
Diazobenzenesulfonic acid TS, **2**, 293
Diazomethane TS, **2**, 293
Diazoxide, **2**, 100
Diazoxide RS, **2**, 292
Diazoxidum, **2**, 100
Dibromomethane R, **1**, 177
Dibutyl ether R, **2**, 293
Dibutyl phthalate R, **2**, 293
Dicainum, *see* Tetracaini hydrochloridum
Dichloroethane R, **2**, 293
Dichlorofluorescein R, TS, **3**, 347
Dichloromethane R, **1**, 177
2,6-Dichloroquinone chlorimide/ethanol TS, **2**, 294
2,6-Dichloroquinone chlorimide R, **2**, 293
Dichromate colour, strong, TS, **1**, 177
Dicloxacillin sodium, **3**, 96
Dicloxacillin sodium RS, **3**, 347
Dicloxacillinum natricum, **3**, 96
Dicoumarol, **2**, 101
Dicoumarol RS, **2**, 294
Dicoumarolum, **2**, 101
Diethoxytetrahydrofuran/acetic acid TS, **2**, 294
Diethoxytetrahydrofuran R, **2**, 294
Diethylamine R, **2**, 294
Diethylaminoethylcellulose R, **3**, 347
Diethylcarbamazine dihydrogen citrate, **2**, 103
Diethylcarbamazine dihydrogen citrate RS, **2**, 294
Diethylcarbamazini dihydrogenocitras, **2**, 103
Diethylene glycol R, **1**, 177
Diethylene glycol succinate R, **2**, 294
Diethyl phthalate R, **3**, 347
Digitonin R, TS, **2**, 294
Digitoxin, **2**, 105
Digitoxin RS, **2**, 294
Digitoxinum, **2**, 105
Digoxin, **2**, 107

Digoxin RS, **2**, 294
Digoxinum, **2**, 107
Diloxanide furoate, **3**, 99
Diloxanide furoate RS, **3**, 347
Diloxanidi furoas, **3**, 99
Dilute arsenic AsTS, **1**, 170
Dilute lead PbTS, **1**, 187
Dimercaprol, **3**, 100
Dimercaprolum, **3**, 100
Dimethylacetamide R, **3**, 347
Dimethylamine/ethanol TS, **2**, 295
Dimethylamine R, **2**, 294
4-Dimethylaminobenzaldehyde R, TS1, TS2, TS3, TS4, **2**, 295; TS5, TS6, **3**, 348
4-Dimethylaminocinnamaldehyde R, TS1, TS2, **2**, 295
N,*N*-Dimethylaniline R, **3**, 348
Dimethylformamide R, **1**, 178
1,4-Di[2-(4-methyl-5-phenyloxazole)]-benzene R, **1**, 178
Dimethyl-POPOP, *see* 1,4-Di[2-(4-methyl-5-phenyloxazole)]benzene R
Dimethyl sulfoxide R, **3**, 348
Dinitrobenzene/ethanol TS, **2**, 296
Dinitrobenzene R, **2**, 296
2,4-Dinitrochlorobenzene R, **3**, 348
Dinonyl phthalate R, **2**, 296
Dioxan R, **1**, 178
Diphenoxylate hydrochloride, **3**, 102
Diphenoxylate hydrochloride RS, **3**, 348
Dyphenoxylati hydrochloridum, **3**, 102
Diphenylamine R, **2**, 296
Diphenylamine/sulfuric acid TS, **3**, 348
Diphenylbenzene, *see* *p*-Terphenyl R
Diphenylbenzidine R, **1**, 178
1,5-Diphenylcarbazide R, **3**, 348
Diphenylcarbazide TS, **3**, 348
Diphenylcarbazone/ethanol TS, **1**, 179
Diphenylcarbazone R, **1**, 179
Diphenyl ether R, **1**, 179
2,5-Diphenyloxazole R, **1**, 179
Dipotassium hydrogen phosphate R, **1**, 179
Diprazinum, *see* Promethazini hydro-chloridum
Disodium chromotropate R, (10 g/l) TS, **2**, 296
Disodium edetate R, (0.05 mol/1) VS, **1**, 179, **3**, 377; (50 g/l) TS, **2**, 296; (0.1 mol/l) VS, **2**, 296, **3**, 385; (20 g/l) TS, (10 g/l) TS, (0.01 mol/l) VS, **3**, 349
Disodium hydrogen phosphate, anhydrous, R, **1**, 179

Disodium hydrogen phosphate R, 296; (40 g/l) TS, **2**, 297; (100 g/l) TS, (28.4 g/l) TS, **3**, 349
Dithizone R, **2**, 297; TS, **3**, 349
Dithizone standard TS, **3**, 349
Dopamine hydrochloride, **3**, 103
Dopamine hydrochloride RS, **3**, 349
Dopamini hydrochloridum, **3**, 103
Doxorubicin hydrochloride, **3**, 105
Doxorubicin hydrochloride RS, **3**, 349
Doxorubicini hydrochloridum, **3**, 105
Doxycycline hyclate, **3**, 107
Doxycyclini hyclas, **3**, 107
Dried peptone R, **1**, 194
Drying, loss on, **1**, 12; **2**, 12

E

Edrophonii chloridum, **3**, 109
Edrophonium chloride, **3**, 109
Emetine hydrochloride, **3**, 111
Emetine hydrochloride RS, **3**, 349
Emetini hydrochloridum, **3**, 111
Eosin Y R, **3**, 349; (5 g/l) TS, **3**, 350
Ephedrine, **3**, 113
Ephedrine hydrochloride, **3**, 115
Ephedrine sulfate, **3**, 117
Ephedrini hydrochloridum, **3**, 115
Ephedrini sulfas, **3**, 117
Ephedrinum, **3**, 113
4-Epianhydrotetracycline hydrochloride RS, **2**, 297
Epinephrine, **2**, 112; **3**, 381
Epinephrine hydrogen tartrate, **2**, 110; **3**, 380
Epinephrine hydrogen tartrate, R, **2**, 297
Epinephrini hydrogenotartras, **2**, 110; **3**, 380
Epinephrinum, **2**, 112; **3**, 381
4-Epitetracycline hydrochloride RS, **2**, 297
Ergocalciferol, **3**, 119
Ergocalciferol RS, **3**, 350
Ergocalciferolum, **3**, 119
Ergometrine hydrogen maleate, **2**, 114
Ergometrine hydrogen maleate RS, **2**, 297
Ergometrini hydrogenomaleas, **2**, 114
Ergosterol R, **3**, 350
Ergotamine tartrate, **2**, 116; **3**, 381
Ergotamine tartrate RS, **2**, 297
Ergotamini tartras, **2**, 116; **3**, 381
Eriochrome Black R, *see* Mordant Black 11 R

Eriochrome Black T, *see* Mordant Black 11 R
Eriochrome Blue Black R, *see* Calcon R
Erythromycin, **3**, 121
Erythromycin RS, **3**, 350
Erythromycin ethylsuccinate, **3**, 123
Erythromycin ethylsuccinate RS, **3**, 350
Erythromycin stearate, **3**, 125
Erythromicyn stearate, RS, **3**, 350
Erythromycini ethylsuccinas, **3**, 123
Erythromycini stearas, **3**, 125
Erythromycinum, **3**, 121
Eserine salicylate, *see* Physostigmine salicylate
Estrone RS, **2**, 297
Ethambutol hydrochloride, **2**, 119
Ethambutol hydrochloride RS, **2**, 297
Ethambutoli hydrochloridum, **2**, 119
2,2′-(Ethanediylidenedinitrilo)diphenol, *see* Glyoxal bis(2-hydroxyanil)R
Ethanol, aldehyde-free, (95 per cent) R *see* Ethanol (~750 g/l), aldehyde-free, TS
Ethanol (95 per cent) R, *see* Ethanol (~750 g/l) TS
Ethanol (~750 g/l) TS, dehydrated, R, **1**, 179; (~750 g/l), sulfate-free, TS, (~710 g/l) TS, (~375 g/l) TS, (~150 g/l) TS, **1**, 180; (~750 g/l), aldehyde-free, TS, neutralized, TS, (~675 g/l) TS, (~600 g/l) TS, **2**, 297
Ether anaesthesicus, **3**, 128
Ether, anaesthetic, **3**, 128
Ether R, **1**, 179
   diphenyl, R, **1**, 179
Ethinylestradiol, **2**, 121
Ethinylestradiol RS, **2**, 297
Ethinylestradiolum, **2**, 121
Ethionamide, **3**, 129
Ethionamide RS, **3**, 350
Ethionamidum, **3**, 129
Ethosuximide, **2**, 123; **3**, 381
Ethosuximide RS, **2**, 297
Ethosuximidum, **2**, 123; **3**, 381
Ethyl acetate R, **1**, 180
Ethyl alcohol, *see* Ethanol
Ethyl aminobenzoate, *see* Benzocaine
Ethylenediamine R, **2**, 298
Ehtylene glycol monoethyl ether R, **1**, 180
Ethylene glycol monomethyl ether R, **3**, 350
Ethyl iodide R, **2**, 298
Ethylmethylketone R, **2**, 298
Examination in ultraviolet light, **2**, 12

F

Ferric ammonium sulfate R, (45 g/l) TS, **1**, 180; TS1, TS2, **2**, 298; (0.1 mol/1) VS, **3**, 350

Ferric chloride R, (25 g/1) TS, **1**, 180; (65 g/l) TS, **3**, 350; (50 g/l) TS, **3**, 351

Ferric chloride/ferricyanide/arsenite TS, **3**, 351

Ferric chloride/potassium ferricyanide TS, **3**, 351

Ferricyanide standard (50 µg/ml) TS, **3**, 351

Ferrocyanide standard (100 µg/ml) TS, **3**, 351

Ferrosi fumaras, **3**, 131

Ferrosi sulfas, **2**, 125

Ferrous ammonium sulfate R, (1 g/l) TS, **1**, 180

Ferrous fumarate, **3**, 131

Ferrous sulfate, **2**, 125

Ferrous sulfate R, (15 g/l) TS, (0.1 mol/l) VS, **1**, 180

Firebrick, pink, R, **2**, 298

Flucytosine, **3**, 133

Flucytosine RS, **3**, 351

Flucytosinum, **3**, 133

Fludrocortisone acetate, **3**, 135

Fludrocortisone acetate RS, **3**, 351

Fludrocortisoni acetas, **3**, 135

Fluorescein sodium, **3**, 138

Fluoresceinum natricum, **3**, 138

Fluorouracil, **3**, 141

Fluorouracil, RS, **3**, 351

Fluorouracilum, **3**, 141

Fluphenazine decanoate, **2**, 127

Fluphenazine decanoate RS, **2**, 298

Fluphenazine enantate, **2**, 129

Fluphenazine enantate RS, **2**, 298

Fluphenazine hydrochloride, **2**, 131

Fluphenazine hydrochloride RS, **2**, 298

Fluphenazini decanoas, **2**, 127

Fluphenazini enantas, **2**, 129

Fluphenazini hydrochloridum, **2**, 131

Folic acid, **2**, 24

Folic acid RS, **2**, 298

Formaldehyde R, *see* Formaldehyde TS

Formaldehyde/sulfuric acid TS, **2**, 298

Formaldehyde TS, **2**, 298

Formamide R, **2**, 298

Formic acid (~1080 g/l) TS, **1**, 181

Formic acid, anhydrous, R, **2**, 299

Formic acid R, *see* Formic acid (~1080 g/l) TS

Formulas, chemical, **2**, 10

3-Formylrifamycin SV RS, **3**, 351

Fradiomycini sulfas, *see* Neomycini sulfas

Fuchsin, basic, R, TS, **2**, 299

  decolorized, TS, **3**, 351

Furadonium, *see* Nitrofurantoinum

Furosemide, **2**, 133

Furosemide RS, **2**, 299

Furosemidum, **2**, 133

G

Gallamine triethiodide, **3**, 143

Gallamine triethiodide RS, **3**, 352

Gallamini triethiodidum, **3**, 143

Gamma benzene hexachloride, *see* Lindane

Gammahexachlorcyclohexane, *see* Lindane

Gelatin R, TS, **1**, 181

General notices, **1**, 10; **2**, 10

Gentamicin sulfate, **3**, 145

Gentamicin sulfate RS, **3**, 352

Gentamicini sulfas, **3**, 145

Glacial acetic acid R, R1, **1**, 168; R1, **2**, 279

Glauber's salt, *see* Sodium sulfate

Glibenclamide, **3**, 147

Glibenclamide RS, **3**, 352

Glibenclamidum, **3**, 147

Glucose, **2**, 135; **3**, 381

Glucose, anhydrous, R, **3**, 352

  hydrate R, **1**, 181

Glucosum, **2**, 135; **3**, 381

Glycerol R, **1**, 181

Glyoxal bis(2-hydroxyanil) R, TS, **1**, 182

Granulated zinc AsR, **1**, 211

Green stock standard TS, **1**, 182

Griseofulvin, **2**, 137

Griseofulvin RS, **2**, 299

Griseofulvinum, **2**, 137

H

Haloperidol, **2**, 139

Haloperidol RS, **2**, 299

Haloperidolum, **2**, 139

Halothane, **2**, 141

Halothanum, **2**, 141

Helium R, **1**, 182

Heparinized saline TS, **1**, 182

Heptane R, **3**, 352
Hermetically closed containers, definition of, **2**, 12
Hexamethyldisilazane R, **3**, 352
Hexamethylene, *see* Cyclohexane
Hexamethylenetetramine, *see* Methenamine
Hexane R, **2**, 299
High performance liquid chromatography, **3**, 373
Histamine dihydrochloride R, **1**, 182
Histamine phosphate R, **1**, 183
Histamine, strong, TS, **1**, 182
Holmium oxide R, **1**, 183
Holmium perchlorate TS, **1**, 183
Homatropine hydrobromide, **3**, 149
Homatropini hydrobromidum, **3**, 149
Hydralazine hydrochloride, **3**, 150
Hydralazini hydrochloridum, **3**, 150
Hydrargyri oxycyanidum, **2**, 143
Hydrated calcium chloride R, **1**, 172
Hydrazine hydrate R, **2**, 300
Hydrazine sulfate R, **3**, 352
Hydriodic acid R, *see* Hydriodic acid (∼970 g/l) TS
Hydriodic acid (∼970 g/l) TS, **1**, 183
Hydrochloric acid, saturated, R, *see* Hydrochloric acid (∼420 g/l) TS
Hydrochloric acid (∼420 g/l) TS, (∼250 g/l) TS, (∼250 g/l) AsTS, **1**, 183; (∼250 g/l), stannated AsTS, (∼70 g/l) TS, ClTS, (2 mol/l) VS, (1 mol/l) VS, (0.5 mol/l) VS, (0.1 mol/l) VS, **1**, 184; (0.015 mol/l) VS, (0.01 mol/l) VS, **1**, 185; (∼250 g/l) FeTS, brominated, AsTS, (5 mol/l) VS, (0.2 mol/l) VS, (0.02 mol/l) VS, (0.001 mol/l) VS, **2**, 300; (∼330 g/l) TS, (0.05 mol/l) VS, **3**, 352; (0.005 mol/l) VS, (0.0001 mol/l) VS, **3**, 353
Hydrochloric acid/methanol (0.01 mol/l) VS, **3**, 353
Hydrochlorothiazide, **2**, 145
Hydrochlorothiazide RS, **2**, 301
Hydrochlorothiazidum, **2**, 145
Hydrocortisone, **2**, 149
Hydrocortisone acetate, **2**, 147
Hydrocortisone acetate RS, **2**, 301
Hydrocortisone R, RS, **2**, 301
Hydrocortisone sodium succinate, **3**, 152
Hydrocortisone sodium succinate RS, **3**, 353
Hydrocortisoni acetas, **2**, 147
Hydrocortisoni natrii succinas, **3**, 152

Hydrocortisonum, **2**, 149
Hydrogen peroxide (30 per cent) R. *see* Hydrogen peroxide (∼330 g/l) TS
Hydrogen peroxide (∼330 g/l) TS, **2**, 301; (∼60 g/l) TS, **1**, 185
Hydrogen sulfide R, TS, **1**, 185
Hydroquinone R, **3**, 353
Hydroxocobalamin, **3**, 154
Hydroxocobalamin chloride, **3**, 158
Hydroxocobalamin sulfate, **3**, 158
Hydroxocobalamini chloridum, **3**, 158
Hydroxocobalamini sulfas, **3**, 158
Hydroxocobalaminum, **3**, 154
Hydroxyethylcellulose R, TS, **2**, 301
Hydroxylamine hydrochloride R, **2**, 302; (200 g/l) TS, **3**, 353
(–)-3-(4-Hydroxy-3-methoxyphenyl)-2-hydrazino-2-methylalanine RS, **3**, 353
(–)-3-(4-Hydroxy-3-methoxyphenyl)-2-methylalanine RS, **2**, 302

I

Ibuprofen, **2**, 151
Ibuprofen RS, **2**, 302
Ibuprofenum, **2**, 151
Identity tests, **2**, 11
Imidazole/mercuric chloride TS, **2**, 302
Imidazole R, crystallized, R, **2**, 302
Iminodibenzyl R, **3**, 353
Impurities, **2**, 11
pH-indicator paper R, **3**, 353
Indicators, visual determination of pH values, **2**, 12
Indometacin, **2**, 154
Indometacin RS, **2**, 302
Indometacinum, **2**, 154
Iodine, **2**, 156
Iodine bromide R, **1**, 185; TS, **1**, 186
Iodine/chloroform TS, **3**, 354
Iodine/ethanol TS, **2**, 302
Iodine R, **1**, 185; TS, (0.1 mol/l) VS, **3**, 377; (0.02 mol/l) VS, (0.01 mol/l) VS, **1**, 185, **3**, 378; (0.05 mol/l) VS, (0.005 mol/l) VS, (0.0001 mol/l) VS, **3**, 354
Iodum, **2**, 156
Ipecacuanhae radix, **3**, 161
Ipecacuanha root, **3**, 161
Iron salicylate TS, **3**, 354
Iron colour, strong, TS, **1**, 186; TS, **1**, 186
Iron standard FeTS, **1**, 186
Isoniazid, **2**, 157

Isoniazid RS, **2**, 302
Isoniazidum, **2**, 157
Isonicotinic acid hydrazide, *see* Isoniazid
Isoprenaline hydrochloride, **2**, 159; **3**, 382
Isoprenaline sulfate, **2**, 161; **3**, 382
Isoprenalini hydrochloridum, **2**, 159; **3**, 382
Isoprenalini sulfas, **2**, 161; **3**, 382
iso-Propanol, *see* 2-Propanol R
Isopropylamine R, **3**, 354

K

Kalii chloridum, **2**, 163; **3**, 382
Kalii citras, **3**, 164
Kalii iodidum, **2**, 165; **3**, 382
Karl Fischer reagent TS, **1**, 186
Kieselguhr R1, **2**, 302; R2, R3, R4, R5, **2**, 303

L

Lanthanum nitrate (30 g/1) TS, **1**, 187
Lead acetate paper R, **3**, 354
Lead acetate R, (80 g/1) TS, **1**, 187
Lead, dilute, PbTS, strong, PbTS, **1**, 187
Lead nitrate R, (0.05 mol/1) VS, **1**, 187; (100 g/1) TS, **3**, 354
Lead(IV) oxide, R, **3**, 355
Leucovorin calcium, *see* Calcium folinate
Levarterenol hydrogen tartrate R, **2**, 303; **3**, 385
Levodopa, **2**, 167
Levodopa RS, **2**, 303
Levodopum, **2**, 167
Levonorgestrel, **3**, 166
Levonorgestrel RS, **3**, 355
Levonorgestrelum, **3**, 166
Levothyroxine sodium, **3**, 168
Levothyroxine sodium RS, **3**, 355
Levothyroxinum natricum, **3**, 168
Lidocaine, **2**, 171
Lidocaine hydrochloride, **2**, 169
Lidocaine RS, **2**, 303
Lidocaini hydrochloridum, **2**, 169
Lidocainum, **2**, 171
Light petroleum R, **1**, 195; R1, **2**, 307
Light, protection from, **1**, 12
Lindane, **2**, 173; **3**, 382
Lindane RS, **2**, 303
Lindanum, **2**, 173; **3**, 382

Liothyronine RS, **3**, 355
Liquid chromatography, high performance, **3**, 373
Liquid paraffin R, **1**, 192
Lithii carbonas, **2**, 175
Lithium carbonate, **2**, 175
Lithium carbonate R, **3**, 355
Lithium carbonate/trinitrophenol TS, **3**, 355
Lithium chloride R, (10 g/1) TS, **3**, 355
Lithium methoxide (0.1 mol/1) VS, **2**, 304; **3**, 386
Lithium perchlorate/acetic acid TS, **1**, 188
Lithium perchlorate R, **1**, 188
Lithium R, **2**, 303
Litmus paper R, **2**, 304
Litmus R. TS **2**, 304
Loperamide hydrochloride, **3**, 170
Loperamide hydrochloride RS, **3**, 355
Loperamidi hydrochloridum, **3**, 170
Loss on drying, **1**, 12; **2**, 12

M

Marcrogol 1000 R, **3**, 355; 400 R, **1**, 188; 20M R, **2**, 304
Macrogol *p*-isooctylphenyl ether R, **3**, 355
Magenta, basic, R. *see* Fuchsin, basic, R
Magnesii hydroxidum, **3**, 172
Magnesii oxidum, **3**, 174
Magnesium acetate R, **3**, 355
Magnesium chloride R, (0.1 mol/1) VS, **3**, 355
Magnesium hydroxide, **3**, 172
Magnesium (0.1 mg/ml Mg) TS, **3**, 356
Magnesium oxide, **3**, 174
Magnesium oxide R, **1**, 169
Magnesium standard (10 µg/ml Mg) TS, **3**, 356
Magnesium sulfate R, **1**, 189; (50 g/l) TS, **2**, 304
Magnesium sulfate/sulfuric acid TS, **3**, 356
Manganese dioxide R, **1**, 189
Manganese/silver paper R, **1**, 189
Manganese sulfate R, (15 g/l) TS, **1**, 190
Mannitol, **2**, 177; **3**, 383
Mannitolum, **2**, 177; **3**, 383
Mebendazole, **3**, 176
Mebendazole RS, **3**, 356
Mebendazolum, **3**, 176
Menadione R, **3**, 356
Meperidine hydrochloride, *see* Pethidine hydrochloride

Mercaptoacetic acid R, **1**, 190
Mercuric acetate/acetic acid TS, **1**, 190
Mercuric acetate R, **1**, 190
Mercuric bromide R, AsTS, paper AsTS, **1**, 190
Mercuric chloride/ethanol TS, **3**, 356
Mercuric chloride R, (65 g/l) TS, (2.7 g/l) TS, **2**, 304
Mercuric nitrate R, (0.01 mol/1) VS, **1**, 190; TS, (0.02 mol/1) VS, **3**, 356
Mercuric oxide, yellow, R, **1**, 191
Mercuric oxycyanide, **2**, 143
Mercuric sulfate TS, **1**, 191
Mercury/nitric acid TS, **3**, 356
Mercury R, **2**, 304
Methanol R, dehydrated, R, **1**, 191
Methenamine R, **1**, 191
Methotrexate, **3**, 178
Methotrexate RS, **3**, 357
Methotrexatum, **3**, 357
Methyl alcohol, *see* Methanol
Methylcyanide, *see* Acetonitrile
Methyldopa, **2**, 179
Methyldopa RS, **2**, 304
Methyldopum, **2**, 179
Methylene blue, *see* Methylthioninium chloride
Methylene bromide, *see* Dibromomethane
Methylene chloride, *see* Dichloromethane
Methylisobutylketone R, **2**, 304
N-Methyl-*N*-nitrosotoluene-4-sulfonamide R, **2**, 304
Methyl orange/acetone TS, **2**, 304
Methyl orange/ethanol TS, **1**, 191
Methyl orange R, **1**, 191
N-Methylpiperazine R, **2**, 305
Methyl red/ethanol TS, **1**, 191
Methyl red/methylthioninium chloride TS, **1**, 192
Methyl red R, **1**, 191
Methyl silicone gum R, **2**, 305
Methyltestosterone, **2**, 181
Methyltestosterone RS, **2**, 305
Methyltestosteronum, **2**, 181
Methylthioninii chloridum, **3**, 180
Methylthioninium chloride, **3**, 180
Methylthioninium chloride R, (0.2 g/l) TS, **1**, 192; (1 g/l) TS, **2**, 305
Methylthymol blue mixture R, **2**, 305
Methylthymol blue R, **2**, 305
Metoclopramide hydrochloride, **3**, 182
Metoclopramide hydrochloride RS, **3**, 357
Metoclopramidi hydrochloridum, **3**, 182

Metrifonate, **3**, 184
Metrifonatum, **3**, 184
Metronidazole, **2**, 183
Metronidazole RS, **2**, 305
Metronidazolum, **2**, 183
Miconazole nitrate, **3**, 186
Miconazole nitrate RS, **3**, 357
Miconazoli nitras, **3**, 186
Molybdenum trioxide R, **3**, 357
Monoethanolamine R, **3**, 357
Monograph nomenclature, **2**, 10
Mordant Black 11 indicator mixture R, **1**, 192
Mordant Black 11 R, **1**, 192
Mordant Black 17, *see* Calcon R
Morphine hydrochloride, **2**, 185
Morphine sulfate, **2**, 187
Morphini hydrochloridum, **2**, 185
Morphini sulfas, **2**, 187
Myelosanum, *see* Busulfanum

N

Nagananinum, *see* Suramin sodium
Naloxone hydrochloride, **3**, 188
Naloxone hydrochloride RS, **3**, 357
Naloxoni hydrochloridum, **3**, 188
Names, chemical, **2**, 10
1-Naphtholbenzein/acetic acid TS, **2**, 305
1-Naphtholbenzein R, **2**, 305
1-Naphthol R, TS1, **2**, 305
2-Naphthol R, TS1, **1**, 192
β-Naphthol, *see* 2-Naphthol R
N-(1-Naphthyl)ethylenediamine hydrochloride/ethanol TS, **2**, 306
N-(1-Naphthyl)ethylenediamine hydrochloride R, **2**, 305; (5 g/l) TS, (1 g/l) TS, **2**, 306
Natrii calcii edetas, **3**, 190
Natrii chloridum, **2**, 189
Natrii citras, **3**, 192
Natrii cromoglicas, **3**, 194
Natrii fluoridum, **3**, 196
Natrii hydrogenocarbonas, **2**, 191
Natrii nitris, **3**, 197
Natrii nitroprussidum, **3**, 199
Natrii salicylas, **2**, 193; **3**, 383
Natrii stibogluconas, **3**, 201
Natrii sulfas, **3**, 203
Natrii sulfas anhydricus, **3**, 205
Natrii thiosulfas, **3**, 207
Natrii valproas, **3**, 209

Neomycin sulfate, **3**, 211
Neomycin B sulfate RS, **3**, 357
Neomycini sulfas, **3**, 211
Neostigmine bromide, **2**, 195
Neostigmini bromidum, **2**, 195
Neostigmine metilsulfate, **3**, 213
Neostigmine metilsulfate RS, **3**, 357
Neostigmini metilsulfas, **3**, 213
Neutral red R, **3**, 357
Neutral red/ethanol TS, **3**, 357
Niclosamide, **2**, 196
Niclosamidum, **2**, 196
Nicotinamide, **2**, 198
Nicotinamide RS, **2**, 306
Nicotinamidum, **2**, 198
Nicotinic acid, **2**, 26
Nicotinic acid RS, **2**, 306
Nifurtimox, **3**, 216
Nifurtimox RS, **3**, 357
Nifurtimoxum, **3**, 216
Niridazole, **3**, 218
Niridazole-chlorethylcarboxamide RS, **3**, 357
Niridazole RS, **3**, 357
Niridazolum, **3**, 218
Nitrazepam, **3**, 220
Nitrazepamum, **3**, 220
Nitric acid (70 per cent) R, *see* Nitric acid (~ 1000 g/l) TS
Nitric acid (~ 1000 g/l) TS, (~ 130 g/l) TS, (15 g/l) TS, (3 g/l) TS, **1**, 192; fuming, R, **2**, 306
4-Nitroaniline R, TS1, TS2, **2**, 306
Nitrobenzene R, **1**, 192
4-Nitrobenzoyl chloride R, **2**, 306
Nitrofurantoin, **3**, 222
Nitrofurantoin RS, **3**, 357
Nitrofurantoinum, **3**, 222
Nitrogen-free sulfuric acid (~ 1760 g/l) TS, **1**, 209
Nitrogen, oxygen-free, R, **2**, 306; R, **1**, 192
Nitromethane R, **3**, 357
1-Nitroso-2-naphthol-3,6-disodium disulfonate R, (2 g/l) TS, **2**, 306
1-Nitroso-2-naphthol-3,6-disodium sulfonate, *see* 1-Nitroso-2-naphthol-3,6-disodium disulfonate
Nomenclature, monograph, **2**, 10
Norethisterone, **2**, 202
Norethisterone acetate, **2**, 200
Norethisterone acetate RS, **2**, 306
Norethisterone RS, **2**, 306
Norethisteroni acetas, **2**, 200
Norethisteronum, **2**, 202
Noroxymorphone hydrochloride RS, **3**, 358
Noscapine, **3**, 224
Noscapine hydrochloride, **3**, 226
Noscapine RS, **3**, 358
Noscapini hydrochloridum, **3**, 226
Noscapinum, **3**, 224
Nystatin, **3**, 228
Nystatin RS, **3**, 358
Nystatinum, **3**, 228

O

iso-Octane, *see* 2,2,4-Trimethylpentane R
Octanoic acid R, **3**, 358
Opalescence standard TS1, **2**, 306; TS2, **2**, 307
Opalescence stock standard TS, **2**, 307
Oracet blue B R, **3**, 358
Oracet blue B/acetic acid TS, **3**, 358
Osmium tetroxide R, **2**, 307
Oxalic acid R, (0.05 g/l) TS, **3**, 358
Oxamniquine, **3**, 229
Oxamniquine RS, **3**, 358
Oxamniquinum, **3**, 229
Oxytetracycline dihydrate, **3**, 231
Oxytetracycline dihydrate RS, **3**, 358
Oxytetracycline hydrochloride, **3**, 234
Oxytetracycline hydrochloride RS, **2**, 307
Oxytetracyclini dihydras, **3**, 231
Oxytetracyclini hydrochloridum, **3**, 234

P

Pancreatic digest of casein R, **1**, 192
Papaic digest of soybean meal R, **1**, 192
Papaverine hydrochloride, **2**, 204
Papaverine hydrochloride RS, **2**, 307
Papaverini hydrochloridum, **2**, 204
Paracetamol, **3**, 237
Paracetamol, 4-aminophenol-free, R, **3**, 358
Paracetamolum, **3**, 237
Paraffin, liquid R, **1**, 192
Paraformaldehyde R, **3**, 358
Paromomycini sulfas, **3**, 239
Paromomycin sulfate, **3**, 239
Paromomycin sulfate RS, **3**, 359
Patents, notice concerning, **1**, 12
Penicillamine, **3**, 241

Penicillaminum, **3**, 241
Penicillinase R, **1**, 192; TS, **1**, 193
Penicillin G benzathine, *see* Benzathine benzylpenicillin
Penicillin G procaine, *see* Procaine benzylpenicillin
Pentamidine isetionate, **3**, 243
Pentamidine mesilate, **3**, 245
Pentamidini isetionas, **3**, 243
Pentamidini mesilas, **3**, 245
1-Pentanesulfonic acid sodium salt R, **3**, 359
1-Pentanesulfonic acid TS, **3**, 359
Peptone R1, (5 g/l) TS, (1 g/l) TS1, (1 g/l) TS2, dried, R, **1**, 194
Perchloric acid (70 per cent w/w) R, *see* Perchloric acid (~1170 g/l) TS
Perchloric acid/dioxan (0.1 mol/l) VS, **3**, 359
Perchloric acid (~1170 g/l) TS, (~140 g/l) TS, **1**, 194; (0.1 mol/l) VS, **1**, 194, **3**, 378; (0.05 mol/l) VS, **2**, 307; (0.02 mol/l) VS, **3**, 359
Pethidine hydrochloride, **3**, 247
Pethidini hydrochloridum, **3**, 247
Petroleum, light, R, **1**, 195; R1, **2**, 307
o-Phenanthroline R, (1 g/l) TS, TS, **1**, 195
Phenobarbital, **2**, 206
Phenobarbital sodium, **2**, 208; **3**, 383
Phenobarbitalum, **2**, 206
Phenobarbitalum natricum, **2**, 208; **3**, 383
Phenolphthalein/ethanol TS, **1**, 195
Phenolphthalein/pyridine TS, **1**, 195
Phenolphthalein R, **1**, 195
Phenol R, **1**, 195
Phenol red/ethanol TS, **1**, 195
Phenol red R, **1**, 195
2-Phenoxyethanol R, **2**, 307
Phenoxymethylpenicillin, **2**, 210
Phenoxymethylpenicillin calcium, **2**, 212
Phenoxymethylpenicillin calcium RS, **2**, 308
Phenoxymethylpenicillin potassium, **2**, 214
Phenoxymethylpenicillin potassium RS, **2**, 308
Phenoxymethylpenicillin RS, **2**, 307
Phenoxymethylpenicillinum, **2**, 210
Phenoxymethylpenicillinum calcicum, **2**, 212
Phenoxymethylpenicillinum kalicum, **2**, 214
1,4-Phenylenediamine dihydrochloride R, **3**, 359

2-Phenylethanol R, TS, **2**, 308
Phenylhydrazine/hydrochloric acid TS, **3**, 360
Phenylhydrazine hydrochloride R, **2**, 308; (10 g/l) TS, **3**, 360
Phenylhydrazine R, **2**, 308
Phenylhydrazine/sulfuric acid TS, **2**, 308
Phenyl/methylpolysiloxane R, **3**, 360
Phenytoin, **2**, 216
Phenytoin RS, **2**, 308
Phenytoin sodium, **2**, 218
Phenytoinum, **2**, 216
Phenytoinum natricum, **2**, 218
Phosphate buffer, pH 7.0, TS, **1**, 196; pH 7.4, TS, pH 7.6, TS, pH 8.0, TS, **3**, 360
Phosphate buffer, sterile, pH 4.5, TS, **1**, 195; pH 6.0, TS1, TS2, TS3, **1**, 196; pH 7.0, TS, pH 7.2, TS, **1**, 196; pH 8.0, TS1, TS2, **1**, 197; pH 7.8, TS, pH 10.5, TS1, **3**, 360
Phosphate/citrate buffer pH 4.5, TS, **2**, 308; pH 6.0, TS, **3**, 361
Phosphate standard buffer, pH 6.8, TS, **1**, 97, 196; pH 7.4, TS, **1**, 97, 197
Phosphate standard (5 µg/ml) TS, **3**, 361
Phosphomolybdic acid R, **2**, 308
Phosphoric acid R, *see* Phosphoric acid (~ 1440 g/l) TS
Phosphoric acid (~ 1440 g/l) TS, **1**, 197; (~ 105 g/l) TS, **3**, 361
Phosphorus pentoxide R, **1**, 197
Phosphorus, red, R, **2**, 308
Phosphotungstic acid TS, **3**, 361
Phthalic anhydride/pyridine TS, **1**, 197
Phthalic anhydride R, **1**, 197
pH values and their precision, **1**, 11
Phyllochinonum, *see* Phytomenadionum
Physostigmine salicylate, **2**, 220
Physostigmini salicylas, **2**, 220
Phytomenadione, **3**, 249
Phytomenadionum, **3**, 249
Phytonadione, *see* Phytomenadione
Pilocarpine hydrochloride, **2**, 222
Pilocarpine nitrate, **2**, 224
Pilocarpini hydrochloridum, **2**, 222
Pilocarpini nitras, **2**, 224
Piperazine adipate, **2**, 226
Piperazine citrate, **2**, 228
Piperazini adipas, **2**, 226
Piperazini citras, **2**, 228
Piperidine R, **3**, 361
Pix lithanthracis, **3**, 251
Platinic chloride R, (60 g/l) TS, **2**, 308

Polyethylene glycol 400, *see* Macrogol 400 R

Polysorbate 80 R, **1**, 197

Potassio-cupric tartrate TS, **2**, 309

Potassio-mercuric iodide TS, alkaline TS, **2**, 309

Potassium acetate R, TS, **1**, 198

Potassium antimonate R, TS, **3**, 361

Potassium bicarbonate R, **1**, 198

Potassium bitartrate, *see* Potassium hydrogen tartrate R

Potassium bromate R, (50 g/l) TS, (0.0167 mol/1) VS, **2**, 309; (0.00833 mol/l) VS, **3**, 361

Potassium bromide R, IR, (100 g/l) TS, **1**, 198; (0.119 g/l) TS, **2**, 309

Potassium carbonate R, **3**, 361
  anhydrous, R, **3**, 362

Potassium chloride, **2**, 163; **3**, 382

Potassium chloride R, IR, (350 g/l) TS, **1**, 198; (100 g/l) TS, **3**, 362

Potassium chromate R, (100 g/l) TS, **2**, 309

Potassium citrate, **3**, 164

Potassium cyanide R, (100 g/l) TS, (50 g/l) TS, **2**, 309; PbTS, **3**, 362

Potassium dichromate R, R1, TS, (0.0167 mol/l) VS, **1**, 198; (100 g/l) TS, **2**, 309; TS2, TS3, **3**, 362

Potassium dihydrogen phosphate R, **1**, 198; (100 g/l) TS, (27.2 g/l) TS, (13.6 g/l) TS, **3**, 362

Potassium ferricyanide R, **1**, 198; (10 g/l) TS, **1**, 199; (50 g/l) TS, **2**, 309

Potassium ferrocyanide R, (45 g/l) TS, **2**, 310

Potassium hydrogen phthalate R, **1**, 199
  standard TS, **1**, 97, 199

Potassium hydrogen tartrate R, **1**, 199
  standard TS, **1**, 97, 199

Potassium hydroxide/ethanol TS1, **1**, 199; (0.5 mol/l) VS, (0.02 mol/l) VS, **1**, 200; TS2, (1 mol/l) VS, **2**, 310

Potassium hydroxide/methanol TS, **2**, 310

Potassium hydroxide R, (~ 110 g/l) TS, (1 mol/l) VS, **1**, 199; (0.5 mol/l) VS, (0.1 mol/l) VS, **1**, 200; (0.01 mol/l) VS, **2**, 310

Potassium iodate R, (0.05 mol/l) VS, (0.01 mol/l) VS, **2**, 310; (3.6 mg/l) TS, **3**, 362

Potassium iodide, **2**, 165; **3**, 382

Potassium iodide R, AsR, (80 g/l) TS, **1**, 200; (400 g/l) TS, (300 g/l) TS, **2**, 310; (60 g/l) TS, **2**, 311; (100 g/l) TS, **3**, 362

Potassium iodide/starch TS1, **2**, 311

Potassium iodobismuthate TS1, TS2, **2**, 311

Potassium iodoplatinate TS, **2**, 311; TS2, **3**, 362

Potassium nitrate R, **1**, 200

Potassium nitrite R, (100 g/l) TS, **1**, 200

Potassium periodate R, TS, **2**, 311

Potassium permanganate R, (10 g/l) TS, (0.02 mol/l) VS, **1**, 201; (0.002 mol/l) VS, **2**, 311; (25 g/l) TS, **3**, 363

Potassium sodium tartrate R, **2**, 311

Potassium sulfate R, (174 mg/l) TS, **1**, 201

Potassium tetraoxalate R, **1**, 201
  standard TS, **1**, 97, 201

Potassium thiocyanate R, **2**, 311 **3**, 386; (200 g/l) TS, **3**, 363

Potato starch R, *see* Starch R

PPO, *see* 2,5-Diphenyloxazole

Praziquantel, **3**, 252

Praziquantel RS, **3**, 363

Praziquantelum, **3**, 252

Precision, pH values, **1**, 11
  quantities, **1**, 10
  temperature measurements, **1**, 11

Prednisolone, **2**, 230

Prednisolone acetate, **3**, 254

Prednisolone acetate RS, **3**, 363

Prednisolone RS, **2**, 312

Prednisolone sodium phosphate RS, **3**, 363

Prednisoloni acetas, **3**, 254

Prednisolonum, **2**, 230

Primaquine diphosphate, **2**, 232

Primaquine diphosphate RS, **2**, 312

Primaquini diphosphas, **2**, 232

Probenecid, **3**, 256

Probenecid RS, **3**, 363

Probenecidum, **3**, 256

Procainamide hydrochloride, **2**, 234

Procainamidi hydrochloridum, **2**, 234

Procaine benzylpenicillin, **3**, 258

Procaine hydrochloride, **2**, 236

Procaine hydrochloride RS, **2**, 312

Procaine penicillin, *see* Procaine benzylpenicillin

Procaini benzylpenicillinum, **3**, 258

Procaini hydrochloridum, **2**, 236

Procarbazine hydrochloride, **3**, 260

Procarbazine hydrochloride RS, **3**, 363

Procarbazini hydrochloridum, **3**, 260

Progesterone, **2**, 238

Progesterone RS, **2**, 312
Progesteronum, **2**, 238
Promethazine hydrochloride, **3**, 262
Promethazini hydrochloridum, **3**, 262
1-Propanol R, **2**, 312
2-Propanol R, **2**, 312
Propranolol hydrochloride, **2**, 240; **3**, 383
Propranolol hydrochloride RS, **2**, 312
Propranololi hydrochloridum, **2**, 240; **3**, 383
Propylene glycol R, **2**, 312
Propylthiouracil, **2**, 242
Propylthiouracilum, **2**, 242
Protection from light, **1**, 12
Protionamide, **3**, 264
Protionamide RS, **3**, 363
Protionamidum, **3**, 264
Provitamin D$_2$, *see* Ergosterol
Pyrantel embonate, **3**, 265
Pyrantel embonate RS, **3**, 363
Pyranteli embonas, **3**, 265
Pyrantel pamoate, *see* Pyrantel embonate
Pyrazinamide, **3**, 268
Pyrazinamide RS, **3**, 363
Pyrazinamidum, **3**, 268
Pyridine R, anhydrous R, **1**, 201
Pyridostigmine bromide, **2**, 244; **3**, 383
Pyridostigmine bromide RS, **2**, 312
Pyridostigmini bromidum, **2**, 244; **3**, 383
Pyridoxine hydrochloride, **2**, 246
Pyridoxini hydrochloridum, **2**, 246
Pyrimethamine, **3**, 269
Pyrimethamine RS, **3**, 363
Pyrimethaminum, **3**, 269
Pyrogallol R, alkaline, TS, **2**, 313

Q

Quantities and their precision, **1**, 10
Quinaldine red/ethanol TS, **2**, 313
Quinaldine red/methanol TS, **2**, 313
Quinaldine red R, **2**, 313
Quinidine sulfate, **3**, 271
Quinidini sulfas, **3**, 271
Quinine bisulfate, **3**, 273
Quinine dihydrochloride, **3**, 276
Quinine hydrochloride, **2**, 248; **3**, 384
Quinine R, **2**, 313
Quinine sulfate, **2**, 250; **3**, 384
Quinini bisulfas, **3**, 273
Quinini dihydrochloridum, **3**, 276
Quinini hydrochloridum, **2**, 248; **3**, 384
Quinini sulfas, **2**, 250; **3**, 384

R

Reagents, **1**, 13
   list of, **1**, 167; **2**, 277; **3**, 337
Red stock standard TS, **1**, 201; **3**, 378
Resazurin sodium R, (1 g/l) TS, **1**, 201
Reserpine, **2**, 252; **3**, 384
Reserpine RS, **2**, 313
Reserpinum, **2**, 252; **3**, 384
Resorcinol R, (20 g/l) TS, **1**, 201
Riboflavin, **2**, 254
Riboflavin RS, **2**, 313
Riboflavinum, **2**, 254
1-β-D-Ribofuranosyluracil, *see* Uridine R
Rifampicin, **3**, 278
Rifampicin quinone RS, **3**, 363
Rifampicin RS, **3**, 363
Rifampicinum, **3**, 278

S

Salazosulfapyridine, *see* Sulfasalazine
Salbutamol, **3**, 280
Salbutamol RS, **3**, 363
Salbutamol sulfate, **3**, 282
Salbutamol sulfate RS, **3**, 363
Salbutamoli sulfas, **3**, 282
Salbutamolum, **3**, 280
Salicylaldehyde R, TS, **3**, 363
Salicylic acid, **2**, 28
Salicylic acid R, **2**, 313
Saline TS, **1**, 202
Selenious acid R, **2**, 313
Selenious acid/sulfuric acid TS, **2**, 314
Selenium R, **1**, 202
Sennae folium, **3**, 284
Sennae fructus, **3**, 286
Senna fruit, **3**, 286
Senna leaf, **3**, 284
Silica gel, desiccant, R, **1**, 202; R1, R2, R3,
   R4, R5, **2**, 314; R6, **3**, 363
Silver nitrate, **3**, 28
Silver nitrate/methanol TS, **3**, 364
Silver nitrate R, (40 g/l) TS, (0.1 mol/l) VS, **1**,
   202; (100 g/l) TS, (0.01 mol/l) VS, **3**,
   364
Silver oxide R, **2**, 314
Soda lime R, **1**, 202
Sodium acetate/glacial acetic acid
   (0.1 mol/l) VS, **3**, 364
Sodium acetate (150 g/l) TS, **1**, 202; R,
   (60 g/l) TS, (50 g/l) TS, **2**, 315
Sodium alizarinsulfonate R, (1 g/l) TS, **1**,
   203; (10 g/l) TS, **3**, 364

Sodium antimonyltartrate, *see* Antimony sodium tartrate

Sodium arsenite (0.1 mol/l) VS, **2**, 316; (0.05 mol/l) VS, **2**, 316; **3**, 386

Sodium bicarbonate, *see also* Sodium hydrogen carbonate

Sodium bicarbonate R, **1**, 203; **2**, 317

Sodium biphosphate, *see* Sodium dihydrogen phosphate

Sodium calcium edetate, **3**, 190

Sodium carbonate R, anhydrous, R, (50 g/l) TS, **1**, 203; anhydrous, FeR, (200 g/l) TS, (75 g/l) TS, (10 g/l) TS, **2**, 316
standard TS, **1**, 97, 203

Sodium chloride, **2**, 189

Sodium chloride R, **1**, 203; pyrogen-free, R, **2**, 316; (400 g/l) TS, (10 g/l) TS, **3**, 364

Sodium citrate, **3**, 192

Sodium citrate R, **1**, 203

Sodium cobaltinitrite R, (100 g/l) TS, **1**, 203

Sodium cromoglicate, **3**, 194

Sodium cromoglicate RS, **3**, 364

Sodium diethyldithiocarbamate R, (0.8 g/l) TS, **2**, 316

Sodium dihydrogen phosphate R, (45 g/l) TS, **2**, 317; (275 g/l) TS, **3**, 364

Sodium fluoride, **3**, 196

Sodium fluoride R, **1**, 203

Sodium formate R, **3**, 364

Sodium hydrogen carbonate, **2**, 191

Sodium hydrogen carbonate R, (40 g/l) TS, **2**, 317

Sodium hydroxide (1 mol/l), carbonate-free, VS, (0.5 mol/l), carbonate-free, VS, (0.2 mol/l), carbonate-free, VS, (0.1 mol/l), carbonate-free, VS, **1**, 205; (0.02 mol/l), carbonate-free, VS, (0.01 mol/l), carbonate-free, VS, **1**, 206

Sodium hydroxide/ethanol TS, **3**, 365

Sodium hydroxide/methanol TS, **2**, 317

Sodium hydroxide R, ($\sim$ 400 g/l) TS, **1**, 203; ($\sim$ 300 g/l) TS, ($\sim$ 200 g/l) TS, ($\sim$ 80 g/l) TS, (1 mol/l) VS, (0.2 mol/l) VS, (0.1 mol/l) VS, (0.05 mol/l) VS, (0.01 mol/l) VS, **1**, 204; ($\sim$ 150 g/l) TS, (10 g/l) TS, (0.5 mol/l) VS, (0.02 mol/l) VS, (0.001 mol/l) VS, **2**, 317; (50 g/l) TS, **3**, 365

Sodium hypochlorite ($\sim$ 40 g/l) TS, **2**, 317; TS1, **2**, 318

Sodium mercaptoacetate R, **1**, 206

Sodium metabisulfite R, **2**, 318

Sodium metaperiodate R, **2**, 318

Sodium methoxide (0.1 mol/l) VS, **2**, 318

Sodium molybdotungstophosphate TS, **2**, 318

Sodium 1,2-naphthoquinone-4-sulfonate R, (5 g/l) TS, **2**, 318

Sodium nitrite, **3**, 197

Sodium nitrite R, (10 g/l) TS, (0.1 mol/l) VS, **1**, 206; (100 g/l) TS, (3 g/l) TS, (1 g/l) TS, **2**, 319; (35 g/l) TS, **3**, 365

Sodium nitroferricyanide, *see* Sodium nitroprusside

Sodium nitroprussiate, *see* Sodium nitroprusside

Sodium nitroprusside, **3**, 199

Sodium nitroprusside R, (45 g/l) TS, **2**, 319; (8.5 g/l) TS, alkaline, TS, **3**, 365

Sodium oxalate R, **1**, 206

Sodium peroxide R, **3**, 365

Sodium phosphate, anhydrous R, *see* Disodium hydrogen phosphate, anhydrous, R

Sodium phosphate R, *see* Disodium hydrogen phosphate R

Sodium potassium tartrate, *see* Potassium sodium tartrate

Sodium R, **2**, 315

Sodium salicylate, **2**, 193; **3**, 383

Sodium salicylate R, (11.5 g/l) TS, **3**, 365

Sodium stibogluconate, **3**, 201

Sodium sulfate, **3**, 203

Sodium sulfate, anhydrous, **3**, 205

Sodium sulfate, anhydrous, R, **1**, 206

Sodium sulfide, R, TS, **1**, 206

Sodium sulfite, R, **3**, 365

Sodium tetraborate R, **1**, 206; (10 g/l) TS, **2**, 319
standard, TS, **1**, 97, 207

Sodium tetrabromofluorescein, *see* Eosin Y R

Sodium tetraphenylborate R, (30 g/l) TS, **1**, 207

Sodium thioglycolate R, *see* Sodium mercaptoacetate R

Sodium thiosulfate, **3**, 207

Sodium thiosulfate R, (0.1 mol/l) VS, **1**, 207; (0.05 mol/l) VS, (0.01 mol/l) VS, **1**, 208; (320 g/l) TS, (0.1 mol/l) VS, (0.02 mol/l) VS, **2**, 319

Sodium tungstate R, **2**, 319

Sodium valproate, **3**, 209

Solochrome Black, *see* Mordant Black 11 R

Solochrome Dark Blue, *see* Calcon R
Solubility, **1**, 11
Soluble starch R, **1**, 208
Solutions, **1**, 11
Solvent blue 19, *see* Oracet blue B R
Sorbitol R, **2**, 319
Spectinomycin hydrochloride, **3**, 288
Spectinomycin hydrochloride RS, **3**, 365
Spectinomycini hydrochloridum, **3**, 288
Spironolactone, **3**, 290
Spironolactone RS, **3**, 365
Spironolactonum, **3**, 290
Squalane R, **3**, 365
Stability information, **2**, 12
Standard buffer solutions, **1**, 97, 98
Standard colour solutions, **1**, 51
Stannated hydrochloric acid ($\sim$ 250 g/1) AsTS, **1**, 184
Stannous chloride R, TS, AsTS, **1**, 208
Starch/iodide paper R, **1**, 208
Starch iodide TS, **2**, 320
Starch R, TS, **1**, 208
Starch, soluble, R, **1**, 208
Sterile phosphate buffer, pH 4.5, TS, **1**, 195; pH 6.0, TS1, TS2, TS3, **1**, 196; pH 7.0, TS, pH 7.2, TS, **1**, 196; pH 8.0, TS1, TS2, **1**, 197; pH 7.8, TS, pH 10.5, TS1, **3**, 360
Stibii natrii tartras, **3**, 293
Stock colour standard solutions, **1**, 51
Streptomycin sulfate, **2**, 256
Streptomycini sulfas, **2**, 256
Strong arsenic AsTS, **1**, 170
Strong cobalt colour TS, **1**, 174
Strong copper colour TS, **1**, 175
Strong dichromate colour RS, **1**, 177
Strong histamine TS, **1**, 182
Strong iron colour TS, **1**, 186
Strong lead PbTS, **1**, 187
Strychnine sulfate R, **2**, 320
Succamethonium chloratum, *see* Suxamethonii chloridum
Succinylcholine chloride, *see* Suxamethonium chloride
Sudan red G R, **3**, 365; TS, **3**, 366
Sulfacetamide, **3**, 294
Sulfacetamide RS, **3**, 366
Sulfacetamide sodium, **3**, 296
Sulfacetamidum, **3**, 294
Sulfacetamidum natricum, **3**, 296
Sulfacylum-natricum, *see* Sulfacetamide sodium
Sulfadimezinum, *see* Sulfadimidinum

Sulfadimidine, **3**, 298
Sulfadimidine RS, **3**, 366
Sulfadimidine sodium, **3**, 300
Sulfadimidinum, **3**, 298
Sulfadimidinum natricum, **3**, 300
Sulfadoxine, **3**, 302
Sulfadoxine RS, **3**, 366
Sulfadoxinum, **3**, 302
Sulfamethazine, *see* Sulfadimidine
Sulfamethoxazole, **2**, 259
Sulfamethoxazole RS, **2**, 320
Sulfamethoxazolum, **2**, 259
Sulfamethoxypyridazine, **2**, 261
Sulfamethoxypyridazine RS, **2**, 320
Sulfamethoxypyridazinum, **2**, 261
Sulfamic acid R, (50 g/l) TS, **2**, 320; (5 g/l) TS, **3**, 366
Sulfanilamide RS, **2**, 320
Sulfanilic acid R, **2**, 320
  diazotized, TS, **3**, 366
Sulfasalazine, **3**, 305
Sulfasalazine RS, **3**, 366
Sulfasalazinum, **3**, 366
Sulfate-free ethanol ($\sim$750 g/l) TS, **1**, 180
Sulfosalicylic acid R, **1**, 208; (175 g/l) TS, **1**, 209
Sulfur dioxide R, **1**, 209
Sulfuric acid/ethanol TS, **2**, 321
Sulfuric acid/methanol TS, **3**, 366
Sulfuric acid R, *see* Sulfuric acid ($\sim$1760 g/l) TS
Sulfuric acid ($\sim$1760 g/l) TS, nitrogen-free, TS, ($\sim$190 g/l) TS, ($\sim$100 g/l) TS, ($\sim$10 g/l) TS, (0.5 mol/l) VS, (0.05 mol/l) VS, (0.01 mol/l) VS, **1**, 209; (0.005 mol/l) VS, **1**, 210; ($\sim$700 g/l) TS, ($\sim$635 g/l) TS, ($\sim$570 g/l) TS, ($\sim$50 g/l) TS, **2**, 320; (0.25 mol/l) VS, (0.1 mol/l) VS, **2**, 321; (0.125 mol/l) VS, **3**, 366
Sulfurous acid R, *see* Sulfurous acid TS
Sulfurous acid TS, **2**, 321
Suramin sodium, **3**, 307
Suraminum natricum, **3**, 307
Suxamethonii chloridum, **3**, 310
Suxamethonium chloride, **3**, 310

T

Tannic acid R, (50 g/l) TS, **3**, 366
Tartaric acid R, (10 g/l) TS, (5 g/l) TS, **2**, 321; (200 g/l) TS, **3**, 366
Temperature measurements, **1**, 11
p-Terphenyl R, **1**, 210

Testosterone enantate, **3**, 312
Testosterone enantate RS, **3**, 366
Testosterone propionate, **2**, 263; **3**, 385
Testosterone propionate RS, **2**, 321
Testosteroni enantas, **3**, 312
Testosteroni propionas, **2**, 263; **3**, 385
Test solutions, **1**, 13
  list of, **1**, 167; **2**, 277; **3**, 337
Tetrabutylammonium hydroxide/methanol
  TS, **3**, 366
Tetrabutylammonium hydroxide (0.1
    mol/l) VS, **2**, 321; TS, **3**, 367
Tetrabutylammonium iodide R, **2**, 322
Tetracaine hydrochloride, **3**, 314
Tetracaini hydrochloridum, **3**, 314
Tetrachloroethane R, **2**, 322
Tetracycline hydrochloride, **2**, 266
Tetracycline hydrochloride RS, **2**, 322
Tetracyclini hydrochloridum, **2**, 266
n-Tetradecane R, **2**, 322
Tetrahydrofuran R, **3**, 367
Tetramethylammonium hydroxide/ethanol
  TS, **2**, 323
Tetramethylammonium hydroxide
  (~100 g/l) TS, **2**, 322
Thiamine hydrobromide, **3**, 316
Thiamine hydrochloride, **3**, 318
Thiamine mononitrate, **3**, 319
Thiamini hydrobromidum, **3**, 316
Thiamini hydrochloridum, **3**, 318
Thiamini mononitras, **3**, 319
Thioacetazone, **3**, 321
Thioacetazone RS, **3**, 367
Thioacetazonum, **3**, 321
4,4′-Thiodianiline RS, **2**, 323
Thioglycolic acid R, see Mercaptoacetic acid
  R
Thiourea R, (0.1 g/l) TS, **2**, 323
Thorin R, (2 g/l) TS, **1**, 210
Thorium nitrate R, (0.005 mol/l) VS, **1**,
  210
Thymol blue/dimethylformanide TS, **2**, 324
Thymol blue/ethanol TS, **2**, 324
Thymol blue/methanol TS, **2**, 324
Thymol blue R, **2**, 323
Thymolphthalein/dimethylformamide TS, **2**,
  324
Thymolphthalein/ethanol TS, **1**, 210
Thymolphthalein R, **1**, 210
Thymol R, TS1, TS2, TS3, **2**, 323
Thyroxine sodium, see Levothyroxine
  sodium
Tiabendazole, **3**, 323

Tiabendazole RS, **3**, 367
Tiabendazolum, **3**, 323
Tightly closed containers, definition of, **1**,
  12
Titanium dioxide R, **2**, 324
Titanium dioxide/sulfuric acid TS, **2**, 324
Titanium trichloride R, (0.1 mol/l) VS, **3**,
  367
Titan yellow R, TS, **3**, 367
Tolbutamide, **2**, 270
Tolbutamide RS, **2**, 324
Tolbutamidum, **2**, 270
Toluene R, **1**, 210
4-Toluenesulfonamide R, **2**, 324
4-Toluenesulfonic acid/ethanol TS, **2**, 324
4-Toluenesulfonic acid R, **2**, 324
Tosylchloramide sodium R, **2**, 325; **3**, 386;
  (15 g/l) TS, **2**, 325
Trademarks and trade names, notices con-
  cerning, **1**, 12, 13
Trichloroacetic acid R, **2**, 325
Trichloroethylene R, **2**, 325
Trichlorotrifluoroethane R, TS, **2**, 325
Trihexyphenidyl hydrochloride, **3**, 325
Trihexyphenidyl hydrochloride RS, **3**, 367
Trihexyphenidyli hydrochloridum, **3**, 325
Triketohydrindene/butanol TS, **3**, 367
Triketohydrindene/cadmium TS, **2**, 325
Triketohydrindene hydrate R, **2**, 325;
  (1 g/l) TS, **3**, 368
Triketohydrindene/methanol TS, **3**, 368
Triketohydrindene/pyridine/acetone TS, **3**,
  368
Triketohydrindene/pyridine/butanol TS, **3**,
  368
Triketohydrindene/stannous chloride TS, **3**,
  368
Trimethadione, **2**, 272; **3**, 385
Trimethadione RS, **2**, 325
Trimethadionum, **2**, 272; **3**, 385
Trimethoprim, **2**, 274
Trimethoprim RS, **2**, 325
Trimethoprimum, **2**, 274
2,2,4-Trimethylpentane R, **3**, 368
Trimethylpyridine R, (50 g/l) TS, **2**, 326
Trinitrophenol R, (7 g/l) TS, **2**, 326
  alkaline, TS, **2**, 326
Triphenylantimony R, **3**, 368
Trisodium orthophosphate R, (2 g/l) TS, **3**,
  368
Tubocurarine chloride, **3**, 326
Tubocurarini chloridum, **3**, 326
Tyrosine R, **2**, 326

U

Ultraviolet light, examination in, **2**, 12
Uranyl acetate R, **1**, 210
Uranyl zinc/acetate TS, **1**, 210
Urea R, **2**, 326
Uridine R, **3**, 368

V

Valproic acid RS, **3**, 368
Vanadium pentoxide R, **3**, 369
Vanadium/sulfuric acid TS, **3**, 369
Vanillin/hydrochloric acid TS, **3**, 369
Vanillin R, (10 g/l) TS, **2**, 326
Verapamil hydrochloride, **3**, 328
Verapamil hydrochloride RS, **3**, 369
Verapamili hydrochloridum, **3**, 328
Vincristine sulfate, **3**, 330
Vincristine sulfate RS, **3**, 369
Vincristini sulfas, **3**, 330
Vitamin B_{12}, *see* Cyanocobalamin
Vitamin B_{12a} and B_{12b}, *see* Hydroxocobalamin
Vitamin D_2, *see* Ergocalciferol
Vitamin K_1, *see* Phytomenadione
Volumetric solutions, **1**, 13
   list of, **1**, 167; **2**, 277; **3**, 337

W

Warfarin sodium, **3**, 332
Warfarin RS, **3**, 369
Warfarinum natricum, **3**, 332
Water, **2**, 11

Water, ammonia-free, R, **2**, 326
Water-bath, **2**, 12
Water, carbon-dioxide-free and ammonia-free, R, **2**, 326
Water, carbon-dioxide-free, R, **1**, 211
Water-soluble yeast extract R, **1**, 211
Water, sterile, R, **2**, 326
Well-closed containers, definition of, **1**, 12

X

Xanthydrol R, TS, **3**, 369
Xylene R, **2**, 326
Xylenol orange indicator mixture R, **1**, 211
Xylenol orange R, **1**, 211

Y

Yeast extract, water-soluble, R, **1**, 211
Yellow mercuric oxide R, **1**, 191
Yellow stock standard TS, **1**, 211

Z

Zinc acetate R, **1**, 211
Zinc AsR, granulated, R, **1**, 211
Zinc bis(dibenzyldithiocarbamate) R, TS, **3**, 369
Zinc chloride R, **2**, 326
Zinci oxydum, **3**, 335
Zinc oxide, **3**, 335
Zinc standard (20 µg/ml Zn) TS, **2**, 327
Zinc sulfate R, **2**, 327
Zirconyl nitrate R, TS, **2**, 327

WHO publications may be obtained, direct or through booksellers, from:

ALGERIA: Entreprise nationale du Livre (ENAL), 3 bd Zirout Youcef, ALGIERS

ARGENTINA: Carlos Hirsch, SRL, Florida 165, Galerías Güemes, Escritorio 453/465, BUENOS AIRES

AUSTRALIA: Hunter Publications, 58A Gipps Street, COLLINGWOOD, VIC 3066.

AUSTRIA: Gerold & Co., Graben 31, 1011 VIENNA I

BAHRAIN: United Schools International, Arab Region Office, P.O. Box 726, BAHRAIN

BANGLADESH: The WHO Representative, G.P.O. Box 250, DHAKA 5

BELGIUM: *For books:* Office International de Librairie s.a., avenue Marnix 30, 1050 BRUSSELS. *For periodicals and subscriptions:* Office International des Périodiques, avenue Louise 485, 1050 BRUSSELS.

BHUTAN: *see* India, WHO Regional Office

BOTSWANA: Botsalo Books (Pty) Ltd., P.O. Box 1532, GABORONE

BRAZIL: Centro Latinoamericano de Informação em Ciencias de Saúde (BIREME), Organização Panamericana de Saúde, Sector de Publicações, C.P. 20381 - Rua Botucatu 862, 04023 SÃO PAULO, SP

BURMA: *see* India, WHO Regional Office

CAMEROON: Cameroon Book Centre, P.O. Box 123, South West Province, VICTORIA

CANADA: Canadian Public Health Association, 1335 Carling Avenue, Suite 210, OTTAWA, Ont. K1Z 8N8. (Tel: (613) 725–3769. Telex: 21–053–3841)

CHINA: China National Publications Import & Export Corporation, P.O. Box 88, BEIJING (PEKING)

DEMOCRATIC PEOPLE'S REPUBLIC OF KOREA: *see* India, WHO Regional Office

DENMARK: Munksgaard Export and Subscription Service, Nørre Søgade 35, 1370 COPENHAGEN K (Tel: + 45 1 12 85 70)

FIJI: The WHO Representative, P.O. Box 113, SUVA

FINLAND: Akateeminen Kirjakauppa, Keskuskatu 2, 00101 HELSINKI 10

FRANCE: Arnette, 2 rue Casimir-Delavigne, 75006 PARIS

GERMAN DEMOCRATIC REPUBLIC: Buchhaus Leipzig, Postfach 140, 701 LEIPZIG

GERMANY FEDERAL REPUBLIC OF: Govi-Verlag GmbH, Ginnheimerstrasse 20, Postfach 5360, 6236 ESCHBORN — Buchhandlung Alexander Horn, Kirchgasse 22, Postfach 3340, 6200 WIESBADEN

GREECE: G.C. Eleftheroudakis S.A., Librairie internationale, rue Nikis 4, 105-63 ATHENS

HONG KONG: Hong Kong Government Information Services, Publication (Sales) Office, Information Services Department, No. 1, Battery Path, Central, HONG KONG.

HUNGARY: Kultura, P.O.B. 149, BUDAPEST 62

ICELAND: Snaebjorn Jonsson & Co., Hafnarstraeti 9, P.O. Box 1131, IS-101 REYKJAVIK

INDIA: WHO Regional Office for South-East Asia, World Health House, Indraprastha Estate, Mahatma Gandhi Road, NEW DELHI 110002

IRAN (ISLAMIC REPUBLIC OF): Iran University Press, 85 Park Avenue, P.O. Box 54/551, TEHERAN

IRELAND: TDC Publishers, 12 North Frederick Street, DUBLIN 1 (Tel: 744835–749677)

ISRAEL: Heiliger & Co., 3 Nathan Strauss Street, JERUSALEM 94227

ITALY: Edizioni Minerva Medica, Corso Bramante 83–85, 10126 TURIN; Via Lamarmora 3, 20100 MILAN; Via Spallanzani 9, 00161 ROME

JAPAN: Maruzen Co. Ltd., P.O. Box 5050, TOKYO International, 100–31

JORDAN: Jordan Book Centre Co. Ltd., University Street, P.O. Box 301 (Al-Jubeiha), AMMAN

KENYA: Text Book Centre Ltd, P.O. Box 47540, NAIROBI

KUWAIT: The Kuwait Bookshops Co. Ltd., Thunayan Al-Ghanem Bldg, P.O. Box 2942, KUWAIT

LAO PEOPLE'S DEMOCRATIC REPUBLIC: The WHO Representative, P.O. Box 343, VIENTIANE

LUXEMBOURG: Librairie du Centre, 49 bd Royal, LUXEMBOURG